Pedophilia, Hebephilia and Sexual Offending against Children

Klaus M. Beier

Editor

Pedophilia, Hebephilia and Sexual Offending against Children

The Berlin Dissexuality Therapy (BEDIT)

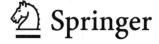 Springer

Editor
Klaus M. Beier
Director, Institute of Sexology and Sexual Medicine
Charité – Universitätsmedizin Berlin
Corporate Member of Freie Universität Berlin
Humboldt-Universität zu Berlin, and Berlin Institute of Health
Center for Human and Health Sciences
Berlin, Germany

ISBN 978-3-030-61264-1   ISBN 978-3-030-61262-7   (eBook)
https://doi.org/10.1007/978-3-030-61262-7

This Springer imprint is published by the registered company Springer Nature Switzerland AG
The registered company address is: Gewerbestrasse 11, 6330 Cham, Switzerland

Preface

Pedophilia is classified in the International Classification of Diseases (ICD-10; World Health Organization, 1992) under disorders of sexual preference (F 65.4) and in the Diagnostic and Statistical Manual of Mental Disorders (DSM-5; American Psychiatric Association 2013) under paraphilias, and, as pedophilic disorder, as a pathological paraphilic disorder. In the ICD-11 (World Health Organization 2018) the generic term is also pedophilic disorder (exclusively specifying prepubescent children and not including early pubescent children, as in the ICD-10).

Under both diagnostic systems, the diagnostic criteria refer to the orientation of sexual preference toward the prepubescent developmental body age of children. Pedophilic orientation manifests itself as fantasies, urges, or behaviors that involve sexual acts with children. The consumption of child sexual abuse images (still frequently referred to as "child pornography," a term that deemphasizes their harmful nature) is likely to be an indicator for pedophilia (Seto et al. 2006). Based on available statistics, it can be assumed that between 30% and 50% of criminal sex offenses carried out on children are committed by people with a pedophilic sexual preference (Beier 1998; Seto 2008). The other part consists of non-pedophilic offenders, who are sexually orientated towards adults and for whom - because of some other ulterior contextual issue (such as a mental disability or a personality disorder) - the sexual abuse of the child serves as a surrogate for a sexual relationship with partners of adequate age. Empirical data reveal very clearly that pedophilic offenders demonstrate a significant higher risk of re-offending (Beier 1995).

According to previous findings, the sexual responsiveness to the child developmental body age that is inherent to pedophilia occurs in up to 1% of men and in very few women (Ahlers et al. 2011; Beier et al. 2005; Dombert et al. 2015). These individuals live largely unnoticed within society and strive to conceal their sexual preference—from others and/or from themselves. Furthermore, the majority of actual incidences involving sexual abuse of children is never reported to the police, is thus not registered by the judiciary and criminal prosecution authorities, and remains in the Dunkelfeld (literally "dark field" which refers to undetected offenses). The Internet Watch Foundation (IWF) identified webpages providing child sexual exploitation material in dramatically increasing numbers: 1,351 webpages in the year 2010 and 105,047 webpages in the year 2018, which reveals a 100 fold increase in only 8 years (IWF 2018).

As we are facing a global health issue here with an increasing impact from the internet concerning the use of child exploitation material, it takes international efforts to reduce the affliction on children and adolescents. Furthermore, there should be no contradiction between law enforcement and the promotion of preventive strategies – both can and should be implemented. Prevention can focus on potential victims as well as potential offenders, who might be liable for the sexual traumatization of children. If it were possible to influence their behaviour before they act out, there would be no offence and no victim – meaning primary prevention at its best.

However, there is a huge lack worldwide regarding the situation for medical and therapeutic care for people with pedophilic disorders within the health care system. Many doctors and psychotherapists refuse to treat these patients because they do not possess the necessary skills, have personal reservations, or shy away from the potential forensic context (for Germany see Jahnke et al., 2015). Furthermore, there are tremendous legal and cultural differences between countries – but despite that, there is a need to react and not only to describe the problem.

Within the context of the Prevention Project Dunkelfeld (Preventionsprojekt Dunkelfeld [PPD]), initiated at the Charité – Universitätsmedizin Berlin at the Institute of Sexology and Sexual Medicine in 2005, it became clear that a significant number of those affected experience distress as a result of a pedophilic sexual preference and are prepared to accept help.

Nevertheless, therapy outside of forensic institutions with pedophilic men who are aware of their problem represents an enormous challenge for clinically practicing therapists. The challenges of establishing concrete procedures and goals for working in this therapeutic area have thus far found little consideration in the relevant literature.

The Berlin Dissexuality Therapy (Berliner Dissexualitätstherapie [BEDIT]) is a therapeutic approach developed for the treatment of people with pedophilia that has existed in manual form since 2013; it is being made available here as part of an overall presentation of this therapeutic area-including the extension program for juveniles established in 2014 (BEDIT-A, i.e., BEDIT for adolescents; see below). Content and interventions that have proven helpful in the context of the Prevention Project Dunkelfeld for adults and juveniles will be introduced accordingly.

The book consists of a theoretical part and a practical part. The theoretical part includes an introduction to the subject areas of pedophilia and hebephilia (the sexual responsiveness to the prepubescent and early pubescent developmental body age) as sexual preference disorders and illuminates their connection with dissexual behaviors (actions that violate the sexual autonomy of others and involve the endangerment of third parties).

The practical part offers background information on treatment rationale and introduces specific therapeutic principles that were put into practice as part of the Prevention Project Dunkelfeld. Prerequisites for the use of the manuals being introduced here are a qualification in the diagnosis and therapy of sexual disorders as well as psychotherapeutic (and/or adolescent psychotherapeutic), forensic, and pharmacological skills. Therapists who decide to put BEDIT or BEDIT-A into practice should be aware that an appropriate level of expertise and advanced training is necessary. A basic knowledge of the relevant risk factors in connection with child sexual abuse is likewise strongly recommended.

BEDIT was developed and continually optimized within the context of the Prevention Project Dunkelfeld, drawing on established diagnostic and therapeutic concepts in sexual medicine (Beier et al. 2005). A variety of therapeutic experiences with treatment approaches for group therapy were also incorporated, such as Dialectic Behavioral Therapy (DBT; Linehan 1996) or Acceptance and Commitment Therapy (ACT; Hayes et al. 2006). Selected therapy manuals for the treatment of sex offenders, such as the Sex Offender Treatment and Evaluation Program (SOTEP; Marques et al. 1989) and the Custody-Based Intensive Treatment Program (CUBIT; New South Wales, Australia), provided additional sources for the conceptualization and further development of BEDIT, and this, in turn, was an important prerequisite for the development of BEDIT-A.

In the beginning, the focus lay on the target group of people who felt a sexual attraction to children and saw themselves as being in danger of committing child sexual abuse. It quickly became apparent, however, that many of these (mostly) male participants were more worried about consuming child abuse images than directly sexually offending against children.

This finding raised the question of whether the project would be able to reach both groups by the same means. With the support of the German Federal Ministry for Family Affairs, Senior Citizens, Women, and Youth, a media campaign was established in the period between 2009 and 2010 that was directed specifically at the group of users of child sexual abuse images in connection with a targeted treatment service. In accordance with recent studies, clinical experiences demonstrated differences between participants who had sexually abused children and those who admitted to having used child sexual abuse images. The latter group exhibited a higher level of education and social integration and also required a different prioritization within the therapy process, such as a focus on emotion-regulation deficits rather than, e.g., deficits in social competency. Further research is required, however, in order to shed light on these differences and draw conclusions for optimal treatment.

Since the beginning of the first therapy groups of the PPD, essential changes to the setup, structure, content, and concrete approaches of the therapy have been necessary. Based on these experiences in the clinical work, important modifications were therefore undertaken. These also proved necessary for the preventative therapy service established at the Institute in Berlin in 2014 for adolescents who have a sexual interest in children and who, because of this, have committed sex offenses, used child sexual abuse images, and/or are experiencing distress. On the one hand, this extension program for adolescents built on the experiences with adults, but on the other hand, necessitated extensive additions and alterations in order to adequately serve the particular living situations of young people and their parents, relatives, teachers, or social youth workers.

This book consists of 10 chapters and a bibliography: Chapter "Pedophilia and Hebephilia" presents the current state of knowledge on the manifestations and prevalence of pedophilia and hebephilia, and also provides information on neurobiological aspects and comorbidities that may be observed in connection with these two preference disorders; the cultural differences in societal evaluation mechanisms that are significant for the establishment of perpetrator-focused prevention services are also addressed.

Chapter "Child Sexual Abuse and the Use of Child Sexual Abuse Images" gives an overview of the state of knowledge on child sexual abuse and the use of child sexual abuse images, including the possibilities for prevention in these areas. Building on this, chapter "Therapeutic Options" addresses in depth the possibilities for perpetrator-oriented prevention through therapy, and chapter "The Berlin Prevention Project Dunkelfeld (PPD)" describes the approach of the Prevention Project Dunkelfeld in detail. Chapters "BEDIT Manual for Adults" and "Modules for Adults" are dedicated to the treatment manual BEDIT for adults (including modules), primarily developed for this version by Anna Konrad, Laura F. Kuhle, Gerold Scherner, Dorit Grundmann, and Till Amelung, building on the work of earlier colleagues. Manuals and modules for the treatment of adolescents are located in chapters "BEDIT-A Manual for Adolescents" and "Modules for Adolescents"; these were primarily based on drafts by Elena Hupp, Eliza Schlinzig, Lea Ludwig, Miriam Schuler, Umut Oezdemir, and Tobias Hellenschmidt, who were also able to draw on their own experience and on preexisting material.

Each module follows the same structure: first, the specific goals of the module are laid out; second, the treatment rationale explains the background information on the subject; third, the content section gives an overview of the relevant themes; and finally, recommendations for concrete interventions with or without the use of specific worksheets are given. These are located separately for adult (chapter "Worksheets BEDIT") and juvenile (chapter "Worksheets BEDIT-A") participants, and are sorted according to the order of the modules and the order in which they appear within the individual modules.

For the sake of readability—and in accordance with Springer Publishing guidelines—this manual has been written using male pronouns when referring to both male and female therapists. When referring to the target group of the project and its participants, who are almost entirely men, male pronouns will be used exclusively.

Berlin, Germany   Klaus M. Beier
December 2020

Acknowledgments

The content presented in this book draws significantly on more than fifteen years of clinical and scientific work with people who, because of a sexual responsiveness to the prepubescent and/or early pubescent developmental body age of children (i.e., pedophilia or hebephilia), took the initiative to seek out help at the Institute of Sexology and Sexual Medicine at the Charité – Univetsitätsmedizin Berlin (i.e., the University Hospital of Berlin) and in the "Don't Offend" ("Kein Täter werden") prevention network. The primary objective of this work was and is to prevent the sexual traumatization of children and teenagers, as well as the consumption of child sexual abuse images.

This pioneering work would not have been possible without the "Prevention of Child Sexual Abuse" research project initiated at the Institute in Berlin, which became well known after a nationwide public awareness campaign under the name "Kein Täter Werden" ("Don't Offend"). The project was funded in its early stages (beginning in 2005) by the Volkswagen Foundation, which thereby became the first funding institution worldwide to make the decision of providing financial support to a therapy program for pedophilic individuals outside of the criminal justice system. This set in motion a process that made a nationally significant perpetrator-focused prevention program possible—one that soon met with increasing interest abroad as well. They had the courage to try out something completely new, and in a highly sensitive, sociopolitically controversial area at that.

Also invaluable in this initial phase was our—to this day, consistent and regular—collaboration with the child protection organization, Hänsel and Gretel, and also with the media agency Scholz & Friends, who understood how to adequately take on public relations in this field in a professional manner and with much engagement and whose media campaign, "lieben sie kinder mehr, als ihnen lieb ist?" ("do you like children in ways you shouldn't") earned them several prizes. Equally important for the concrete implementation of the clinical and scientific work was the support of the Charité as a University Hospital.

A deciding factor in the success of the project was without a doubt the unwavering support of the German Federal Ministry of Justice (BMJV) when the Volkswagen Foundation's funds ran out in 2008. To the then-Federal Minister of Justice, Brigitte Zypries and her colleagues, we owe special thanks—but also respect, as they stood behind the causer-related prevention approach and advocated for it at a time when its trial was still in its infancy and skepticism was still the overwhelming position for many in the public sphere. The establishment of the Germany-wide network "Kein Täter werden" ("Don't Offend") was also made possible through the financial contributions of the Federal Ministry of Justice, which were maintained until the end of 2016 under the leadership of the later Federal Minister Sabine Leutheusser-Schnarrenberger and, subsequently, Federal Minster of Justice and Consumer Protection Heiko Maas. The Federal Ministry of Justice and Consumer Protection continues to show its commitment to the network by financing the public relations work that is so important for the project.

The Berlin Senate eventually secured last-minute financing for the Berlin location for 2017 in order to guarantee a seamless transition. Because beginning in 2018, a new statutory regulation would be implemented according to § 65 d of Book 5 of the Social Code (SGB)[1], whereby the anonymous use of preventative help for pedophilic individuals was defined as the responsibility of the statutory health insurers, who have earmarked financing as part of a pilot project for the next five years. This new regulation in the Social Code came about due to the tremendous dedication of the Federal Ministries of Health (BMG) and of Justice and Consumer Protection (BMJV), as well as the Federal Ministry of Family Affairs, Senior Citizens, Women and Youth (BMFSFJ).

Many thanks are owed to the BMFSFJ and to then-Federal Minister Manuela Schwesig and her State Secretary, Dr. Ralf Kleindiek for making possible the start of the "Prevention of Child Sexual Abuse by Juveniles" project—a collaboration between the Institute of Sexology and Sexual Medicine and the Vivantes Klinikum am Friedrichshain in Berlin. This project offered confidential therapeutic services to 12- to 18-year-olds with a sexual responsiveness to children and will also be financed by the statutory health insurers (in accordance with § 65 d of SGB V) as part of the pilot program starting in 2018.

It is an exceptional stroke of good luck for a team of scientists and therapists to have the continual and constructive support of funding institutions and ministries over an extended period of time—this is precisely what happened in the case of the Prevention Project Dunkelfeld ("Kein Täter werden" ["Don't Offend"]). We were exceptionally fortunate as well to be afforded the experience of receiving the targeted support of legislators, as was the case with the new statutory regulation in the Social Code.

This reinforcement always encouraged the employees involved in the project at the Institute for Sexology and Sexual Medicine of the Charité – University Hospital Berlin to contribute to its success with great motivation and readiness for duty. Since 2005, these included (in alphabetical order): Christoph J. Ahlers, Rainer Alisch, Till Amelung, Madelaine Dimitrowa, Stefan Faistbauer, Steven Feelgood, Torsten Freitag, David Goecker, Hannes Gieseler, Anna Groll, Dorit Grundmann, Franz Henkel, Elena Hupp, Corinne Kaszner, Anna Konrad, Stephanie Kossow, Laura Kuhle, Lea Ludwig, Ingrid Mundt, Janina Neutze, Pierre Pantazidis, Alfred Pauls,

---

[1]All statements are exclusively with regard to German Criminal Law. The Justice System in other countries is, in parts, often very different.

Karl Pauls, Andreas Peter, Umut Oezdemir, Gerard A. Schaefer, Gerold Scherner, Eliza Schlinzig, Horst Schütz, Miriam Schuler, Stefan Siegel, Sabine Teßner, Hannes Ulrich, Maximilian von Heyden, Katharina Schweder, and Jens Wagner.

For the extraordinarily fruitful and informative collaboration on this new preventative approach to improving child protection, I owe a heavy debt of gratitude to all participants named here, but also to all of the other individuals, institutions, and organizations active in this field, who, many of them for decades, have dedicated themselves to the prevention of the sexual traumatization of children and adolescents. The fact that these efforts are having an increasing effect on the most diverse spheres of society can be seen in the fact that, since the last German Doctors' Day in May 2018, sexual medicine has been adopted as part of the model specialty-training regulations of the German Medical Association (*Bundesärztekammer*). The justification for this was, among other things, the significance of sexual traumatization on health and thereby the medical care system.

The English translation of the BEDIT-manual was supported by the funding programme "Hospital Partnerships" which was established by Germany's Federal Ministry for Economic Cooperation and Development (BMZ) and the "Else Kröner-Fresenius Foundation" as an important contribution for global health and granted in the context of the international collaboration between the Institute of Sexology and Sexual Medicine of the Charité – Universitätsmedizin Berlin and the King Edwards Memorial Hospital of Pune (Maharashtra) in order to establish a causer-related primary prevention programme in India (see www.pppsv.org).

Finally, we would like to thank the employees of Springer-Verlag for their professional guidance on the German version of the book, particularly Renate Scheddin (planning) and Axel Treiber (project management), as well as the external reader, Gabriele Siese, for her careful editing of the texts, as well as Dave Youssef for the translation work and Sylvana Freyberg for organizing the English version, not forgetting—the current co-workers of the Prevention Projects in Berlin for reading the final proofs.

Berlin, Germany   Klaus M. Beier
December 2020

Contents

Contributors

Till Amelung, Dr. med. Charité – Universitätsmedizin Berlin, Corporate Member of Freie Universität Berlin, Humboldt-Universität zu Berlin, and Berlin Institute of Health, Center for Human and Health Sciences, Institute of Sexology and Sexual Medicine, Department of Psychiatry and Psychotherapy, Charité Campus Mitte, Berlin, Germany

Klaus M. Beier, Prof. Dr. med. Dr. phil. Charité – Universitätsmedizin Berlin, Corporate Member of Freie Universität Berlin, Humboldt-Universität zu Berlin, and Berlin Institute of Health, Center for Human and Health Sciences, Institute of Sexology and Sexual Medicine, Berlin, Germany

Hannes Gieseler Charité – Universitätsmedizin Berlin, Corporate Member of Freie Universität Berlin, Humboldt-Universität zu Berlin, and Berlin Institute of Health, Center for Human and Health Sciences, Institute of Sexology and Sexual Medicine, Berlin, Germany

Dorit Grundmann, Dr. rer. medic. Dipl.-Psych. Charité – Universitätsmedizin Berlin, Corporate Member of Freie Universität Berlin, Humboldt-Universität zu Berlin, and Berlin Institute of Health, Center for Human and Health Sciences, Institute of Sexology and Sexual Medicine, Berlin, Germany

Anna Konrad, Dr. rer. medic. Dipl.-Psych. Charité – Universitätsmedizin Berlin, Corporate Member of Freie Universität Berlin, Humboldt-Universität zu Berlin, and Berlin Institute of Health, Center for Human and Health Sciences, Institute of Sexology and Sexual Medicine, Berlin, Germany

Stephanie Kossow, Dr. med. Charité – Universitätsmedizin Berlin, Corporate Member of Freie Universität Berlin, Humboldt-Universität zu Berlin, and Berlin Institute of Health, Center for Human and Health Sciences, Institute of Sexology and Sexual Medicine, Berlin, Germany

Laura F. Kuhle, Dr. rer. medic. Dipl.-Psych. Charité – Universitätsmedizin Berlin, Corporate Member of Freie Universität Berlin, Humboldt-Universität zu Berlin, and Berlin Institute of Health, Center for Human and Health Sciences, Institute of Sexology and Sexual Medicine, Berlin, Germany

Umut Oezdemir, Dipl.-Psych. Charité – Universitätsmedizin Berlin, Corporate Member of Freie Universität Berlin, Humboldt-Universität zu Berlin, and Berlin Institute of Health, Center for Human and Health Sciences, Institute of Sexology and Sexual Medicine, Berlin, Germany

Gerold Scherner, Dipl.-Psych. Charité – Universitätsmedizin Berlin, Corporate Member of Freie Universität Berlin, Humboldt-Universität zu Berlin, and Berlin Institute of Health, Center for Human and Health Sciences, Institute of Sexology and Sexual Medicine, Berlin, Germany

Eliza Schlinzig, Dipl.-Psych. Charité – Universitätsmedizin Berlin, Corporate Member of Freie Universität Berlin, Humboldt-Universität zu Berlin, and Berlin Institute of Health, Center for Human and Health Sciences, Institute of Sexology and Sexual Medicine, Berlin, Germany

Miriam Schuler, M.Sc. Charité – Universitätsmedizin Berlin, Corporate Member of Freie Universität Berlin, Humboldt-Universität zu Berlin, and Berlin Institute of Health, Center for Human and Health Sciences, Institute of Sexology and Sexual Medicine, Berlin, Germany

Stefan Siegel, Prof. Dr. med. Charité – Universitätsmedizin Berlin, Corporate Member of Freie Universität Berlin, Humboldt-Universität zu Berlin, and Berlin Institute of Health, Center for Human and Health Sciences, Institute of Sexology and Sexual Medicine, Berlin, Germany

Hannes Ulrich, M.Sc. Charité – Universitätsmedizin Berlin, Corporate Member of Freie Universität Berlin, Humboldt-Universität zu Berlin, and Berlin Institute of Health, Center for Human and Health Sciences, Institute of Sexology and Sexual Medicine, Berlin, Germany

About the Author

Klaus M. Beier born 1961, studied Medicine (beginning in 1979) and Philosophy (beginning in 1980) at the Freie Universität Berlin. From 1988, Research Associate; from 1994 Assistant Professor for Sexual Medicine at the hospital of the Universität Kiel; specialist for psychosomatic medicine and psychoanalyst; since 1996, director of the newly established Institute for Sexology and Sexual Medicine at the Charité – Universitätsmedizin Berlin (University Hospital in Berlin) (with a connected university outpatient clinic); since 2005, occupied with the establishment of the research project "Prevention of Child Sexual Abuse in the Dunkelfeld" with subsequent nationwide extension (see www.kein-taeter-werden.de); and, since 2014, with an extension program for adolescents (www.du-traeumst-von-ihnen.de); as well as, since 2017, an international expansion with an internet-based diagnostic and therapy service (www.troubled-desire.com) following his activities to build up prevention programme in India (since 2015; see www.pppsv.org). In the year 2020 he established the first online (remote) treatment project for pedophilically and/or hebephilically inclined individuals – financed by the Ministry of Labor, Social Affairs and Integration of the State of Saxony-Anhalt. He was one of the Principal Investigators of the research consortium "Neural Mechanisms Underlying Pedophilia and Sexual Offending Against Children: Origins, Assessment, and Therapies" funded by the German Ministry of Education and Health (www.nemup.de). At the Charité, Prof. Beier is responsible for the "Sexuality and Endocrine System" module that all medical school students (more than 600 per year) must go through, and leads the curricular development program for the further-specialization area of Sexual Medicine (authorized by the Berlin Chamber of Physicians).

Abbreviations

ACT	Acceptance and commitment therapy
ACTH	Adrenocorticotropic hormone
ADT	Androgen deprivation therapy
APA	American Psychiatric Association
BEDIT	The Berlin dissexuality therapy
BKiSchG	Bundeskinderschutzgesetz (Federal Child Protection Act)
COPINE	Combating Pedophile Information Networks in Europe
CSA	Child Sexual Abuse
CSAI	Child Sexual Abuse Images
CUBIT	Custody-Based Intensive Treatment Program
DHT	Dihydrotestosterone
GnRH	Gonadotropin-releasing hormone
DBT	Dialectical behavior therapy
DSM-5	Diagnostic and Statistical Manual of Mental Disorders, 5th Edition
ICD-10	International Classification of Diseases and Related Health Problems, 10th Edition
ICD-11	International Classification of Diseases and Related Health Problems, 11th Edition
KKG	Gesetz zur Kooperation und Information im Kinderschutz (Child Protection, Cooperation and Information Act)
LH	Luteinizing hormone
LHRH	Luteinizing hormone-releasing hormone
PCS	Police Crime Statistics
PPD	Prevention Project Dunkelfeld
RNR	Risk-need-responsivity
SOTEP	Sex Offender Treatment and Evaluation Program
SSRI	Selective serotonin reuptake inhibitor
StGB	Strafgesetzbuch (criminal code)
WHO	World Health Organization

Pedophilia and Hebephilia

Gerold Scherner, Till Amelung, Miriam Schuler,
Dorit Grundmann, and Klaus M. Beier

Sexual Attraction to Prepubescent and/or Early Pubescent Children: Pedophilia and Hebephilia

Sexual attraction to children who are in the stages of physical development before the onset of puberty (Tanner stage I) or in an early stage of puberty (Tanner stages II and III) has increasingly become the focus of scientific research in recent years. Even if the etiology of these non-normative sexual particularities has not yet been sufficiently explained, their existence can nonetheless be verified both physiologically and neurobiologically (Freund et al. 1972; Banse et al. 2010; Ponseti et al. 2012). Meta-analytical studies were able to demonstrate the significance of a corresponding sexual preference in the prognosis and treatment of sex offenders (Hanson and Morton-Bourgon 2005).

Sexual attraction to the prepubescent developmental body age is designated as pedophilia, and sexual attraction to the early pubescent body age is designated as hebephilia. Both terms refer to clinical diagnoses and are not intended in a criminological or legal sense. Generally speaking, a person must be at least 16 years of age and at least 5 years older than the child in question in order to fulfill the criteria of either pedophilia or hebephilia. In cases where the category of pedophilia or hebephilia is applied to a juvenile (at least 16 years old), emotional, cognitive, and sexual maturity should be taken into consideration before the appropriate diagnosis is determined (Diagnostic and Statistical Manual of Mental Disorders, Fifth Edition [DSM-5]; American Psychiatric Association [APA] 2013). The diagnostic criteria of the DSM-5 require the presence of recurring, intense sexually arousing fantasies, sexual urges, and/or sexual behaviors involving prepubescent children for a period of at least 6 months conceptualized as "pedophilic sexual orientation." Cases of "pedophilic disorder" require the additional criterion that these fantasies and/or behavioral patterns are accompanied by psychological distress, interpersonal difficulties, or functional impairments. In cases

G. Scherner · M. Schuler · D. Grundmann
K. M. Beier (✉)
Charité – Universitätsmedizin Berlin, Corporate Member of Freie Universität Berlin, Humboldt-Universität zu Berlin, and Berlin Institute of Health, Center for Human and Health Sciences, Institute of Sexology and Sexual Medicine, Berlin, Germany
e-mail: klaus.beier@charite.de

T. Amelung
Charité – Universitätsmedizin Berlin, Corporate Member of Freie Universität Berlin, Humboldt-Universität zu Berlin, and Berlin Institute of Health, Center for Human and Health Sciences, Institute of Sexology and Sexual Medicine, Department of Psychiatry and Psychotherapy, Charité Campus Mitte, Berlin, Germany

where actual child sexual abuse (CSA) has taken place, the diagnosis of "pedophilic disorder" is also possible even when no psychological distress has occurred because abusive acts are a danger to and can cause harm to others, and thus by definition violate social norms. Individuals who act on their sexual fantasies and impulses directed toward prepubescent children thus fulfill the criteria of the diagnosis "pedophilic disorder," even if they do not consider their behavior as problematic. On the other hand, individuals who do not experience significant distress as a result of their fantasies about prepubescent children, who are not functionally impaired, and who have never acted upon their sexual impulses have a "pedophilic sexual orientation" but do not have a "pedophilic disorder" according to the DSM-5.

Excursus

Concerning the terminology in denoting pedophilia (as sexual preference, sexual orientation, or sexual interest), the current situation is far from clear. There are some researchers suggesting the acknowledgement of pedophilia as a form of sexual orientation (Seto 2012) which had been implemented in the DSM-5, but it was criticized later proposing a change toward "sexual interest" (statement APA October 2013) – mainly for political reasons because of the close proximity to the expressions "homosexual orientation" or "heterosexual orientation" – demonstrating once more the moral stigmatization of pedophilia: because no one would ever appreciate being compared here on the basis of even one single criterion, which may explain that some people go as far as claiming that pedophilically inclined persons are not even human beings.

In this manual, the term "sexual preference for prepubescent children" is a description for pedophilia which could be replaced by the term "sexual interest for

children" or "sexual orientation toward children" because of the synonymous meaning – a person who experiences sexual arousal through the occurrence of children in his fantasies, particularly during masturbation. The evaluation of data from the Prevention Project Dunkelfeld (PPD) documents the early onset of this preference, the obvious romantic dimension (falling in love with children), and the high stability thereof (Grundmann et al. 2016), i.e., criteria for the definition of sexual orientation (Seto 2012).

Independent of these terminological uncertainties, there is no doubt about the significance of the two criteria for diagnosis according to DSM-5 differentiating between pedophilia and pedophilic disorder (cf. chapter "Pedophilia and Hebephilia").

In cases of hebephilia, the early pubertal body age of a child is the focus of sexual fantasies, impulses, and behavior. The difference between pedophilic and hebephilic individuals thus lies, psycho-physiologically and clinically, in the parameters of the sexually preferred body age (Beier et al. 2015b; Blanchard et al. 2009). In the opinion of the authors of this book, hebephilia can thus be regarded from a clinical perspective as a non-normative type of sexual preference with the potential character of a disorder (for more detail, see Beier et al. 2015b). It is nevertheless important to note that the concept of hebephilia, as well as its features as a disorder, is a subject of controversy frequently discussed in the professional community (see Hames and Blanchard 2012), a controversy which is also reflected in the diagnostic criteria of the two most relevant classification systems, DSM-5 (APA 2013) and ICD-10 (the International Statistical Classification of Diseases and Related Health Problems, 10th edition; World Health Organization [WHO] 1992). While in the DSM-5 the diagnostic criteria for pedophilia refer explicitly to prepubescent children, the clinical description of pedophilia in the ICD-10 refers to "A sexual preference for children, usually of prepubertal or early pubertal age. Some paedophiles are attracted only to girls, others only to boys, and others again are interested in both sexes" and a differentiation to the diagnostic criteria for research in the same edition can be noted (see Table 1). In the ICD-10, the term pedophilia is used to describe the responsiveness to the prepubescent and/or early pubescent body age, whereas in the DSM-5, the term pedophilia focuses on the prepubescent body age. The term hebephilia or the responsiveness to the early pubescent body age is not listed as a separate category in DSM-5, but it does meet the criteria for the diagnosis

"unspecified paraphilic disorder" (APA 2013; Blanchard et al. 2009).

1 Definition and Manifestations

To provide a summary of the similarities and differences between the classification systems of the ICD-10, DSM-5, and the ICD-11, they are compared and contrasted in Table 1. In addition to the main criteria (A, B, C), the diagnostic assessment must take into account whether pedophilia, in the sense of a sexual preference disorder and its corresponding need for treatment, is an exclusive

Table 1 Diagnostic Criteria according to ICD-10 (International Classification of Diseases and Related Health Problems, 10th edition, Diagnostic criteria for research), DSM-5 (Diagnostic and Statistical Manual of Mental Disorders, 5th edition), and ICD-11 (International Classification of Diseases and Related Health Problems, 11th edition)

ICD-10	DSM-5	ICD-11
Pedophilia F65.4	Pedophilic disorder 302.2	6D32 Pedophilic disorder
A. The general criteria for disorders of sexual preference (F65) must be met G1 Recurrent intense sexual urges and fantasies involving unusual objects or activities G2 Acts on the urges or is markedly distressed by them G3 The disorder must have been present for at least 6 months	A. Over a period of at least 6 months, recurrent, intense sexually arousing fantasies, sexual urges, or behaviors involving sexual activity with a prepubescent child or children (generally age 13 years or younger)	Pedophilic disorder is characterized by a sustained, focused, and intense pattern of sexual arousal – as manifested by persistent sexual thoughts, fantasies, urges, or behaviors – involving pre-pubertal children. In addition, in order for pedophilic disorder to be diagnosed, the individual must have acted on these thoughts, fantasies, or urges or be markedly distressed by them. This diagnosis does not apply to sexual behaviors among pre- or post-pubertal children with peers who are close in age
B. A persistent or a predominant preference for sexual activity with a prepubescent child or children	B. The individual has acted on these sexual urges, or the sexual urges or fantasies cause marked distress or interpersonal difficulty	
C. The person is at least 16 years old and at least 5 years older than the child or children	C. The individual is at least 16 years and at least 5 years older than the child or children in criterion A **Note:** Do not include an individual in late adolescence involved in an ongoing sexual relationship with a 12- or 13-year-old. *Specify* whether: **Exclusive type** (attracted only to children) **Nonexclusive type** *Specify* whether: **Sexually attracted to males** **Sexually attracted to females** **Sexually attracted to both** *Specify* whether: **Limited to incest**	

type in which sexual attraction occurs only with regard to the prepubescent and/or early pubescent body age referred to in the literature as "exclusive pedophilia" or a nonexclusive type where sexual attraction extends not only to a child's prepubescent and/or early pubescent body age but also to the late-pubescent/adult body age. This has consequences for the clinical assessment and the therapeutic approach which is based on it, especially regarding risk-assessment and possible beneficial resources. It is also necessary to determine which sex is considered to be sexually attractive.

In the ICD-11, as well as in the DSM-5, the generic term is "paraphilic disorders." In the ICD-11 the term "paraphilic disorders" explicitly covers "exhibitionistic disorder," "voyeuristic disorder," "pedophilic disorder" (exclusively specifying prepubescent children and not including also early pubescent children, as in the ICD-10), "frotteuristic disorder," and the "coercive sexual sadism disorder," as well as a separate category concerning the "paraphilic disorder involving solitary behavior or consenting individuals".

Not explicitly taken up are the "fetishistic disorder," the "transvestic-fetishistic disorder," the "sexual masochistic disorder," and the "sexual sadistic disorder." The reasoning is based on the recognition that a diagnosis is generally of no significance regarding the health care system and that there is no connection to the degree of suffering and loss of function. Also taken into account is the frequency of particular sexual practices (e.g., "bondage") which cause no psychological distress and would not benefit from any diagnostic term in the health care system.

It is obvious that this point of view is not stringently followed up in the ICD-11, looking at the rest categories allowing for the code "other paraphilic disorder involving non-consenting individuals" – this allowing for all sorts of paraphilias which can be ascribed to the sadistic spectrum (e.g., the desire for sexual contact with disabled or drugged individuals or with animals) – and also mentioning the category "paraphilic disorder involving solitary behavior or consenting individuals." This, of course, would cover such terms as "fetishism" and "transvestic fetishism," pro-

viding that significant distress is involved or that the practice might lead to permanently endangering oneself or (consenting) others (e.g., asphyxiophilia, that is, inducing oxygen deprivation in order to increase sexual arousal).

It is particularly important to diagnostically assess the different axes of the structure of sexual preference, the different forms of sexual experience and behavior, as well as the concrete forms of sexual activity (cf. Beier et al. 2005; Beier and Loewit 2013).

Human sexual preference can be described along three different axes:

- The responsiveness to the gender of the preferred partner (the male partner, the female, both sexes etc.)
- The relevant developmental body age of the preferred partner (prepubescent [Tanner stage I], early pubescent [Tanner stages II and III], late pubescent [Tanner stage IV], or postpubescent [Tanner stage V] body age)
- The desired practices with the preferred partner (sexually preferred interactions/behaviors)

Sexual experience and behavior can also be characterized according to three levels:

- The level of the concrete sexual behavior
- The level of the sexual fantasy (especially during masturbation and regarding the concrete, orgasm-triggering fantasies)
- The level of the sexual self-concept

Regarding sexual activity, three forms can be distinguished:

- Masturbation (self-stimulation and self-gratification)
- Extragenital sexual interactions (e.g., caressing, stroking, cuddling)
- Genital stimulation (manual, oral, or other stimulation, e.g., petting, vaginal, anal penetration)

Regarding sexual attraction to a body age, the differentiation between sexual interest in prepubescent children (pedophilia) and/or early pubescent children (hebephilia), in contrast to late pubescent or adult (teleiophilia) body age, is significant.

Regarding developmental biological processes during puberty, it should be noted that 20 years ago in Germany, the beginning of pubescent development (genital development in boys and breast development in girls) was determined to be roughly around age 11 (Engelhardt et al. 1995; Willers et al. 1996). Recent studies indicate an earlier onset of pubescent development and an acceleration of physical maturity. At the age of ten, about half of the girls and more than a third of the boys reported the onset of pubic hair development. The average age for reaching late-pubescent and adult pubic hair development (Tanner stages IV and V) is, respectively, 12.3 and 13.4 years for girls and 13.4 and 14.1 years for boys (Kahl et al. 2007). In addition to the differences in the preferred body age, persons may be exclusively (pedophilia, hebephilia, pedo-hebephilia) or non-exclusively (pedo-teleiophilia, hebe-teleiophilia, pedo-hebe-teleiophilia) responsive to certain body age. The sexual preference for prepubescent and/or early pubescent children can also have impacts upon sociosexual relationships with adults. As shown in Fig. 1, phenomenologically, responsiveness to one or more developmental body age (physical stages of development) is possible.

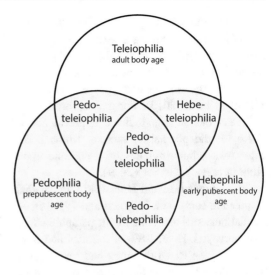

Fig. 1 Schematic representation of the phenomenology of sexual attraction with regard to developmental body ages according to Beier et al. 2013

2   Prevalence

There is even less reliable data on the prevalence of pedophilia in women, and the available literature consists predominantly of descriptions of individual cases. According to the most recent literature, the entire spectrum of sexual paraphilia appears to be a primarily male domain, which is also the case for pedophilia/hebephilia. Additionally, in the few existing special outpatient centers for people who feel sexually attracted to children and who are seeking therapeutic assistance, it is predominantly men who register. Studies to determine prevalence are generally difficult to conduct. In the studies to date, it should be taken into account that some of these have been conducted on selected population samples, in which the definitions of pedophilia and its diagnostic criteria were not uniformly or consistently operationalized, and that in addition to other methodological problems, the generalizability of the results in each case remains questionable. In a twin study conducted in Finland with 1310 participants, 0.2% of the participants stated that they had a sexual interest in children between the ages of 7 and 12. In total, 3.3% of respondents said they had a sexual interest in children under the age of 15. In this study, sexual interest was surveyed over the previous 12 months, so that the timescale criterion was also included (Alanko et al. 2013). Out of 367 men from a representative sample from Berlin, 9.5% stated that prepubescent children's bodies appeared in their sexual fantasies, 6% reported the occurrence of children in their masturbation fantasies, and 3.8% stated that they had already sexually abused a child (Ahlers et al. 2011). In a recent study conducted as part of an online survey of 8718 male participants in Germany, 4.1% of the participants reported sexual fantasies in which prepubescent children played a role, 3.2% reported sexual abuse of prepubescent children, of which 1.7% exclusively used sexual abuse images, and 0.1% of the participants reported having a sexual preference in terms of pedophilia. The authors interpret this value as a conservative estimate of the prevalence of the exclusive type of pedophilia (Dombert et al. 2015). For a less conservative estimate, the authors indicate a prevalence of 5.4% for the population sample, which correlates with other estimates of a possible upper limit of prevalence (Seto 2009).

In a study on sexual fantasies in a Canadian population sample of 717 men and 799 women, sexual fantasies associated with paraphilia were also surveyed. Here, 1.8% of the men and 0.8% of the women stated that they had sexual fantasies about children under the age of 12 in the course of their lives. The diagnostic criteria for pedophilia were not further investigated in this study (Joyal et al. 2015).

The number of persons with pedophilia among those convicted of sexual abuse of children is supported by much more reliable figures and better research. It is estimated that about 40–50% of men who have committed sexual assault on children are pedophilic (Beier et al. 2005; see Seto 2008 for an overview). Pedophilia is therefore by no means synonymous with child sexual abuse (CSA), although these terms are often used synonymously in public discourse, politics, and the media. Therefore, there are men with pedophilia who have not yet committed child sexual abuse (Beier et al. 2007, 2009; Riegel 2004) and, conversely, there are many perpetrators who sexually abuse children even though they are not pedophilic (Beier 1998; Beier et al. 2005; Seto 2008).

Nonetheless, a clear connection can be established between deviant sexual interests and sexual abuse of children (Hanson and Bussière 1998; Mann et al. 2010). This involves both sexual abuse of children and the use, distribution, or production of child sexual abuse images (CSAI). Perpetrators of child sexual abuse differ from other men (sex offenders with adult victims, perpetrators of nonsexual offences, control population samples without criminal charges) in terms of their sexual responsiveness to stimuli in phallometric studies in which prepubescent and/or early pubescent children were displayed (see,

e.g., Blanchard et al. 2001, 2006). Furthermore, indicators of sexual interest in children in population samples with identified sex offenders are a strong predictor for reoffending (Hanson and Morton-Bourgon 2005). The recidivism rate among pedophilic sex offenders is between 50% and 80%, whereas among offenders who sexually abuse children but have no pedophilic sexual preference, it is between 10% and 25%, i.e., significantly lower (Beier 1998).

With regard to the consumption of CSAI, most pedophilic men state that they find such materials sexually exciting and have already used them in their lives (Neutze et al. 2011; Quayle and Taylor 2002; Riegel 2004). Criminals convicted of the use of CSAI, on the other hand, often show a responsiveness to the child-like body age along the lines of pedophilia/hebephilia (Seto et al. 2006). The use of CSAI can therefore be regarded as an indicator of the existence of pedophilia. This also seems plausible in light of the background assumption that people use pornographic materials which correspond to their own sexual fantasies and experience them as sexually arousing.

Since people with a pedophilic sexual preference have a higher risk of repeatedly committing child sexual abuse or using CSAI (Eke et al. 2011), it must be assumed that these persons also exhibit a higher lifetime risk of committing first-time offences. This makes them an important target group for the prevention of child sexual abuse and the use of CSAI. For those affected, constant confrontation with sexual fantasies and impulses directed toward children can go hand in hand with their own self-humiliation and lack of acceptance (Schaefer et al. 2010). Furthermore, they have to deal with possible legal and social consequences if they act on their sexual desires (ibid.). This may explain the frequent occurrence of symptoms of psychological distress (e.g., anxiety and depression) in this indication group. Corresponding psychological distress would be preference-related and can be found both in the DSM-5 (APA 2013) and in the ICD-10 (World Health Organization [WHO] 1992), where this distress is explicitly listed as a diagnostic criterion for pedophilia.

In summary, it can be assumed that nondelinquent pedophilic and hebephilic individuals, as well as pedophilic/hebephilic perpetrators in the *Dunkelfeld* (i.e., perpetrators whose actions either remain undetected or have not been reported to the authorities) represent an important target group for the prevention of child sexual abuse, since their subjectively experienced psychological distress motivates them to undergo treatment and makes them receptive to preventive approaches (Beier et al. 2009; Schaefer et al. 2010; for an in-depth explanation on the subject, see Beier et al. 2015a, d; Kuhle, Grundmann and Beier 2015).

3 Etiology and Neurobiology

Since Krafft-Ebing, "pedophilia erotica" has been understood as a psychological disease (*psychopathologia sexualis*). Based on the relatively unspecific auto- and alloerotic behavior of children, early theorists of human sexual behavior assumed that a maturation of the psyche was a precondition for the adult sexual behavior of humans. Deviations from the ever-changing norm—which has been observed over the decades—were accordingly regarded as disorders within this development. This notion continues to influence empirical research on biological and developmental causes of pedophilia and child sexual abuse to this day. In recent years, two major explanatory models have been competing for interpretative primacy regarding the development of non-normative sexual particularities and sexual behavior disorders. Based on the considerations of the cognitive turn in behavioral therapy, one of the models of pedophilic sexual fantasy assumes it to be a learned behavior. According to this school, the primary characteristics of pedophilic men lie in their capacity to respond sexually to children. A second school assumes that the above-mentioned abnormal sexual development occurs as result of malfunctioning biological processes. Following this school, deeper biological changes can be found in connection with pedophilia.

3.1 Learning Theory Models

Conditioning

On the basis of learning theory models, both classical and operational conditioning processes have been connected with pedophilic sexual preference. McGuire and colleagues formulated a theory of "sexual deviance as conditioned behavior" (McGuire et al. 1964), according to which sexual arousal represents an unconditioned reaction which, coupled with an initially non-arousing stimulus, can lead to sexual arousal and, under certain circumstances, to sexual behavior (see also Laws and Marshall 1990).

According to this theory, sexual experience with children of the same age can connect a previously neutral stimulus (childlike body age to sexual arousal). Through the experience of sexual gratification (reinforcement stimulus), a lasting sexual interest in the childlike body age develops. The few existing studies on the topic do suggest that the sexual reaction of mammals and specifically of humans can be conditioned (O'Donohue and Plaud 1994; Pfaus et al. 2001). The survey work by O'Donohue and Plaud (1994) includes experiments in which originally neutral visual stimuli were paired with sexually arousing stimuli, such as images of naked women, in order to trigger sexual arousal by means of neutral visual stimuli. The results showed that stimuli that in principle have sexually salient characteristics (e.g., signal colors ["eye-catching colors"], surface texture, odor) are better suited for conditioning than less-salient stimuli (e.g., geometric figures). This is associated with the evolutionary predisposition for conditioning (preparedness; Seligman 1970), which indicates that certain stimuli are better suited for conditioning than others.

According to this theory, the principle of extinction should also apply to sexual arousal. This means that the conditioned reaction might be extinguished if the conditioned stimulus is repeatedly performed without the unconditioned reaction. The temporary changes in arousal profiles through deconditioning presented by

Marshall (1997, 2008) cannot be regarded as generalizable due to methodological weaknesses. The proof of a permanent change in sexual preference for body age is still lacking. Grundmann et al. (2016) also demonstrated a high stability in sexual preference for pedophilic and hebephilic sexual interests after puberty.

With Conditioning Theory, it still remains unclear as to why child sexual behavior is preserved only in a minority of all men as pedophilic fantasies after puberty. The predisposing factors to be considered are experiences of sexual abuse, lack of education, and a high propensity for aggression (Ward et al. 2006; see also section "From Victim to Perpetrator").

Exotic Becomes Erotic

In his theory "Exotic Becomes Erotic," Bem also emphasizes the relevance of experience for the development of sexual preferences (Bem 1996). According to the "Exotic Becomes Erotic" theory, adult sexual preference is influenced by prepubescent play behavior. In the prepubescent phase, it can be observed that children, in accordance with their preferences for "gender-typical" or "gender-atypical" activities, feel closer to their own or the opposite sex, respectively, and experience the other sex as strange or "exotic." This exoticism in the prepubescent phase generates feelings such as antipathy, fear, or disgust, coupled with increased physiological excitement. According to the "Exotic Becomes Erotic" theory, the physiological and emotional excitement triggered by the "exotic sex" is sexualized by hormonal influences and leads to an opposite- or same-sex sexual orientation. As a result, men and women with gender-typical play behavior in childhood tend to develop an opposite-sex orientation, whereas adults with gender-atypical play behavior in childhood tend to develop a same-sex orientation. There are also findings that support this theory as an explanation for the content of pedophilic fantasy. Using qualitative interviews, Bundschuh (2001) found that pedophilic men describe their relationship to their peers in childhood and adolescence as problematic. (Banse 2013) was also able to show that pedophilic men exhibited inadequate or dysfunctional peer rela-

tionships in childhood. This correlation also remained under the influence of other suspected risk factors (e.g., traumatic experiences). Other features associated with sexual interest in children along the lines of pedophilia (lower IQ, experiences of abuse, traumatization) also fit well into Bem's theory, as these factors can complicate relationships with peers. It remains unclear why some men are sexually attracted only to children and others to both children and adults (Banse 2013). The question of why it is mainly men (and not women) who develop a pedophilic sexual preference also remains unresolved. These questions require further research.

From Victim to Perpetrator

"From Victim to Perpetrator" is a much-discussed theory on the emergence of sexual preference disorders. Some studies show an increased incidence of experiences of abuse among persons who offend sexually (Jespersen et al. 2009; Seto and Lalumière 2010). In a longitudinal study, Salter et al. (2003) found that out of 224 men who were victims of sexual abuse during childhood, 12% committed sexual offenses themselves after 7–19 years—mainly against children. Because sex crimes do not allow conclusions to be drawn about sexual fantasies, these studies also do not allow conclusions to be drawn about the etiology of pedophilic interests.

3.2 Neuroendocrine and Genetic Factors

To date, there is little data to explain the relationship between neuroendocrine and genetic factors and pedophilia. From the results of a Finnish study of twins with over 4000 male twins and their siblings, the authors concluded that a certain percentage of pedophilia is hereditary (Alanko et al. 2013). Although the effect is minimal, this suggests a certain genetic component. Clinical similarities between pedophilia and diseases of the compulsive spectrum, attention deficit syndrome, personality and affective disorders, as well as addiction disorders with correspondingly high comorbidities (Grubin 2008) suggest disorders in the serotonergic and dopaminergic systems and the hypothalamic-pituitary adrenal (HPA) axis. (Gaffney and Berlin 1984) also suspect that there may be an altered activity of the hypothalamus-pituitary gonad (HPG) axis, which controls the regulation of sex hormones via a feedback mechanism. However, the data on sex hormone homeostasis in pedophilia and child sexual abuse remains inconsistent (Grubin 2008).

3.3 Neurobiological Correlates of Pedophilia and Child Sexual Abuse

Neurobiological research on pedophilia has largely been conducted on pedophilic sexual offenders (Mohnke et al. 2014). Findings from this research primarily allow conclusions to be drawn about the neurobiological particularities of those men with pedophilic sexual preference who have committed acts of child sexual abuse and to a much lesser extent about those who use CSAI. Neurobiological research results on pedophilia can be divided into neuroanatomical and neurofunctional investigations.

Neuroanatomical Research Results on Pedophilia and Child Sexual Abuse
At the root of all neurobiological research are individual case reports on behavioral disorders in connection with structural changes in the brain (for a summary, see Mohnke et al. 2014). Published case reports pointing to neuroanatomical changes associated with pedophilia or child sexual abuse consistently refer to the onset of new sexual behavior with children or the desire to do so. Case reports in which patients report emerging genuine sexual fantasies with children after having brain lesions have not been published. From the locations of lesions, shown in the published case reports, it can be deduced that pedophilia or sexually abusive behavior is associated with frontotemporal, orbitofrontal, and frontocentral structures. The structural changes in the brain were never exclusively associated with sexually assaultive behavior toward children. Rather, the patients suffered more from personal-

ity changes, generally sexual or general disinhibition, changes in intelligence, or dementia. This constellation indicates that these neuroanatomical changes predisposed patients primarily to sexually assaultive behavior and not so much to genuine sexual interest in children.

Early structural MRI studies on pedophilic men who had committed sexual assault on children were only marginally conclusive and replicable due to the small number of cases concerning deficiencies found in the gray matter. The first study, which examined both pedophilic sexual offenders and pedophilic men who had not committed acts of abuse, came from the NeMUP consortium (www.nemup.de) and replicated minor differences between pedophilic men who had sexually abused children and nonviolent teleophiles (= sexual attraction to an adult body age). Differences in gray matter between pedophilic offenders and pedophilic non-offenders were particularly pronounced. Here, more gray matter was found in the temporal pole area in pedophilic non-offenders in comparison to pedophilic offenders (Schiffer et al. 2017). This finding fits into the existing literature on the function of the temporal pole, the experimental removal of which in rhesus monkeys leads to the so-called Klüver-Bucy syndrome—a behavioral disorder characterized by generally unusual social behavior and sexual disinhibition (Klüver and Bucy 1939).

Regarding changes in the white matter, the findings are still divergent. To date, only three studies on this topic have been published. Two studies show deficits in the integrity of fronto-occipital and fronto-thalamic fiber bundles in pedophilic offenders and users of abuse images compared to normal random samples (Cantor et al. 2008, 2015). However, a study from Germany could not replicate these deficits (Gerwinn et al. 2015).

In view of the still widespread inconsistency of the results, no clinical implications can yet be drawn from neuroanatomical investigations. In the case of emergent sexual behavior involving children or corresponding behavioral impulses in older age groups, however, one should seek to rule out the presence of a brain organic disorder.

Neurofunctional Correlates of Pedophilia and Child Sexual Abuse

Neurofunctional data on pedophilia and child sexual abuse were initially collected as part of clinical investigations of convicted sexual offenders. Here, various indications of brain-functional particularities associated with child sexual abuse were found. Pedophilic sexual offenders showed lower intelligence quotients than their non-pedophilic counterparts and the normal population. There was also an increase in non-right-handedness (left-handedness and ambidexterity) and minor craniofacial malformations (Blanchard et al. 2008; Dyshniku et al. 2015), which the authors interpreted as indications of prenatal developmental disorders.

The findings from quantitative studies on neurofunctional correlates of pedophilia and child sexual abuse are more complex than those with regard to neuroanatomy, and a differentiation between a sexual preference disorder (pedophilia) and a behavioral disorder (sexual abuse) is not always possible (Tenbergen et al. 2015). In measurements of the behavior of frontal-brain functions (executive functions), sexual offenders who had abused children exhibited deficits in impulse control; deficits in verbal fluency, verbal memory, and processing; and deficits in sustained concentration. More detailed studies, distinguishing between pedophilic and non-pedophilic abusers, found evidence that these impairments are more pronounced in non-pedophilic offenders (who had sexually abused children). However, this data varies widely between individual studies with different forensic and non-forensic samples. Tenbergen et al. (2015) therefore suspect that comorbid disorders such as depression or antisociality significantly affect disorders of executive function. Data from the NeMUP consortium, on the other hand, suggests that while there certainly are corresponding deficits—which primarily differentiate between pedophilic offenders and pedophilic non-offenders—the discrepancy between them and a sample of the normal population is minimal. This also entails that the variability of the above-mentioned results could once again constitute a problem of a lack of statistical power.

On the other hand, findings regarding the processing of sexual stimuli are much less ambiguous. Here, consistent differences between pedophilic and non-pedophilic men can be found throughout a large number of studies with a wide variety of methodologies, regardless of their history of abusive behavior (Mohnke et al. 2014). Pedophilic men process stimuli with children as sexual, and this is not surprising. This phenomenon is also used in various diagnostic procedures, e.g., in phallometry (the measurement of the penile reaction to sensory stimuli), as well as for indirect approaches such as Viewing Reaction Time, implicit association tests, Snake-in-the-Grass paradigms, etc., or Attentional Blink Procedure (Schmidt et al. 2015). These indirect approaches repeatedly prove to be less precise in their application when used individually. A well-proven approach, on the other hand, is a method that makes diagnostic use of these neurofunctional particularities related to pedophilia by combining two indirect methods and a questionnaire (Explicit and Implicit Sexual Interest Profile [EISIP]; see Banse et al. 2010). However, this procedure, like other indirect methods, is also susceptible to arbitrary manipulation by the person tested. Ponseti and colleagues succeeded in developing a highly sensitive and specific classification of pedophilic and non-pedophilic men based on their brain activity when viewing child and adult sexual stimuli (Ponseti et al. 2012). The brain areas recruited for the processing of child-related stimuli in pedophilic men seem to correspond to those used for the processing of sexual stimuli for adults in teleiophilic men (Polisois-Keating and Joyal 2013). Initial data indicates that these activations are not subject to arbitrary control, making manipulation of the test results considerably more difficult. The replication of the study by Ponseti et al. is still pending.

While neuroanatomical changes in connection with pedophilia and child sexual abuse have no clinical significance, important clinical conclusions can be drawn from neurofunctional changes. Thus, phallometry, implicit methods, and, possibly in the future, MRI provide important tools for objectifying the diagnosis of pedophilia. The importance of impaired executive function and possible comorbidities with affective or personality disorders should be taken into account when planning treatment.

Biopsychosocial Approach
None of the explanatory approaches described above has so far been sufficiently verified empirically to establish an evidence-based etiological model. The emergence of pedophilic fantasy activity cannot therefore be explained in a monocausal fashion. Only a multidimensional approach, which integrates biological, social, and psychological factors, can help to understand potential factors in the emergence of a particular sexual preference (see Sect. 4 in chapter "Child Sexual Abuse and the Use of Abuse Images").

4　Comorbidity

Various studies indicate that comorbidities are the rule rather than the exception among pedophilic men and men convicted of child sexual abuse (Dunsieth et al. 2004; Kafka and Hennen 2002; Raymond et al. 1999). In a study by Raymond et al. (1999), the majority of clinical samples of outpatient pedophilic sexual offenders that were examined showed comorbid psychiatric disorders of axes I and II of the DSM-IV. The most frequent additional diagnoses on axis I were present-day affective disorders (31.1%) and anxiety disorders (5.3%). In addition, 60% fulfilled the criteria of having a personality disorder on axis II. These and other results related to comorbidities are consistent with the experience of clinical work conducted within the framework of the Prevention Project Dunkelfeld (PPD). In addition, subclinical dysfunctions or abnormalities that do not meet the criteria of psychiatric disorders appear to be even more common. In a study by Konrad et al. (2017b), the general psychological distress of 455 PPD participants was recorded using the Brief Symptom Inventory (BSI; Franke 2000). The results showed that 59% of the survey sample had clinically relevant psychological distress that was comparable to that of inpatients. The high frequency of comorbid disorders in pedophilic and hebephilic individuals

has an influence on the planning and implementation of therapy for this specific target group (for a more detailed description, see Sect. 6 in chapter "Therapeutic Options").

5　Societal Assessment and Cultural Differences

Society reacts to pedophilic individuals with intensely negative emotions, social exclusion, and stigmatization (Jahnke et al. 2015). More than 95% of the outpatient psychotherapists in Germany are not willing to work with pedophilic patients (Stiels-Glenn 2010). More than 60% of psychotherapists in training cannot imagine working with a pedophilic who has already assaulted someone (Jahnke et al. 2015). Accordingly, the majority of pedophilic individuals say that fear of stigmatization by therapists is the main reason for not seeking therapeutic help (Kramer 2011).

Beyond the context of Germany, there is also no society or culture that would not prohibit the sexual abuse of children. This is most likely also the case historically speaking. Contrary to the frequently mentioned assumption that in ancient Greece sexual acts involving children were a common and thus customary practice, there is no plausible evidence for this. Rather, we find many more descriptions of exclusive relationships between young men and men who belonged to the upper class that served the purpose of an initiation process to prepare the younger generation for their later tasks as leading (military) figures of society.

Similar initiation rites are still found today in different ethnic groups, e.g., with the Sambia in Papua New Guinea. In this case, it is stipulated that the pubescent young men as future warriors will perform oral intercourse on the older warriors up until sexual climax in order to imbibe their semen, the idea being that their martial strength will be transferred to the younger generation, and this is consequently to be seen as completely independent from the sexual responsiveness of the participants (Herdt 1982). It is a well-established ritual practice that nobody would classify as sexual abuse, considering that sexual acts with children outside this frame of reference are strictly prohibited.

Yet at the same time, there is little evidence that the various (both past and present) cultures differentiate between the fantasy level (where sexual preference is revealed) and the behavioral level (where the realization of sexual acts against children because of various motives is made explicit). This speaks against an in-depth discussion of the possible underlying causes of child sexual abuse, although the available figures show that it is a widespread problem that has arisen in a wide variety of countries and cultures (cf. Stoltenborgh et al. 2011). This is all the more true since most sexual assaults on children take place in the *Dunkelfeld*, and the cases known to the justice system (the *Hellfeld*) represent only a small fraction of all incidents.

With regard to pedophilia and hebephilia, the situation is further complicated by the fact that these two non-normative sexual particularities are largely unknown not only to the general population but also to professionals in national health systems. If the term pedophilia is used at all, it is equated with child sexual abuse, i.e., as a description of one and the same phenomenon. As a result, there is no differentiated analysis of the causes of child sexual abuse and thus no framework for perpetrator-oriented primary preventive measures.

Community involvement is more visible with regard to the victims, although this also only affects primary prevention measures to a limited extent. Efforts to provide assistance for victims (i.e., to alleviate the effects of sexual trauma) are more likely to be found, as long as those who need help are willing to reveal themselves as victims of sexual abuse. Cultural norms can prevent this from happening. For example, to avoid any loss of reputation for the victim's family, the victim may be silenced in the event that reporting abuse would threaten disgrace for the family, and in this way the perpetrators (especially if they are family members) are "protected" by the victims themselves.

The fear of a loss of reputation may also affect the victim himself or herself. For some, the chances of getting married would decrease if it became publicly known that the bride had been the victim of sexual abuse—which, in some cases, can be so stigmatized that marriage would no longer even be considered (cf. for example on the situation in India in this regard: Carson et al. 2013). Such difficulties are particularly prevalent in many countries where the marriage is arranged by the parents. This makes the dysfunctional behavior of the families at least more understandable, but it clearly comes at the victim's expense and ultimately protects the perpetrator. It is remarkable how little victim-empathy there is, because the priority they give to the well-being of the family is also of paramount importance. This is underscored by a case study from the work of the Institute for Sexual Science and Sexual Medicine of the Charité in India, which has since 2015 worked to establish perpetrator-oriented, culturally adapted measures for the primary prevention of child sexual abuse (see "Programme for Primary Prevention of Sexual Violence" at www.pppsv.org).

Case Study

This 14-year-old teenager lives in Mumbai (India) and is considered an attentive and conscientious student. He asked for medication to subdue his sexual needs, which, according to the study, were directed primarily at girls of prepubescent age. During masturbation, he fantasized about touching a child's vagina and observing the discharge of urine. During this fantasy, he reached orgasm. However, this condition concerned him less than the distraction it caused him from his goal of obtaining the best possible graduation degree. This was necessary for him to receive good vocational training that promised a high income, which he wanted to earn above all to finance his sister's dowry. He was the oldest son in a poor family and sought to elevate his family's reputation, and hence the social acceptance they received, which depended on his sister's marital status. He was not bothered by the fact that it was precisely this sister, still of prepubescent age, who was the object of his sexual fantasies. He had ambushed her along with other girls from the neighborhood several times to watch them urinate. As it turned out, this was also the activity that cost him the most time and kept him from studying, which is why he was seeking medication.

The extent to which a society confronts the sexual traumatization of children depends significantly on the extent to which that culture is individualized: the more the individual is compelled to withdraw behind collective interests or to yield to the pressures of conformity, the less attention is paid to victims' interests, a phenomenon which is reflected in a low rate of reported complaints and a diminished willingness to take preventive measures.

International Prevention with Online Services
Nevertheless, the multiple inquiries received by the Institute for Sexology and Sexual Medicine of the Charité from all over the world (inquiries from Africa, Asia, Australia, and North, Central, and South America, as well as from various European countries) make it clear that also within other countries, there are some very young people who have already recognized that they have a pedophilic tendency, which causes them suffering, and would like assistance in coping with the problem.

For example, a 28-year-old from Costa Rica writes that he already knows that he is a person with pedophilia, but he has never sexually abused a child. He goes on to say in his e-mail: "I really need help, I have been dealing with these feelings since I was 11 years old. This disease really depresses me. It has made my life a nightmare. I do not know what to do. I haven't had any sexual experiences because of this pedophilia."

And a 22-year-old Australian writes via e-mail: "I have tried to give myself therapy and to gain control over my thoughts and impulses because I do not want to harm any child. I am sure that I am a pedophilic, even though I have never contacted a specialist, which I would be afraid to do, as there is an obligatory reporting requirement in Australia, which makes it difficult to find help."

A man from Portugal (no age reported) in turn writes: "I watch child pornography very often. It has taken on enormous significance in my life.

Sometimes I can stop watching it for a few days, but I always end up on these sites again. What can you do to help me?"

As a result of the large number of requests and a special cooperation between the Berlin Institute and a network of therapists in India (especially in Mumbai and Pune, see www.PPPSV.org.), where therapists are obliged to report cases to the police and encounter patients who report that they have committed a crime or used abuse images, an online self-management program was developed, which contains diagnostic and therapeutic elements (see www.troubled-desire.com).

This has been available online since October 25, 2017, and was initially published in English. Since April 25, 2018, it has also been available in German. It is an anonymous, free-of-charge service, which is equipped with special security standards. It is intended not only for adults and adolescents (as well as for their relatives), who exhibit sexual responsiveness to the childlike prepubescent and/or early pubescent body age, but also for therapists or professional caregivers who would like to inform themselves about the problems of pedophilia or hebephilia.

As long as there is a cooperation between a network of therapists in the respective country (as is the case in India), this program makes it possible to refer those individuals with a pedophilic inclination, who have not yet committed a crime or do not have to be reported to the authorities, to therapists within the network. By the time of April 2020, this program is available in additional languages (Spanish, French, Marathi, Hindi, Russian and Turkish Portuguese) in order to provide globally effective prevention measures. The data will be evaluated for research purposes and should make it possible to understand the national and cultural specificities more precisely, in order to be able to respond to them adequately. The first extensive evaluation of Troubled Desire revealed that within the first 30 months, the self-assessment was completed by more than 4000 users from more than 80 countries (Schuler et al., forthcoming/in press).

Child Sexual Abuse and the Use of Child Sexual Abuse Images

Laura F. Kuhle, Umut Oezdemir,
and Klaus M. Beier

1   Child Sexual Abuse

According to police statistics, 12,019 cases of child sexual abuse with 14,051 victims were recorded by police in Germany in 2016 (Bundeskriminalamt 2017). Those cases that are brought to the attention of the judicial authorities and are located within the so-called *Hellfeld* (lit. "light field"), however, represent merely a fraction of the actual magnitude (Beier et al. 2015d). By and large, there is little willingness on the part of those affected to report to the police (between 11.7% and 18%); this has however increased in recent years. Abusive acts with vaginal, anal, or oral penetration and those that have taken place over a long period of time have the greatest likelihood of being reported (Bieneck et al. 2011). It is estimated that the number of unreported cases is up to 30 times higher than those included in police crime statistics (Stoltenborgh et al. 2011). Of the participants at the Berlin location of the *Prevention Project Dunkelfeld* (Präventionsprojekt

Dunkelfeld [PPD]), 43% admitted to having committed child sexual abuse, the significant majority of which (83%) were unknown to the judicial authorities (Kuhle, Kossow and Beier 2015). A similar picture emerged from the *Juvenile Prevention Project* (Präventionsprojekt Jugendliche [PPJ]): 45% of the 12- 18-year-olds who expressed interest in the project admitted to having committed child sexual abuse. Approximately 60% of these cases were unknown to the judicial authorities (Schlinzig et al. 2017).

Under German law, the sexual abuse of children is classified under criminal offenses "against sexual autonomy" (*gegen die sexuelle Selbstbestimmung* – §§ 174 ff. of the German Penal Code; Bundesministerium der Justiz und für Verbraucherschutz 2016). This refers to sex acts that are entered into against the will of the victim, as well as those in which the perpetrator induces ostensible consent by exploiting the victim's inability to consent and/or his own position of power. Acts without physical contact are also punishable, meaning that the use of force in the narrower sense is not a prerequisite for a criminal offense to have taken place.

The ostensible consent of the child in question is meaningless as a defining criterion, as, due to the cognitive, psychological, physical, and structural power imbalance in relation to the adult perpetrator, the child cannot agree to such an act with autonomy. This is also expressed in § 176 of

L. F. Kuhle · U. Oezdemir · K. M. Beier (✉)
Charité – Universitätsmedizin Berlin, Corporate Member of Freie Universität Berlin, Humboldt-Universität zu Berlin, and Berlin Institute of Health, Center for Human and Health Sciences, Institute of Sexology and Sexual Medicine, Berlin, Germany
e-mail: klaus.beier@charite.de

the German Penal Code on the criminal offense of the sexual abuse of children, which makes the deed punishable by law irrespective of the consent of the victim. The German Penal Code defines as child sexual abuse all sexual acts performed on or in front of a child under 14 years of age or the instigation of sexual acts by a child on oneself or a third person. Child sexual abuse also occurs when an offender attempts to influence a victim by showing pornographic images or representations, playing recorded media with pornographic content, making pornographic content available by means of information and communication technology, or by applicable acts of speech (German Penal Code, § 176). Additional differentiations that take into account, above all, the extent of the short- and long-term consequences for the victim are useful. Relevant factors in this respect are the initiation and duration of the abuse (one-time vs. repeated abuse), the relationship of the offender to the victim (e.g., intra- vs. extrafamilial), the extent of the severity of the act (e.g., with or without physical contact, with or without penetration), and the use or threat of violence. According the WHO's current analyses of the prevalence of child sexual abuse in Europe, 9.6% of all children and adolescents under 18 years of age become victims of sexual abuse (13.4% of girls and 5.7% of boys; WHO Regional Office for Europe 2013). According to the first representative survey of the German general population, 8.6% of girls and 2.8% of boys will become victims of sexual assault with direct physical contact by an adult perpetrator over the course of childhood and adolescence (Wetzels 1997). More recent, equally representative studies in Germany gave, on the one hand, lower (Bieneck et al. 2011) and, on the other, higher rates of prevalence (Häuser et al. 2011), although a correlation with the age distribution of the random sample under study may be observed: the more comprehensive the range of ages that was being surveyed for experiences of abuse (e.g., up to the age of 14, 16, or 18), the higher the prevalence of reported instances of sexual abuse.

The experience of sexual abuse can have far-reaching consequences for the psychological and social development of a child or adolescent.

Immediate and long-term psychological, social, physical, and/or behavioral problems may require professional support (Leeb et al. 2011). Immediate effects of sexual abuse include physical injuries or infections, as well as psychological symptoms of a more nonspecific nature, that manifest themselves, for example, as diffuse physical complaints, eating or sleep disorders, attention disorders, depression, and suicide attempts (Beier et al. 2005; Görgen et al. 2012). In regard to long-term physical effects, studies show correlations between the experience of sexual abuse and the later appearance of cardiopulmonary and gynecological illnesses, functional gastrointestinal problems, chronic pain, psychogenic seizures, and obesity, as well as an increased risk of becoming infected with HIV and developing AIDS (Bensley et al. 2000; Irish et al. 2010; Görgen et al. 2012; Paras et al. 2009; Trickett et al. 2011). A reduction in gray matter in the area of the brain's somatosensory cortex that controls the genital region has just recently been demonstrated (Heim et al. 2013). In regard to psychological illnesses, the experience of sexual abuse is considered a risk factor for a number of psychopathological symptoms and illnesses, such as self-harming behavior; suicide attempts; depression; posttraumatic stress disorders; and eating, anxiety, and sleep disorders (Brezo et al. 2008; Chen et al. 2010; Cougle et al. 2010; Noll et al. 2006; Paolucci et al. 2001; Steine et al. 2012). The consequences resulting from an experience of sexual abuse typically represent an intense burden for the affected child or adolescent that often has a lasting effect over the course of her or his remaining lifespan. Furthermore, they also have an effect on society as a whole. For example, the socioeconomic costs of posttraumatic disorders as a result of child maltreatment, abuse, or neglect amount to an estimated sum of roughly 11 billion Euros per year (Habetha et al. 2012). Added to that are the so-called intangible costs of the impact on quality of life. Yet for many victims of sexual violence, it is their faith in their ability to have successful relationships that are shaken, that is, in that experiential dimension of human sexuality that has an immediate effect on life satisfaction; this can facilitate the formation of sexual impairments and failures in relationships (Berthelot et al. 2014). This in turn explains the difficulties often experienced by those affected in actualizing romantic and familial relationships and underlines the urgent imperative to make every effort to prevent the sexual abuse of children from happening in the first place, as well as to expand the available options for (preventative) therapy (Beier et al. 2015d).

2   Consumption of Child Sexual Abuse Images

From a legal perspective, the consumption of images of child sexual abuse is not considered child sexual abuse, although the production of the materials in question necessitates sexual exploitation and in many cases is the result of sexual abuse of children that has taken place. The acquisition, distribution, and use of images of child sexual abuse therefore cannot be considered victimless crimes. The procurement of the so-called "child pornography" can increase the demand for more material. In addition, the victims of these production processes are forced to suffer the continuation of their traumatization through the knowledge that the documentation of the sexual abuse enacted upon them was made public and is still accessible (cf. Beier, Amelung, Grundmann et al. Beier et al. 2015a).

§ 184b of the German Penal Code defines child pornography as "pornographic materials" (*pornografische Schriften*), the subject of which are as follows: (a) sexual acts by, on, or in front of a person under 14 years of age (child); (b) the representation of an entirely or partially unclothed child in an unnaturally sexually suggestive posture; or (c) the sexually provocative representation of the unclothed genitalia or unclothed rear of a child (§ 184c of the Penal Code defines "juvenile pornographic materials" in a similar fashion with regard to persons of "fourteen, but not yet eighteen years of age"). Clinical experience has shown that representations that are used for sexual arousal and for masturbatory purposes vary significantly in their degree of ambiguity and explicitness, such that some people may use

images that do not feature any overt representations of abuse and are therefore not illegal (Wortley and Smallbone 2006). Research and preventative work must therefore take into account the entire spectrum of sexually explicit and non-explicit representations of children that are used for the purposes of sexual gratification (Beier et al. 2015d).

A differentiated categorization of the wide range of sexually explicit and non-explicit representations of children was achieved through the further development of Lanning's (2001) classification attempts in the context of the COPINE (Combating Pedophilic Information Networks in Europe) project. The 10-stage COPINE scale was thereafter frequently used as the basis for international scientific comparison (Taylor et al. 2001). It differentiates the degrees of severity of the depictions based on the expected harm caused to the victims. The spectrum of images available on the Internet ranges from depictions of completely clothed children, e.g., in mail order catalogs, to the gravest sexual violence toward children. Many consumers use the so-called pose images and attempt to relativize their use of them by downplaying the depictions as harmless, since the children depicted are shown smiling. This however dismisses the fact that children are also abused in the production of the so-called erotic and explicit pose images. Moreover, these images are often part of the so-called series that start off as ostensibly harmless and over the course of which the gravest sexual abuse can be seen.

In Germany in 2016, police crime statistics recorded a total of 5687 cases of distribution, acquisition, and possession of photographic or filmic representations of child sexual abuse or the explicit depiction of the unclothed genitalia of children (Bundeskriminalamt 2017). Here, too, it must be assumed that the significant majority of cases remain undiscovered and thereby take place within the *Dunkelfeld* (Beier et al. 2005, 2009; Wetzels 1997). In a representative study of German men, 2.4% of those surveyed claimed to have already used abuse images (Dombert et al. 2015). Of the PPD participants at the Berlin location, 71% claimed to have used abuse images. The significant majority (89%) was not known to the justice system for this offence (Kuhle, Kossow and Beier). In addition, a closer analysis of the usage behavior of the PPD participants indicated that, at the time of the initial interview (including the preceding 6 months), participants had in large part consumed non-explicit as well as explicit sexual depictions of children. Roughly a third of participants used indicative pictures: 65% images within the categories of "nudity," "erotica," and "(erotic) posing;" 59% within the categories of "explicit erotic posing" and "explicit sexual activity;" 51% within the category of "(grave) sexual assault;" and 27% within the category of "sadism/zoophilia" (Kuhle et al. 2011). A significant difference can be seen when looking at the PPJ results. Here, approximately one-fifth (18%) of those expressing interest in the project claimed to have used depictions of child abuse (Schlinzig et al. 2017).

In regard to the consumption of abuse images, most pedophilic men claim that they find the respective materials sexually arousing and that they have already used them in their lives (Neutze et al. 2011; Quayle and Taylor 2002; Riegel 2004). Offenders who have been convicted of using abuse images often exhibit an attraction to the child developmental body age along the lines of pedophilia/hebephilia (Seto et al. 2006). The use of abuse images can therefore be considered as an indicator for the presence of pedophilia. This is also plausible due to the fact that men primarily use pornographic materials that correspond to their sexual fantasies.

3   Dissexuality

While the possible forms of sexual expression are diverse, sexual activities can be roughly subdivided into three forms of sexual interactions:

- Genital interactions
- Non-genital interactions
- Masturbation

Generally speaking, all behaviors that are sexually motivated may be seen as sexual behaviors. A behavior is sexually motivated when it is in the service of sexual arousal and/or the preparation for sexual activity—including by means of the use of text or image materials.

The concept of dissexuality came about in reference to the definition of dissociality as social failure, as sexual misconduct is in principle primarily an expression of a dysfunctional social dimension of sexuality. As a—as morally neutral as possible—signifier of this central aspect, the term dissexuality offers itself as a "social failure that expresses itself in the area of the sexual," defined as a failure of the (historically and socio-culturally determined and therefore mutable) average expectable partner interests (Beier 1995). It is irrelevant whether this failure is prosecuted or provides grounds for prosecution. The linguistic analogy with the concept of dissociality as an "advanced and general social failure" is intentional: dissexuality and dissociality not only can overlap with one another (in that dissexual behaviors, such as rape, are part of dissociality) but can also stand alone. Dissexuality also always represents a relational process, as the disregard for the autonomy of another person is an essential aspect. In this sense, sexual behavior can be classified as dissexual when the integrity and individuality of another person is infringed upon and/or if it includes people who have not given consent. Although dissexuality predominantly represents a clinical and not a legal construct, it intersects with legal aspects to a large degree, due to its inherent potential for the endangerment of others. The lack of consent and free will of a person may be determined by the fact that their ability to consent to sexual activities is absent or impossible due to age and/or lack of knowledge. Adult persons (over 18 years of age) are equal sexual partners insofar as they are informed about the content, execution, and consequences/alternatives of sexual interactions and to the extent that their physical, mental, and economic situation enables them to make independent, free, and unconstrained decisions to take part in these sexual interactions. Only under these conditions can an "informed consent" or knowing agreement to sexual acts take place (Finkelhor 1997). Determining what constitutes informed consent may be additionally challenging due to the difficulty in differentiating it from passive cooperation without open resistance. The so-called cooperation or compliance may exist in spite of feelings that would actually be more in line with the opposite behavior. No (outward or inward) consent is therefore necessary for one—contrary to one's own feelings—to take part in sexual activities. As such, the objective behavior may be the same, while the intention, motivation, and perception may be very different. In the case of child sexual abuse, these complex but extremely relevant conceptualizations of (lack of) volition, informed consent, or knowing agreement mean that a careful assessment of the motivations and affective side effects of the children involved is essential. It is evident that the question of volition is not simply to be determined by referring to a child's supposed "participation."

Due to the psychological-developmental immaturity or incapability of children to fully comprehend sexual activities and to agree to them, it is impossible for children to realistically assess their consent in terms of the execution and possible consequences of their behavior or the behavior of others for themselves or for others. Cerebro-physiologically speaking, too, due to their incomplete brain development, they do not possess the necessary prospective abilities that would allow them to estimate the consequences of decisions.

Of great significance to preventative and therapeutic measures with regard to dissexual behaviors is the motivation of the (potential) perpetrator. This may consist in the child being abused as a replacement for the actual desired adult sexual partner, as in the case of perpetrators with mental disabilities or personality disorders, for instance, as well as in cases of sociosexual inexperience, and also in the context of particular familial constellations that are marked by a general violation of boundaries. Alternatively, the motivation behind the abuse may consist in the presence of a sexual preference for the child developmental body age in the sense of pedophilia or hebephilia.

According to estimates, approximately 40–50% of men who have committed sexual assault on children are pedophilically inclined individuals (Beier et al. 2005; for an overview, see Seto 2008).

As previously emphasized, pedophilia must not be equated with child sexual abuse, although this often occurs in public discourse and in the media. Not everyone who is pedophilic sexually abuses children and not everyone who commits child sexual abuse is pedophilic (Sect. 2).

Because people with a pedophilic sexual preference exhibit a higher risk of repeatedly committing child sexual abuse or using abuse images (Eke et al. 2011), one must presume that these persons also exhibit a higher lifetime risk for first-time offences. They thereby represent a meaningful target group for the prevention of child sexual abuse and the use of abuse images. For those affected, the constant confrontation with sexual fantasies and impulses directed toward children can go hand in hand with self-denigration and lack of self-acceptance (Schaefer et al. 2010). Furthermore, they must concern themselves with the potential consequences, should they live out their sexual preference (ibid.). This can explain the common occurrence of psychological stress symptoms (e.g., anxiety and depression; Sect. 4) in this indication group. Corresponding psychological distress would be related to the preference and is to be found both in the DSM-5 (APA 2013) and in the ICD-10 (World Health Organization [WHO] 1992), where this distress is listed explicitly as a diagnostic criterion for pedophilia.

In this context and in consideration of these numbers and the resulting estimates of a considerable *Dunkelfeld* for both child sexual abuse and offenses related to abuse images, it must be assumed that the majority of perpetrators are never prosecuted and therefore can never profit from the therapeutic offerings available within the *Hellfeld* (e.g., in social therapy institutions or in forensic-therapeutic outpatient centers). People in the *Dunkelfeld* with a sexual interest in children therefore represent a meaningful target group for the prevention of child sexual abuse, as their subjectively experienced psychological distress motivates them to seek out treatment and makes them receptive to preventative approaches

(Beier et al. 2009; Schaefer et al. 2010; for more in-depth commentaries on the subject, see Beier et al. 2015a; Beier et al. 2015d; Kuhle, Grundmann and Beier 2015; Scherner et al. 2015).

4 Explanatory Models for the Sexual Abuse of Children

There are several single-factorial and multifactorial etiological models for sexual abuse. Exemplary instances named here are *Finkelhor's Model of Preconditions* (Finkelhor 1984), the *Integrated Model* by Marshall and Barbaree (1990), the *Quadripartite Model of child sexual abuse* (Hall and Hirschmann 1992), or the *Pathways Model* (Ward and Siegert 2002). In order to be able to offer a more comprehensive explanation of the initiation, development, and maintenance of sexual abuse, these various models of sexual abuse were brought together into an *Integrative Theory of sexual abuse* (Ward and Beech 2006).

4.1 Integrative Theory of Sexual Abuse

The Integrative Theory of sexual abuse combines different biopsychosocial factors to explicate a case of sexual abuse (Fig. 1). A fundamental assumption is that the different weight given to individual risk factors or vulnerabilities, as well as how they interact in an individual case, lead to different constellations of interdependent conditions and therefore to different trajectories of sexually abusive behavior. In general, it can be said that the probability of a case of sexual abuse increases with the number (quantity) and the severity (quality) of the offender's clinical symptoms (Thornton and Beech 2002). In spite of the authors' efforts, even this theory cannot adequately illustrate the complexity of the various forms of sexual abuse, but rather serves solely as a set of guidelines. The model is too imprecise, for instance, not only with respect to victims but also with respect to specific subgroups of offenders, such as men outside of the criminal justice system who use abuse images or who have a pedophilic preference.

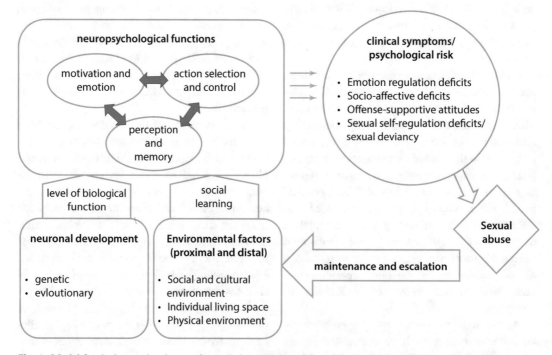

Fig. 1 Model for the integrative theory of sexual abuse. (Adapted from Ward and Beech 2006)

With regard to pedophilia, one may notice that it is seen more as a consequence than a point of departure, which at most can apply to the expression of the dissexual behavior itself (Sect. 4.3).

The psychological risk factors and clinical symptoms identified in the model are etiological and, as starting points for interventions, are important elements of therapeutic work with persons who offend sexually. Research has shown four clusters of significant risk factors:

- Emotional regulation issues
- Socio-affective deficits
- Offense-supportive attitudes
- Deficits in sexual self-regulation or deviant sexual interests (Hanson and Harris 2000; Hanson et al. 2007)

Emotional regulation issues manifest themselves in the form of a limited perception of one's own emotions, a dysfunctional regulation of uncomfortable emotional states, and/or the inability to seek out social support in times of emotional stress (Feelgood et al. 2005; Marshall et al. 2000; Ward et al. 1998; Ward and Siegert 2002).

Socio-affective deficits are characterized by, among other things, intimacy issues such as loneliness, the absence of or difficulty establishing intimate relationships (Bumby and Hansen 1997; Marsa et al. 2004; Seidman et al. 1994); a sense of one's own inadequacy; externalizing attributional styles; mistrust (Elliott et al. 2009; Laulik et al. 2007; Raymond et al. 1999; Stinson et al. 2005; Dennison et al. 2001; Fagan et al. 1991; Wilson and Cox 1983); and emotional identification with children (Wilson 1999). It is understood that issues with establishing socio-sexual relationships arise because of socio-affective deficits, and as a consequence, the sexual abuse of children takes place as a compensation for the non-existent socio-sexual relationships (cf. Ward et al. 1996; Ward and Siegert 2002). However, social isolation and intimacy problems in connection with disinhibiting factors such as substance abuse can also lead to the dysfunctional attempt to bring about emotional intimacy by means of sexual intimacy (Marshall et al. 1993; Ward et al. 1996; Ward et al. 1995). Analogously

to this second explanatory approach, a sexual interest in children can, on the one hand, be the cause of the lack of socio-sexual relationships with adults and, on the other hand, reinforce the desire for sexual intimacy with children.

Offense-supportive attitudes are cognitive distortions that are defined as attitudes that excuse or defend sexual abuse (Abel et al. 1984). They are relatively common among sexual abusers of children (Arkowitz and Vess 2003; Feelgood et al. 2005; Hanson and Harris 2000; Marshall et al. 2001). Offense-supportive attitudes can be roughly categorized into the following basic assumptions:

- Children are sexual beings.
- Sexual activities between children and adults are not harmful.
- One's own sexual needs are impossible to control.
- The offender feels entitled to use children for his own sexual gratification because of his superiority (Ward 2000).

Before an act of sexual abuse, offense-supportive attitudes influence how information is perceived and processed and reduce inhibition thresholds for the offense (cf. Ward and Siegert 2002). After the offense, these convictions facilitate the justification of the offense by means of minimizing the harm caused, as well as reducing one's own feelings of guilt and shame. In addition, they lead to false attribution of consequences, to denial, to shifting of responsibility by means of denigrating the victim, and to a rationalization of the behavior (Hayashino et al. 1995). It is in this manner that sexual abuse of children can be initiated or sustained (Bumby 1996; Prentky and Knight 1991).

Although a pedophilic sexual preference represents a significant influencing factor on the perpetration of an act of child sexual abuse, it does not receive explicit mention from Ward and Beech (2006). It is accompanied by fantasies and (relationship) desires involving children, as well as compulsive sexual behaviors (see Sect. 2 in chapter "Pedophilia and Hebephilia"). Meta-analyses confirm sexual deviance in general as being a significant risk factor for sexual abuse (Hanson and

Morton-Bourgon 2005). An existing sexual interest in children in particular increases the risk of first-time and repeated child sexual abuse (Hanson and Morton-Bourgon 2004). In the literature, the relationship between the occurrence of deviant sexual fantasies (about sexual acts with minors, for example) and the resulting sexual behaviors is predominantly discussed. Relevant in this context is the degree of *sexual self-regulation*—in the sense of a noticeably high interest in sexuality in general, the ability to distance oneself from sexual fantasies or impulses, as well as to refrain from utilizing sexual behavior (e.g., masturbation, pornography consumption, sexual contact) to a problematic degree as a means of reducing negative emotional states (Cortoni and Marshall 2001; Mann et al. 2010; Marshall et al. 2008).

The psychological and social consequences of an act of child sexual abuse have an influence on the offender, the victim, as well as the immediate living environment and can thereby contribute to either the maintenance or even the escalation or cessation of the abuse behavior.

An act of child sexual abuse is all the more likely to be repeated if *clinical symptoms/psychological risk factors* are maintained or reinforced because of the following: offense (e.g., increased social isolation and continued activation of offense-supportive attitudes); the victim does not have the opportunity to remove themselves from the abuse (e.g., threats, shame, and guilt); and the social environment does not or is unable to have an intervening effect. In terms of the risk of reoffending, it is also significant whether there is an existing pedophilic and/or hebephilic preference—an influencing factor of high stability (Grundmann et al. 2016) that receives only insufficient attention in the Integrative Theory of sexual abuse by Ward and Beech (2006) and that also plays a significant role in the consumption of abuse images (Sect. 4.2).

4.2   Theories on the Use of Child Sexual Abuse Images

There are but few sufficient explanatory models that refer to the development and maintenance of the use of child sexual abuse images. Existing models proceed from differing basic assump-

tions. Depending on the model, the use of abuse images can be explained by the following:

- The same factors that explain direct child sexual abuse
- Factors that are specific to the use of child sexual abuse images and are associated with problematic internet use
- Factors that are specific to the use of child sexual abuse images and are associated with addictive sexual behaviors and compulsivity

Also under discussion is whether the use of child sexual abuse images is a delimitable abuse behavior that is completely different from the direct sexual abuse of children and for which new explanatory models must be found.

However, these different approaches also have common hypotheses:

- General emotional mood and the use of child sexual abuse images have a mutual effect on each other.
- The use of child sexual abuse images can be positively reinforced by means of the accompanying sexual arousal, masturbation, and fantasy, as well as through like-minded people.
- Attitudes and convictions, as well as online behavior and the use of child sexual abuse images, have a mutual effect on each other.
- Familiarization in the sense of habituation leads to reinforced and more intensive use of child sexual abuse images.
- Some individuals, due to increasing boredom with respect to the use of pictures or by being actively addressed by contacts on the Internet, may transition over to the direct sexual abuse of children (cf. Seto 2013).

In a comparison of phallometric results from convicted users of abuse images and offenders convicted of child sexual abuse, the group of users of child sexual abuse images demonstrated a significantly stronger sexual arousal in response to children than the offender group (Seto et al. 2006). In total, 61% of the users of abuse images demonstrated a sexual preference for images of children as opposed to images of adults. Seto et al. (2006) thereby conclude that the use of abuse images rep-

Fig. 2 Biopsychosocial causal model for dissexual acts toward children

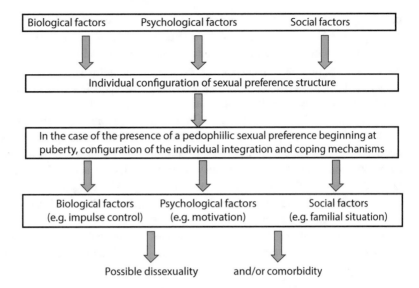

resents a valid indicator for the presence of a sexual preference for children. This aspect was adopted into the diagnostic system of the DSM-5: "The extensive use of pornography depicting prepubescent children is a useful diagnostic indicator of pedophilic disorder" (APA 2013, p. 698). Accordingly, sexual preference for children must receive stronger consideration in causal models.

4.3 Biopsychosocial Causal Model for Dissexual Acts Toward Children

The Integrative Theory of sexual abuse according to Ward and Beech (2006) does not sufficiently take into account the potential influence of existing sexual particularities along the lines of pedophilia or hebephilia. This sexual preference likely manifests itself under the influence of sex hormones and other biopsychosocial factors in the course of an individual's psychosexual development, beginning in adolescence. The process of this development is still largely scientifically unexplained, however. In the absence of evidence of a lasting change in sexual preference for a particular body age, some authors surmise that it is essentially stable (cf. Beckstead 2012; Seto 2009, 2012), while others do not see this fixity, at least not in individual cases, as a given (cf. Müller et al.

2014; Marshall 2008). If one takes as a basis that the preference for children develops during adolescence, one must assume that this has an influence on personality development and also on the psychological risk factors mentioned by Ward and Beech (2006) (in terms of deficits of emotional regulation and socioaffectivity, offense-supportive attitudes, as well as deficits of sexual self-regulation). In a biopsychosocial causal model, this must be adequately taken into account (Fig. 2).

5 Perpetrator-Oriented Prevention of Child Sexual Abuse

Typically, preventative approaches focus on children, families, teachers, and social workers in youth care, or other groups of people who are in a position to intervene. These are usually successfully administered through schools (Finkelhor 2009). The chief goal of these pedagogical programs consists in teaching how to distinguish between appropriate and inappropriate touching and how to notify a trusted adult when sexual touching has taken place. The focus is consequently often directed at children and adolescents as (potential) victims.

Prevention can also be concentrated, however, on persons who exhibit an increased risk of becoming sexually abusive. According to the existing research literature, a sexual preference for children is one of the most significant risk factors for first-time and repeated sexual offenses (Beier 1998; Hanson and Bussière 1998; Hanson and Morton-Bourgon 2005; Mann et al. 2010). One possibility for the prevention of child sexual abuse consists in turning directly to the group of pedophilic and/or hebephilic individuals who, in an autonomous and self-motivated way, want to take advantage of therapeutic help in order to receive support in dealing with their sexual impulses responsibly and who want to avoid the (renewed) loss of their present control over their behavior. Those affected should receive therapeutic support in their efforts to refrain from committing (repeated) child sexual abuse or consuming (additional) abuse images. The treatment of people with a sexual preference for children who exhibit the risk of committing first-time offenses can therefore be understood as a proactive primary preventative measure (Beier et al. 2009). In this context, secondary prevention means preventing a relapse if sexual abuse has already taken place—even if this was never prosecuted and took place within the *Dunkelfeld.*

According to the Integrative Model of sexual abuse, a multidimensional treatment approach that includes pharmacological, psychological, and sexological intervention strategies is required for (potential) perpetrators of child sexual abuse (cf. Ward and Beech 2006). The therapeutic approach of the Berlin Dissexuality Therapy (Berliner Dissexualitätstherapie) (BEDIT 2013), with which the PPD was initiated in Berlin, is based on models and already-established therapeutic approaches for the reduction of recidivism risk in persons who offend sexually who are known to the criminal justice system and have been accordingly convicted. Notably, the successive treatment approaches are also used for those affected within the *Dunkelfeld* (for an overview, see Scherner et al. 2015). It seems useful to consider here the Relapse Prevention model, the Good Lives model, the Risk-Need-Responsivity model, cognitive behavioral therapy, as well as pharmacological approaches. In order to prohibit relapses, the Relapse Prevention approach

focuses on teaching self-regulating skills (Pithers 1990; Ward et al. 1998; Ward and Hudson 2000). The Good Lives approach is a positive therapeutic approach that understands crimes as socially inadequate attempts at fulfilling general and basic human needs (e.g., attachment, community, and autonomy). It therefore aims to help those affected build worthwhile and fulfilling lives in which individual basic needs can be realized by socially acceptable means (Ward and Gannon 2006). Programs that work in accordance with the Risk-Need-Responsivity (RNR) principle (Andrews and Bonta 2006) orient their treatment based on the questions of who is in need of intensive care ("risk"), which problems must be addressed ("need"), and how the treatment can best be structured ("responsivity"). RNR programs make use of cognitive behavioral techniques while taking into account contextual factors such as motivation, intellectual abilities, personality features, and aspects of learning theory. Cognitive therapy is based on the hypothesis that certain thought patterns determine behaviors and that modifying them can bring about a change in behavior. Behavioral therapy assumes that behavior is learned and can also be unlearned by means of various conditioning mechanisms.

Although the results of empirical studies on the effectiveness of pharmacological treatment with respect to relapse prophylaxes are the subject of controversial discussion (for an overview, see Rice and Harris 2011; according to the meta-analysis of Lösel and Schmucker 2005, however, they have the highest effect size), pharmacological support—by means of treatment with androgen deprivation therapy (ADT), selective serotonin reuptake inhibitors (SSRIs), and other medications (e.g., opioid antagonists)—is capable of meeting the demands of the RNR principles. The additional use of medications can be beneficial and important within the larger therapeutic concept. Sexual preference and sexual behavior have a biopsychosocial foundation in which various biological systems also play a role—such as the endocrine system with the male- or female-typical sex hormones or the dopaminergic and serotonergic reward systems (Sect. 3 in chapter "Pedophilia and Hebephilia"; Sect. 4.3). Via these systems, medications can directly influence an individual's sexual experience, e.g., by reducing urgent sexual behavioral impulses and fantasies that are experienced as distressing (cf. Amelung et al. 2012; Siegel et al. 2015).

Although the results are heterogeneous, different meta-analyses on the efficacy of therapy programs for persons who offend sexually were able to show that therapeutic interventions can successfully reduce the risk of renewed sexual offenses (Lösel and Schmucker 2005; Schmucker and Lösel 2015). The efficacy of therapy programs that work according to the RNR principles (Andrews and Bonta 2006) and with cognitive behavioral approaches (Hanson et al. 2002) is the best proven empirically. McGrath et al. (2010) emphasize that in practice no specific approach should be used, but rather a combination of various approaches and models (on this, see also Scherner et al. 2015).

Therapeutic Options

Anna Konrad, Eliza Schlinzig, Stefan Siegel,
Stephanie Kossow, and Klaus M. Beier

1 Specific Conditions for the Treatment of People with Pedophilia and Hebephilia

The treatment program BEDIT is based on three pillars representative of the biopsychosocial character of the preventative approach:

- Sex-therapeutic interventions support participants in accepting their sexual preference, integrating their fantasies into their self-concept, and taking responsibility for their sexual behavior.
- Cognitive behavioral therapy serves to improve the general and sexual self-regulation mechanisms of the patients by questioning offense-supportive attitudes and strengthening both positive coping strategies and social competences.
- Sexual impulses and fantasies can additionally be reduced with the help of pharmacotherapy (Beier et al. 2010).

A. Konrad · E. Schlinzig · S. Siegel · S. Kossow
K. M. Beier (✉)
Charité – Universitätsmedizin Berlin, Corporate Member of Freie Universität Berlin, Humboldt-Universität zu Berlin, and Berlin Institute of Health, Center for Human and Health Sciences, Institute of Sexology and Sexual Medicine, Berlin, Germany
e-mail: klaus.beier@charite.de

These interventions take place against the background of a clear therapeutic approach and substantive principles: pedophilic or hebephilic fantasies and other potential deviant sexual fantasies are not valued morally, as they are not governed by free choice. Inseparable from this, all forms of sexual contact with children, as well as the use of CSAI, are clearly laid out as sexually transgressive and not tolerated. Originally stemming from Client-Centered Psychotherapy (Rogers 1999), the conditions of congruence/authenticity of the therapist, empathy, and unconditional positive esteem of the client have proven themselves just as helpful as the fundamental concepts of the *Good Lives Approach* (Ward and Gannon 2006), according to which all humans strive to fulfill fundamental human needs, and sexual offenses can be understood as the attempt to fulfill legitimate needs by illegitimate means.

While numerous similarities are to be found between BEDIT and sex-offender programs like *Core STOP or i-STOP* (Middleton et al. 2009) (such as the modular structure, therapy goals, and group meetings), the differences lie principally in the selection of participants and the focus on sexual deviance in the sense of pedophilia/hebephilia. This affects the definition and emphasis of therapy goals and therapeutic interventions, for example self-observation of sexual fantasies and paraphilic interests, as well as the monitoring of sexual arousal and impulses. BEDIT is directed especially toward persons normally allocated to the high-deviance cluster (Ward and Siegert 2002). Assuming that pedophilia and hebephilia manifest themselves in the course of puberty and remain relatively stable throughout one's lifespan, this sexual preference can be compared with the construct of sexual orientation. It can accordingly be conceptually organized like gynephilia, the sexual attraction to female partners, or androphilia, the sexual attraction to male partners (for a detailed discussion, see Seto 2012) and is expressed in the DSM-5 as "pedophilic sexual orientation." The confrontation with sexual feelings toward children poses a great and sometimes permanent challenge in the individual development of a person that can impinge on their day-to-day life. Furthermore, men in the *Dunkelfeld* display another underlying motivation. It is assumed that persons not being prosecuted display a greater awareness of the problem, a greater motivation to change, and responsiveness to treatment (Beier et al. 2009). Accordingly, the following sections will serve to clarify the characteristics of the target groups and their respective significances to the therapeutic approach of BEDIT.

2 Specific Conditions for the Treatment of Juveniles with Sexual Attraction to Prepubescent or Early Pubescent Body Ages

BEDIT-A is based on the same principles and therapeutic rationales as BEDIT, on the basis of which it was developed, but is directed instead at a juvenile target group with a sexual attraction to the prepubescent and/or early pubescent body age. Accompanying the change in target group are two challenges in particular:

- Working with the diagnosis of "pedophilia" as such
- The inclusion of caregivers, specifically with regard to therapeutic confidentiality

The great and sometimes permanent challenge of being confronted with sexual feelings toward

children often begins in the adolescent years. A major task in individual development is the perception and corresponding acceptance of one's own sexual preference. This manifests itself during puberty or adolescence as affected persons first perceive sexual fantasies and impulses, as well as the desire to act upon these out, on the behavioral level are first perceived during adolescence, and increasingly differentiate themselves in early adulthood (Beier et al. 2005). This pertains not only to the sexual attraction to the sex of the preferred partner (male, female, both sexes) but also to the relevant body age of the preferred partner (see Sect. 1 in chapter "Pedophilia and Hebephilia"): affected adolescents must already engage during puberty with their sexual fantasies regarding the prepubescent and/or early pubescent body age and find a means of dealing with them. This presents individuals already in the thick of physical, psychic, and emotional development with an extremely difficult developmental task that can be associated with aspects of endangerment of the self and of others. The mere existence of sexual fantasies about children can be as debilitating an experience as the understanding of the significance of this preference can be for adults. Every reaction is thus conceivable, from the avoidance of any thoughts regarding sexual desires to acting on one's preference—the realization of which is made easier by the smaller age difference to children than it would be for adults. Moreover, possible developments such as social withdrawal and the emergence of suicidal thoughts make therapeutic support indispensable.

However, following the ICD-10 (WHO 1992) and the DSM-5 (APA 2013), the diagnosis of *pedophilia* can be applied beginning at the age of 16, in order to avoid incorrectly pathologizing sexual interest in those of a similar age or sexual curiosity (APA 2013). This strategy should be maintained in the face of the extreme societal stigmatization of pedophilic sexual preference, as well as the individually variable developmental processes at work in adolescents. Nevertheless, empirical data on adults has shown that sexual preference manifested in adolescence remains categorically stable (for an overview, see Seto 2008). In order to both counteract early—and unnecessary—stigmatization, as well as work in accordance with empirical results, the term *sexual particularities* should rather be used regarding adolescents. This can be used as a diagnostic assessment at the time of the preferences' emergence and can trace their development or course in an open-ended manner. This should accordingly be explained to the adolescent patient as well as their caregiver (e.g., parents).

The continuing implementation of an accompanying clinical sexual diagnosis with a focus on current sexual fantasies during treatment of adolescents is thus all the more important regarding a sexual non-normative preference for the prepubescent and/or early pubescent body schema. Clinical experience shows that adolescents already possess a high introspective capability when it comes to their own sexual fantasies, supposing a viable therapeutic relationship adheres to a nonjudgmental and trust-based framework (Beier et al. 2015c). It must be noted that adolescents also have an acute awareness of non-conformity, so the perceived threat of social sanctions produces socially desirable answers above all else. In clinical psychotherapeutic contact, adolescents possess a limited autonomy relative to adults and are often predominately motivated by external forces, which have great significance in the process of building a viable therapeutic relationship (see Sect. 4.3 in chapter "BEDIT-A Manual for Adolescents").

A further characteristic in the counseling and therapy of adolescents with non-normative sexual particularities is the necessary incorporation of caregivers into therapeutic work, as they can check in on the generalization of therapeutic goals in day-to-day life, particulary in regard to relapse prevention— they are of immense importance. Primary caregivers are most often the parents. The social network can however additionally extend to care supervisors from various institutions, grandparents, other relatives, friends, assistants for individual cases, youth welfare officers, etc. It should be worked out with the patient who can and/or must be brought into the process. It is important that the primary caregivers act as resources and support the patient in achievement of goals, as well as serve as points of contact in critical situations. At the same time, this places

adolescents in the situation of opening up to adults whom they possibly do not fully trust. Therapeutic confidentiality under all circumstances must be discussed with the patient and all caregivers, but boundaries must also be worked out in depth, as not only the protection of the patient but also the mandated reporter status of those in the custody of the patient must be maintained (see Sect. 4.4 in chapter "BEDIT-A Manual for Adolescents"). Work with the caregivers of patients with sexual particularities requires not just a great degree of flexibility but also transparency above all else. As adolescents with non-normative sexual particularities for children are often already known to child welfare systems and persons beyond the parents/caregivers are generally involved, the disclosure of information must remain clearly and fundamentally contingent upon a release from the obligation to confidentiality. Supporting the adolescent's autonomy is key. The desires and needs of the patient must be kept in mind, as action in accordance with child protective laws must be taken in the context of acute moments of endangerment (see Sect. 8.5 in chapter "The Berlin Prevention Project Dunkelfeld (PPD)"). It must generally be taken into account that, given the explosive nature of the subject, upset is common within the social network. This must be dealt with, but focus on the patient cannot be lost. Decisions cannot be made by the therapist—they are there to help facilitate reflection and can under certain circumstances make recommendations. But they are generally the main contact for the patient, who must trust them. Should the patient develop the impression of complicity between the therapist and the adult caregivers, it should be assumed that they will no longer be able to fully express themselves in the context of the therapy.

A therapeutic relationship with an individual under the age of 18 generally requires the permission of the legal guardian. Should the patient make their participation in a diagnostic and/or therapeutic process conditional on their parents not being informed of the therapy, decisions must be made on an individual basis. Given the sensitivity of the subject, potentially denying the adolescent help must be considered against the backdrop of German jurisprudence (Beier et al. 2015c). From the age of 16 onward in particular, it seems prudent from a medical and therapeutic perspective to support an adolescent without the permission of their parents, though (retroactive) disclosure to the parents is to be sought, per therapeutic considerations.

3   Pedophilia and Hebephilia as Sexual Orientations

It has been recently suggested that pedophilia can be understood as a construct comparable to sexual orientation toward one or both sexes (Seto 2012; Grundmann et al. 2016); the DSM-5 also uses the phrase "pedophilic sexual orientation" (APA 2013). Seto (2012) identifies the onset around puberty, sexual and romantic behaviors with the desired partner, and stability over time as the core characteristics of sexual orientation with regard to the sex of the partner (defined as sexual gender orientation). It can be shown based on empirical data that pedophilia shares these characteristics with sexual orientation toward one sex. Grundmann et al. (2016) support this hypothesis with data from the Prevention Project Dunkelfeld (PPD). In a sample of 494 PPD participants with a pedophilic and/or hebephilic sexual preference, onset and stability of the preference(s) over time were studied based on self-reports. Between 58.2% and 72.3% of the participants retroactively reported sexual arousal since their own puberty from the content of fantasies involving prepubescent and/or early pubescent children. A prospective study of a subsample of 121 male participants in the PPD therapy program showed a medium- to high-rank correlation of self-reported arousal from pedophilic/hebephilic content to a simultaneous absence of significant median differences of reported arousal in an observation period of about 2 years. Taken together, these initial empirical findings suggest that pedophilic and/or hebephilic sexual attraction in the majority of those affected first emerges or is perceived during puberty or adolescence and can be viewed as a relatively stable clinical phenomenon. Conceiving of sexual attraction to children in the sense of a sexual orientation (APA 2013; Seto 2012) has wide-reaching implications for work with this specific population, to which the following will refer.

4   Sexual Attraction to Children and Sexual Identity

Sexual identity is part of the general identity of a person. The concept of sexual identity was explored first in connection with homosexuality but later also with heterosexuality (Beier et al. 2005). Models of sexual identity generally include social norms and values as influences on the development of one's identity. A person who feels sexual attraction to prepubescent and/or early pubescent children will experience an external conflict between their sexual needs and desires, on the one hand, and societal values, on the other. Western society condemns sexual behavior with children with varying degrees of severity. Public discourse around pedophilia and hebephilia is widely informed by stigmatization, which has to do with the degree to which pedophilia and child sexual abuse are mistakenly conflated (Jahnke, Imhoff, and Hoyer 2015).

While social circles generally discuss sexual feelings and experiences with age-appropriate partners more or less openly, fear of rejection and exclusion makes open discussion of sexual attraction to children only rarely possible. This is also the case even when no corresponding actions have occurred. For a person who identifies their sexual attraction to children during puberty or (late) adolescence, models for the development of their sexual identity are chiefly to be found in images of those convicted of child sexual abuse. In most cases, these individuals are depicted as socially isolated sex offenders who have been cast off by society. The experience of learning about sexual feelings toward children thus entails guilt, shame, and rejection. Also important to the development of a self-conception is the minimized possibility of experiencing understanding from others in discussions of sexual needs.

Consequently, a significant goal of BEDIT and BEDIT-A consists of enabling the patient to perceive and communicate sexual needs and feelings such as guilt or shame that can accompany them. Here, it is of the utmost importance to differentiate between guilt and shame for sexual fantasies, on the one hand, and illegal and/or inappropriate sexual behavior, on the other. Following the Good Lives Approach (Ward and Gannon 2006), sexual fantasies and the desire for sexual satisfaction can be understood as a legitimate need, while their direct realization in the form of sexual contact with children or the use of CSAI necessarily always represent an inadequate and transgressive means of fulfilling these needs.

Additional paraphilias often occur in pedophilic/hebephilic men that can intensify feelings of shame and guilt. The so-called paraphilic burdens are common, of which non-exclusive pedophilic patients would be found at the top end, and polyparaphilic pedophilic patients would be found at the lower end. One reason for this is the recurrent discussion in the treatment groups about the possibility of living out a sexuality that does not hurt anyone and is experienced as fulfilling in spite of a sexual attraction to children. This is more easily achieved by those who, alongside deviant sexual fantasies, also have fantasies whose realization in the context of appropriate sexual contact with an adult partner would be principally possible. It is thus of great importance to seek to reduce feelings of shame and guilt, and foster an approach of acceptance regarding sexual preference and sexual particularities that also clearly condemn sexual behavior toward children. For this, a thorough sexual history and diagnostic are essential.

4.1 Egosyntonic and Egodystonic Sexual Attraction to Prepubescent and Early Pubescent Body Ages

Consistent with the concept of egosyntonic and egodystonic sexual orientation, strategies to help pedophilic and hebephilic persons manage experiences of sexual attraction to a pre- or early-pubescent body age can also be categorized as egosyntonic or egodystonic. Patients who display egosyntonic sexual attraction to children under-

stand it as an integral part of their personality. This part does not need to be positively viewed, but the attraction is understood as fact, and the corresponding burdens can be reflected upon and verbalized. An egosyntonic integration of the sexual preference thus facilitates an active engagement with the burdens this sort of preference may bring with it.

For patients with an egodystonic attraction to children, on the other hand, sexual feelings toward children are rejected as not belonging to their personality. This rejection is a result of the incompatibility of sexual attraction to children with normative social values in the self-conception. Among the factors that hinder the integration of a sexual attraction to children are concepts of romantic relationships with adult partners, family, one's own children, presumptions and prejudices about pedophilic and hebephilic persons, and fear of engagement with one's own sexual fantasies. Patients with an egdystonic conception of their own sexual attraction to children would deny that this attraction plays any role in their daily lives. Externalizing explanations for high-risk situations or dissexual behavior (e.g., nonrecognition of one's own role in frequent occurrences of contact with unknown children in the train) then become more likely. Against this background, the development of active strategies for the avoidance of high-risk situations is accordingly less likely.

The concepts of the egosyntonic and the egodystonic thus play an important role in the planning of therapeutic processes. For patients with an egosyntonic conception of their own sexual preference, therapy can concentrate directly on relevant dynamic risk factors that encourage abusive behavior. For patients with an egodystonic conception, a greater amount of time in therapy must be dedicated to motivational work.

4.2 Realistic vs. Unrealistic Therapy Goals

It is still disputed today as to whether a person's sexual preference can be therapeutically influenced—whether, for example, a sexual attraction to children can be transformed into a sexual attraction to adult partners. According to the DSM-5, pedophilia implies a lifelong characteristic or sexual orientation, while the disorder aspect of pedophilia (for which subjective distress is a prerequisite, for instance) can undergo fluctuations throughout a person's life (APA 2013). Some patients accept—at least to some extent—the idea that their sexual attraction has not changed thus far and may remain constant for the rest of their life. Meanwhile others seek help with the aim of changing their sexual preference for children into a sexual preference for partners with an adult body age.

In the view of research up to this point, the therapeutic goal of a lasting change to sexual preference—in particular in people with an exclusive attraction to the prepubesent and/or early pubescent body ages—is held to be unrealistic (for more on interventions toward the acceptance of sexual attraction to children, see Module 2, "Acceptance").

Realistic therapy goals, on the other hand, could include strengthening of an existing sexual attraction to the adult body age, integration of sexual attraction to children in a way that preserves the patient's self-esteem, or the identification and restructuring of problematic attitudes to social interactions with children as well as adults. These would entail exploring empathy toward and assuming the perspective of potential victims, the identification of individually relevant high-risk situations, as well as the learning and implementation of self-control strategies for different situations. Another realistic therapy goal would be to enhance self-efficacy expectations with respect to sexual behaviors. This could be achieved through building up experiences of control, abstention from problematic sexual behavior, and the development of strategies for the maintenance and improvement of general quality of life.

4.3   Social and Sexual Perception

The conceptual differentiation between normative social perception and cognitive distortion is difficult to establish conclusively. Similarly, the etiological connections between social perception deficits, cognitive distortions, and sexual attraction to children remain largely unclear (for an overview, see Blake and Gannon 2008). However, a connection seems to exist between sexual preference and social/sexual perception. Men with and men without sexual attraction to children seem to differ from each other in their informational processing procedures. If sexual orientation fulfills the function of initiating sociosexual interactions with potential partners, then it also directs interpretations of social interactions on the interpersonal level. If pedophilia or hebephilia does in fact correspond to a sexual orientation, then pedophilic and hebephilic men might tend to understand successful social interactions between a child and an adult as an expression of affection with sexual potential. This can in turn be understood as a social perception emerging from a sexual preference for children. From a clinical perspective, this resembles automatic thinking as it is understood within the framework of other psychiatric disorders.

The (unreflected) interpretation of interactions between children and adults as dictated by a pedophilic or hebephilic sexual preference bears considerable influence on dealing with sexual impulses toward children as well as available self-regulatory capabilities. The influence of the individual sexual preference of participants on their social perception represents a central component of therapy that can be worked on through cognitive techniques such as reality testing (see Modules 4, "Perception", and 10, "Social Relationships," of BEDIT, and Modules 2 and 7 of BEDIT-A)

A helpful illustration of this phenomenon are the so-called rose-tinted glasses of lovers: a person who feels attracted to another person will eagerly interpret their social signals as directed toward them. Based on clinical experience, as well as the assumption that sexual preference remains more or less stable and conditions social perception, it is quite likely that ongoing spontaneous and sexualized interpretations of child-adult interactions, as well as children's behavior, occur in pedophilic and hebephilic men.

The scale of these distortions is difficult to ascertain. Through the assessment of exemplary situations, the therapist can evaluate whether the patient understands the principle of cognitive distortion. It is however possible that a new situation will leave him completely unaware of his misinterpretation. It is important in this case to confront patients with the fact that under no circumstances do social signals from a child correspond to the patients' sexual interest.

From the therapist's perspective, it is especially important to keep in mind that perceptional biases are not only necessarily the result of trying to make excuses for problematic behavior, but they could also have emerged from the necessity of coping with one's own sexual preference.

Case Study
A patient describes a situation in which he watched a child of his preferred body age playing at the playground. The child interrupted his play multiple times to look in the direction of the patient.

1. Automatic perception and interpretation (through the rose-tinted glasses): The boy is playing alone and looks at me continually. He wants someone to play with and would like me to join in.
2. Alternative interpretation (from a neutral point of view): The boy is playing alone and looks multiple times at the man who is obviously watching him.

4.4 Cognitive Distortions

Somewhat different from the phenomenon described above, cognitive distortions may also be understood as perpetuated social perception bias (Blake and Gannon 2008). Given the highly taboo nature of the sexual needs of pedophilic and hebephilic persons, confrontation with these needs can lead to cognitive dissonance. Cognitive distortions may thus present the possibility to reduce this dissonance, in that they may allow sexual needs regarding children to appear rational and morally acceptable. While cognitive distortions were previously discussed as rationalizations, it may also be that they result not from punishable sexual behaviors, but rather emerge solely through the presence of pedophilic or hebephilic fantasies as a means of reducing dissonance and maintaining the self-concept.

Cognitive distortions thus typically offer subjective explanations as to why sexual interest in and sexual interactions with a child are not so problematic as they are generally held to be. Some of these explanations seek to minimize the damages to children caused by sexual abuse, pointing for example to the supposedly widespread ancient Greek pederasty (which modern scholarship suggests involved postpubescent adolescents), or to the fact that sex criminals commit extreme acts of sexual abuse, while they themselves would never turn to any kind of force. Other attitudes serve to legitimize interactions between adults and children through claiming, for instance, that society denies the sexual needs of children, or that sexual contact initiated by an adult can be ascribed to youthful sexual curiosity and consequent exploratory behaviors. These distortions can furthermore serve to shift focus away from one's own sexual interest in interactions with children. These explanations tend to revolve around the supposed needs of the child, such as taking responsibility for a neglected child (who may in fact actually be neglected) through building a relationship with them. Alternatively, one may also explain his behavior as trying to give the child a positive start to their adolescence through bringing them into sexual conversations on equal footing.

To preserve an empathetic, nonjudgmental, and productive relationship between therapist and patient, it is important in this case not to regard any statements of this nature as malicious. In the context of this approach to cognitive distortions, explanations like these serve a self-stabilizing function.

In some patients, the contents of perceptional bias and cognitive distortion manifest themselves as firm convictions. These convictions are maintained in an almost religious or ideological manner. Convictions internalized to this degree cannot necessarily be affected by therapeutic interventions, or the therapist may find that discussions with patients like these continually drift into political or moral territory. It can be helpful in such cases to question the patient's motivations for change as well as their motivation for seeking therapy in the first place (see Module 3, "Motivation").

Excursus—Pedophilia and Romantic Love

From a clinical perspective, it can be assumed that pedophilic men experience love like other people. However, there is little empirical data on this topic. The only important difference between pedophilic/hebephilic men and teleiphilic men appears to be in the body age of the desired partner. Here the above-mentioned biased social perceptions—as dictated by the individual sexual preference—can be particularly pronounced. The feeling of love can elevate the desired partner into an idealized fulfillment of one's own needs and hopes. In the process, one's own sexual motivations are drowned out by subjectively influenced perceptions.

A variety of cross-cultural experiences imply that existing values and views can be markedly impaired in these situations. Even when the patient possesses good self-perception and self-control, feelings of love for a child represent an enormous challenge to the maintenance of these capabilities. Love for a child can accordingly lead to a situation with a massive risk of abuse or assault. Although the child's well-being is the prime concern, the therapist should confront the patient carefully, as a harsh confrontation can endanger the therapeutic relationship if the patient has not yet assessed the danger for themselves (for more information, see Sect. 5.2 in chapter "Therapeutic Options").

An Example of Cognitive Distortions

M. is a 53 year-old, hetero-pedo-hebe-teleiophilic man who sexually abused, a child by being repeatedly masturbated by an (pre-pubescent) 8-year-old girl. In his account, M. gives an external explanation for his actions by making the sexual curiosity of the girl responsible for what happened: "Her interest in my penis got the best of me. She just had to touch it and masturbate me; I couldn't forbid her from doing it." On his

teenage friends: "I just feel better around young people. There's nothing sexual about it." And further: "It's just more lively with young people. We talk about everything: friendship, school, goals in life, and sex."

5   Critical Situations

5.1   Diagnostic Assessment Instead of Moral Assessment

The process of pedophilic and hebephilic men getting close to children of their preferred age and body age often follows typical patterns. These do not however correspond to widely held clichés, like the image of a man lying in wait for a potential victim in a dark alley. Rather, they tend to resemble the ways that teleiophilic people come into contact with a desired person. Pedophilic and hebephilic men often react sensitively to children's need for bonding. Children, especially those in emotionally disadvantaged circumstances, sometimes crave intensive relationships of trust with someone who seems to take their needs seriously, gives them attention and affection, and enjoys spending time with them. In a study of the participants of the PPD, it was shown that some of the subjects felt more emotionally connected to children than to adults, a phenomenon which can be associated with past abusive behaviors toward children (Konrad et al. 2018b).

To aid in reflection on these processes, it is important that the therapist offers as nonjudgmental an environment as possible. Patients commonly assume that the therapists condemn all interactions between pedophilic men and children. Social interactions may certainly represent a concrete risk for sexually abusive behaviors; however, it is vital that these interactions are also accessible to the therapeutic process. Otherwise information about risky patterns of behavior, needs of the patient, perceptions of the patient, and social factors could be missed. An initial therapeutic success might consist of establishing an appropriate vocabulary and atmosphere to discuss these mechanisms. Many patients have their first experience of a nonjudgmental and open discussion of their socio-sexual desires and impulses toward children in therapy. This experience can help differentiate between desires and wishes, on the one hand, and sexual behavior, on the other, and to work out the necessity of building up self-regulatory mechanisms together with the patient.

From a therapist's perspective, the use of the classic approaches of cognitive therapy, such as guided discovery or different forms of disputation in the Socratic dialogue, is needed. Away from judgment, toward diagnostic evaluation, this fundamental principle of the therapist-patient relationship can facilitate an open analysis of the behavior and perceptions of the patient. Through guided discovery and Socratic dialogue, the conflicting background motivations of sexual interest and social norms, as well as the desire not to harm children, can be reflected upon. This technique can help strengthen the will of the patient toward behavioral control and solidify their resistance to sexual impulses.

In the framework of German jurisprudence, the disclosure of past criminal sexual acts against children in the context of therapy is protected by therapeutic confidentiality. A patient may reveal past sexual acts with children during therapy. In these situations, it can be especially difficult to stick to the previously mentioned principles of diagnostic evaluation rather than moral judgment. Although abusive behavior is not to be tolerated under any circumstances and special precautions must be taken for these cases, it is of utmost importance to maintain esteem toward the patient. The therapist must clearly condemn sexual behaviors with children or the use of CSAI, at the same time, they must not judge the patients themselves.

5.2 High-Risk Situations

In the therapeutic context of working with pedophilic and hebephilic men from the *Dunkelfeld* who display a risk for a first or repeated instance of child sexual abuse, situations of immediate risk may occur. These situations represent the most difficult tasks in the completion of a therapeutic program in the legal *Dunkelfeld*. As previously mentioned, therapists should weigh different options in high-risk situations to minimize the chances of child sexual abuse or to stop a potential crime. Breaking therapeutic confidentiality by alerting the authorities should be the last option. Initially, it must be considered by what means the danger can be avoided and the potential victim can best be protected.

With the offer of therapy in the *Dunkelfeld* that appeals to self-motivated people aware of their problem, it is to be expected that different measures to avert the danger of a case of child abuse could be discussed and developed together with the patient. As participation in the program is voluntary, it can be assumed that—unlike in the forensic context—patients are ready to work together with therapists.

Within the prevention network *Dunkelfeld*, regarding therapy with adult participants (the methodology for therapy with juveniles deviates at a number of points from that of therapy with adults; see: chapters "BEDIT-A Manual for Adolescents" and "Modules for Adolescents"), the following steps have been established for the prevention of imminent abusive behavior:

1. Maintenance of transparency regarding risk prognosis and possible options: The patient's and the therapist's assessment of risk may deviate. Patients can overlook important steps in the prevention of abusive behaviors. Any deviating estimations of risk that the therapist regards as more serious than the patients do must be discussed with the patients themselves in order to seek solutions together and to be able to speak with transparency about a further course of action.

2. Concrete measures toward minimization of risk for the child: If, for example, the child lives in the same area as the (potential) offender, the inclusion of the patient's partner (or other person) for the heightening of social supervision or the removal of the (potential) offender from the shared domicile should be considered. This course of action corresponds to the Law on Cooperation and Information in Child Protection of the Federal Child Protection Law

Bundeskinderschutzgesetz=German Federal Child Protection Act, Article 1 § 4 (1)).[1]

3. Evaluation of pharmaceutical options for the attenuation of sexual impulses (not as an alternative, but rather in parallel to step 2 above.): At this point, an androgen-deprivation therapy, perhaps in combination with an antidepressant, is generally appropriate (see Sect. 7).

The course described in steps 1–3 above is guided by the following questions: Is the patient's awareness of the problem a certainty? Is the willingness to give up on the risk behavior present in the patient? If this is in question or not present, further explanation in conversation and in writing is appropriate (with any documents safeguarded by the therapists). In the event of the behavior's persistence, a written agreement must be met that the therapeutic confidentiality agreement will be terminated and continuation of the therapy cannot be guaranteed.

4. Assessment of the possibility of employing appropriately experienced specialists by the child welfare provider, per specific German Federal Child Protection Act, Article 1, Paragraph 4(2). According to this law the information of the involved parties is to be made pseudonymized. Any contact will serve to assess endangerment to the child's welfare and work toward a collective evaluation of possible measures in any further course of action.

5. As applicable, self-referral (into a psychiatric clinic with care mandate, where psychiatric council and inpatient admission are available) to increase the child's safety: this is protected by therapeutic confidentiality, which also applies to any work with the psychiatric clinic.

6. Check and, as necessary, implement procedures in accordance with the specific German Federal Child Protection Act, Article 1, Paragraph 4(3). Patients are to be informed in advance, unless it could call into question the effective protection of the child or adolescent. A breach of confidentiality can be announced in the event that steps 1–5 fail, the person in question proves unreasonable, and adequate evidence is present to justify the request for a court-ordered forced confinement on this basis—even when the person in question denies everything. The hurdle before a forced confinement is exceptionally high.

6   Working with Comorbid Impairments in Therapy

Different studies have shown that in cases of paraphilias, and pedophilia specifically, comorbidity with other psychic disorders represents a norm rather than an exception (see Sect. 4 in chapter "Pedophilia and Hebephilia", as well as Modules 8 [Treatment of Comorbid Disorders] and 9 [Drug-Based Treatment Options with BEDIT-A]). The general psychological distress of 455 PPD participants was assessed using the Brief Symptom Inventory (BIS; Franke 2000). The results showed that 59% of the test group displayed a clinically relevant distress comparable with that of patients receiving inpatient psychiatric care (Konrad et al. 2017). Two-thirds of the participants indicated in their introductory sessions that they had already been in psychiatric or psychotherapeutic treatment at least once in their lives (Kuhle et al. 2016).

Based on the high rate of comorbidities within the target group, it cannot be considered a criterion for exclusion for the treatment of pedophilic and hebephilic people in a group setting. At the same time, however, comorbidity could lead to conflict in group therapeutic work—in that it could make the focus on risk factors or patients' problematic behavior more difficult, for example. It is thus vital to systematically account for comorbid mental disorders in order to factor them into the planning of the therapy. In the framework of the disorder model and the indi-

---

[1] In Germany, since 2012, a specific Child Protection Law ensures that health care professionals who, having noticed child sexual abuse concerning a known child, can inform the youth welfare services in a defined staged procedure. From a legal point of view, it is a form of authorization alongside the general pledge of confidentiality to enable health care professionals to take action in order to immediately stop child endangerment. The last step in the sequence of stages is the denomination of the child to the child protection services, i.e., in Germany the Youth Welfare Offices.

vidual delinquency and risk models established at the beginning of treatment, it must also be factored in to what extent further psychological illnesses may be present or may even have contributed to past dissexual behaviors. Based on the disorder and risk model, it is then decided if participation in dissexuality therapy is possible in spite of comorbid illnesses.

Even when the question of the precise cause-effect relationship cannot be definitively answered, some patients consider their depressive symptoms an effect of their pedophilic and/or hebephilic sexual preference. In the framework of a microanalytic observation of the problematic behaviors, a corresponding vicious cycle can often be observed. Patients also report, for instance, that they react to negative emotional states (e.g., depression and feelings of inadequacy) with sexual behaviors (e.g., use of CSAI), so that they feel relieved (in the sense of negative reinforcement) in the short term but an increase in depression and feelings of inadequacy in the long term. This leads then to the desire to escape this aversive feeling and to the impulse to further use CSAI. In this case a close association between depressive symptoms and the problematic behavior can be recognized. It is possible that a focus on the problematic behavior (use of CSAI) and the development of other forms of behavior to deal with aversive feelings can lead to an improvement in depressive symptoms, so that this comorbid mental disorder may not represent a contraindication for dissexuality therapy in an individual or group setting. In the Good Lives model, an important part of therapy is similarly based on addressing dysfunctional fundamental schemata, as these may stand in conflict with the fulfillment of basic needs. According to the basic principles of group therapy, participants' preference- and risk-related issues that are relevant to the group should be addressed first. A thematization of basic schemata or general psychological distress can enable a conscious and open approach to dealing with sexual preference, risk factors, or problematic behaviors.

In opposition to this integrable comorbidity, there may be others so prominent and acutely in need of treatment that a focus on sexuality, risk factors, and problematic behavior is hardly pos-

sible. In these instances, it may also be the case that there is a connection between the pedophilic or hebephilic disorder and the comorbid mental disorder. However, in some cases, the severity of the comorbid mental illness may make participation in weekly outpatient group therapy impossible, as necessary psychological stability is a prerequisite. Comorbid conditions and impairments acutely requiring treatment (e.g., florid substance addictions, acute psychotic symptoms, severe depressive symptoms, and suicidal tendencies) represent on these grounds criteria for exclusion from standardized dissexuality therapy (see Sect. 2 in chapter "The Berlin Prevention Project Dunkelfeld (PPD)"). In these cases, a standard psychiatric/psychotherapeutic treatment of the comorbid conditions is prioritized (in the case of acute substance addiction, for example, begin with long-term cessation therapy after stabilization and then at least 3 months abstinence before admission into dissexuality therapy) or the patient is treated in an individual setting, where greater individualization and flexibility are possible.

Patients with comorbid personality disorders or severe interaction disorders present a particular challenge in the group setting. This does not indicate a categorical unsuitability of these patients, as the completion of a focused dissexuality therapy in a controlled group setting and good group cohesion is also possible with individual patients with interaction disorders. In patients with very pronounced personality traits (e.g., antisocial personality traits and severe narcissistic or borderline personality disorders) who may run into conflict in a structured group dissexuality therapy, an individual therapeutic treatment must be undertaken. This is especially necessary when the more stable personality traits represent a central component of the patient's disorder and delinquency hypothesis.

7 Drug Treatment to Increase Sexual Impulse Control

In accordance with a fundamental biopsychosocial understanding of human sexuality, BEDIT regards pharmacotherapy as an important supplemental pillar of an all-encompassing therapeutic treatment plan. Sexual preference and sexual behavior of an individual have a biological basis, in which diverse neurobiological systems appear to be relevant (see Sect. 3 in chapter "Pedophilia and Hebephilia"). Certain medications can influence these systems. The goal of pharmacological intervention is to directly influence the sexual experiencing of the person concerned, e.g., helping to reduce urgent, burdensome sexual impulses, thereby directly effecting consequential changes to sexual behavior.

Drug therapy alone will not, in the long term, lead to any change in behavior, as long as fundamental sex-related psychosocial needs remain unaddressed and cannot be adequately fulfilled. Nevertheless, a pharmacological modification of impulses under therapeutic care and based on a detailed explanation and the informed consent can be a great relief to the patient. In practice, different groups of medications play a role in the different biological mechanisms by which they work (Hill et al. 2003). There are medical guidelines for both English- and German-speaking countries offering important information and orientation for patients and practitioners about suitable medications (Berner et al. 2007; Thibaut et al. 2010). Initial experiences with drug-based support from the project "Kein Täter Werden" have already been scientifically analyzed. It was generally concluded, for instance, that participants' confidence in their capacity for regulation of sexual impulses increased with pharmacological treatment (Amelung et al. 2012).

One medication group either directly blocks receptors for the sex hormone testosterone (antiandrogens, e.g., cyproterone acetate) or reduces the body's production of testosterone in the testicles by targeting the hormonal control centers in the brain (GnRH-analogues, e.g., triptorelin). This is known as androgen deprivation treatment (ADT). The sex hormone testosterone in humans is not only responsible for the development of the typical male body (growth of body hair, deeper voice, typical distribution of fat, and development of muscle mass), but it also has effects on the psychic level—alongside general urges—in relation to stamina, "lust for life," and both domi-

nant and aggressive behavior patterns such as sexual urges and interests, as well as the occurrence of sexual fantasies, thoughts, and desires. The above-mentioned medications lead to a decrease in testosterone levels and a reduction of the effects of testosterone, thereby modifying the said psychic factors.

Another group of medications are those that affect the serotonergic reward system. This refers principally to drugs used to treat depression, anxiety, and obsessive-compulsive disorders. The so-called selective serotonin reuptake inhibitors (SSRIs) produce an increase in the concentration of the naturally occurring messenger substance serotonin in the brain. Serotonin is known for its effect on sexual excitability and climax (including ejaculation) and a high level of serotonin can reduce sexual urges. It is additionally known that in the case of obsessive-compulsive disorders, medication that increases serotonin levels can also help to better control impulsive behavior. Unlike the first group of medication, the SSRIs do not effect a change in sexual urges through testosterone balance, but rather through a modification of inner experiential and emotional states.

In individual cases, the biological basis of human sexuality can also be affected through medications from other groups. The central-nervous reward system seems to be important to problematic sexual behavior. This is the rational basis for the implementation of drugs from the realm of addiction therapy that affects the body's own opioid system (e.g., naltrexone). Clinical experience shows that these can make compulsive sexual urges more controllable and influence both gratifying sexual experiences and aversive states in the absence of sexual activity.

Considering pharmacological options can take time and a final decision is a participatory process, not spontaneously resolved. The decision of a project participant for or against medication can take place at any point during the therapy. Therapists support the decision-making process by making information available and through motivating interventions. An initial probation period with adjunctive pharmacological therapy can help with the individual decision, because both the positive effects and uses, as well as the unwanted side effects, can hardly be foreseen from case to case. A typical positive effect of drug treatment can be the experience that it becomes easier to interest onself in other things and to achieve greater serenity in day-to-day life. Thereby, more personal freedoms emerge and contact to other peoople is perceived as less stressful. Patients also report that with impulse-inhibiting medication they experience sexuality as less burdensome and have fewer or no disruptive sexual fantasies, so the general risk of further sexual offenses is decreased. Possible negative effects identified include impairment of self-gratification (decreased capacity for erection and orgasm) and the impairment of sexuality with an adult partner, as the drugs do not only reduce sexual interest in children. It is also to be expected that sexuality will be experienced as less intense and exciting. This, in any case, applies only to the part of intimacy leading to sexual arousal, while non-genital sexuality, including physical intimacy with an adult partner, can feel like a new, positive realm of experience that has a relationship-strengthening function. However, unwanted physical side effects of the drugs such as gynecomastia, fatigue, and weight gain can present themselves.

All medications utilized have been in use for many years and are generally well tolerated (Turner et al. 2013). As one medication can have very different effects on the individual body, care must be taken regarding the following known clinical conditions: a known risk of developing thrombosis, liver cancer, hematopoiesis disorders, bone marrow illnesses, osteoporosis, certain brain tumors (meningioma, pituitary tumors), blood sugar illnesses (diabetes mellitus), dyslipidemia, high blood pressure (arterial hypertonia), obesity (adiposity), and coronary heart disease.

From a medical perspective, routine checkups should be performed prior to the prescription of appropriate medication as well as throughout the course of therapeutic observation. If other medications are being taken, instances of adverse drug interactions—though uncommon—must be watched out for. Physical exercise, especially endurance sports and outdoor activities, can help minimize unwanted physical effects, many of which are generally only temporary.

8 Couples Counseling, Involvement of Relatives, and Follow-Up Care

The state of data on couples relationships involving people with pedophilic/hebephilic tendencies is unsatisfactory. Existing studies on sex offenders can only be used conditionally. One study on intra-familial offenders (whose sexual preferences are not specified) showed significant social and relationship deficits in 30–40% of those studied (Smith & Sanders 1995). They had difficulties building and maintaining emotionally intimate and trusting relationships and were anxious about contact to others. A study of couples relationships involving sex offenders also showed the burden felt by female partners (Iffland et al. 2015). The women interviewed characterized a more uncertain form of attachment, downplayed the offenses of their partners, and were socially isolated.

The partner who had committed an offense was described as being unstable in his self-esteem, but sought dominance and could be socially aggressive. On the basis of mutual support, however, both partners would benefit from weathering a difficult time together, as well as from the experience of mutual acceptance (Iffland et al. 2015). Some results of a meta-analysis show that convicted sex offenders with personal resources and who are in long-term relationships have a lower risk of relapse than those who cannot look to these resources (Hanson and Bussière 1998). Relationship status (being single) is also a proven risk factor for recidivism according to Static-99's assessment of static risk factors (Harris et al. 2003) or Stable-2007's assessment of dynamic risk factors (Fernandez et al. 2012). Problematic couple relationships, on the other hand, can increase the risk of further offenses. This is all the more the case when dependencies or cognitive distortions on the part of the female partner result in insufficient awareness of endangerment to the child and, consequently, to not reckoning with necessary precautionary measures.

About 40% of the participants in the Berlin Prevention Project are in a partner relationship, and about one-third are caregivers to one or more children. Participants who live in a partnership have a significantly higher instance of non-exclusive sexual preference (on the definitions of exclusive vs. non-exclusive sexual preference, see Beier et al. 2013).

One of the fundamental therapeutic premises of the Prevention Project works from the assumption that alongside the dimension of sexual pleasure, pedophilic/hebephilic patients are also motivated by their relationship needs, so that both couples counseling and therapy and, since 2014, a relatives' group are offered. Here, sexual preference, pedophilia, as well as functions and expressions of sexuality are worked through in a psychoeducational framework.

Successful social relationships and the associated personal contact have a direct effect on physical well-being and health. They strengthen resilience in the broadest sense: they improve the immune system, lower heart rate and blood pressure, and reduce feelings of anxiety. Mortality rates are higher in socially isolated people than socially well-integrated people (Holt-Lunstad et al. 2010), and the health of married persons is better than that of unmarried (Liu and Umberson 2008). According to Ainsworth and Bowlby, "secure attachment behavior" belongs to the empirically proven protection factors that hinder mental and psychosomatic disorders (cited in Egle et al. 1997).

It makes sense then to involve relatives and partners of pedophilic/hebephilic people in therapy and in no small part to counteract social stigmatization (Jahnke, Imhoff, and Hoyer 2015). It should be added that relationships work against the isolation of patients and can thus further decrease the risk of the use of CSAI and sexual offenses against children.

8.1   Working with Couples

Sessions in a couples' setting are oriented by need: they are voluntary and designed variably. They range from a single counseling session to about 20 sessions, are free of charge within the PPD, and are subject to therapeutic confidentiality. The therapeutic process that couples go through can be reminiscent of the mourning process (Kast 1982), with a phase of denial, a phase of intense outburst of emotion, a phase of seeking, finding, and letting go, on to reorientation and acceptance. It can be helpful for both partners to steer the focus from the dimension of lust and the corresponding frustration regarding non-preferred body ages to the attachment dimension of the relationship. Even when the partner does not correspond with the pedophilia-specific ideal of the patient, it is still possible to experience sexuality in a satisfying way, so long as closeness, intimacy, and emotional security are brought to the foreground.

With the help of Basson's model (see Fig. 1, Basson et al. 2004), couples can come to understand the sexual reaction cycle, in which the lust and relationship dimensions are bound: a positive cycle emerges from emotionally satisfying sexuality, without the key sexual stimulus being the main motivator for sexual contact. Patients experience this as a relief, the partners can be close to one another without the "pressure to succeed," and sexual function can be improved. Similarly, Basson's model can serve as the basis for a better mutual understanding of shared sexual interaction.

This approach is successful when attention is paid to the limits of focusing on the relationship dimension (cf. Beier 2010), not least because it is itself dictated by the preference structure of both partners. A limitation can be, for example, the "significance of paraphilic stimulus on inner experience" (Beier 2010, p. 28), when alongside the pleasure gain, desire for connection and the experience of connection are also obscured by the paraphilic stimulus, so that "a real partner falls away in the inner assignment of meaning and this tightly limits couples-based interventions" (ibid.) Additionally, "it makes a great difference if the paraphilic experience marks the entire preference structure, or if non-paraphilic parts of the experience exist alongside the paraphilic that can be realized with a partner" (ibid.)

Insofar as a shared perspective connects the two partners, focusing on the relationship dimension can improve the partnership. In the best case scenario, the counseling can lead to a mutual

Fig. 1 The sexual
reaction cycle. (Adapted
from Basson et al. 2004)

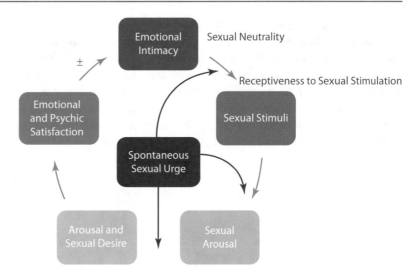

acceptance of the sexual tendencies and a reorientation to a shared identity as a couple, in which the tendencies can be dealt with responsibly, and basic emotional needs can be mutually perceived and fulfilled (cf. Konrad et al. 2018a).

8.2 Working with Relatives

The open relatives' group within the PPD offers information, counseling, and communication for partners, parents, adult children, siblings, and other relatives. The group meets as necessary from twice a year to multiple times per quarter, and the number of participants ranges from two to six persons. The group thematically orients itself to the needs and wishes of the participants and is similar in its concerns and topics to the work of couples therapy. One focal point lies in dealing with anxieties, fears, and negatives emotions such as guilt and shame. These may include anxieties and insecurities about interactions with the partner, a wish to eventually have children, or interactions with children (of the relationship or brought into the relationship) of the preferred age of the participant. Similarly cumbersome can be the navigation of what feels like a stigmatizing society and fear of one's own stigmatization as an individual. Partners have the feeling of being in "competition" with the desired children in terms of sexual attractiveness. Feelings of guilt develop

among parents of participants from the feeling of "having done something wrong." Depressive reactions, feelings of guilt and self-doubt, and even suicidal tendencies may occur, as well as additional psychosomatic symptoms. In the group, relatives can learn from and with each other how concerns and anxieties can be dealt with. Relationships to individual participants can be strengthened through this process, and the isolation of both participants and partners/relatives can be counteracted.

8.3 Follow-Up Care

Based on the multidimensional understanding of sexuality (in its pleasure, reproductive, and relationship dimensions), it must be kept in mind that some people with pedophilic tendencies attempt to fulfill the relationship dimension (with a focus on the biopsychosocial needs for acceptance, security, and warmth) with a child as partner, which is of course impossible in the sense of an equal partnership. It is thus necessary to establish other relationships in order to receive the emotionally stabilizing factors of a close and intimate relationship, even when these persons are not perceived as attractive in the pleasure/lust dimension. Nevertheless a pedophilic person will most likely not feel the same intensity for an adult partner or friend that they would for a child.

People with this tendency must therefore learn to live and deal with an unfulfilled desire. The situation as a whole may be seen as a chronic burden on the individual that requires qualified follow-up care after the end of therapy. It is thus necessary to make follow-up care available in order to support the patient both therapeutically and with counseling. In a flexible process, help tailored to the specific needs and situation of the person should be available. Accordingly, in the context of the PPD, opportunities remain available for all participants to take advantage of follow-up care after the completion of therapy. This serves to stabilize and consolidate the achieved therapeutic goals, and is completed in a group or individual setting.

The Berlin Prevention Project Dunkelfeld (PPD)

Klaus M. Beier, Hannes Gieseler, Hannes Ulrich, Gerold Scherner, and Eliza Schlinzig

1 The Medical Care Situation and the Project's Development

The *Präventionsprojekt Dunkelfeld* ("Prevention Project Dunkelfeld" or PPD) was officially launched on June 6, 2005—World Children's Day—during a media briefing at the Federal Press Conference in Berlin. The date was chosen to highlight the main goal of the project: to make an active contribution to child protection. The project's goal is to hinder sex abuse of minors by offering special treatment options to people who feel sexually attracted to children and are seeking help in controlling their behavior.

Clinical experience had shown that a portion of pedophilic men freely sought professional help in order to stop further abusive behavior. At the same time, there was a notable lack of qualified treatment and counseling services for this group of people. Existing therapeutic services for pedophilic/hebephilic men were, at that point, directed almost exclusively toward convicted sex offenders—that is, offenders currently living under non-confined or confined correctional authority (the so-called *Hellfeld* [Translator's note: literally "bright field," connoting "visible" or "in the open"]). This meant, however, that men sexually attracted to children who were unknown to the authorities remained unconsidered. Belonging to this group are both men who have committed sexual offenses against children but have not yet or ever become known to the criminal justice system and men who have never acted in accordance with their sexual interests toward children and had never sexually abused a child. As the term *Dunkelfeld* was applied to both unknown and unreported crimes (Pfäfflin and Ross 2007), the name Prevention Project Dunkelfeld was chosen (see Fig. 1). As mentioned, a great discrepancy is assumed to exist between the number of sexual offenses against children and the number that get reported. This often leads to distorted research and results, as studies of causes for child sexual abuse are based far more on research samples from forensic contexts than non-forensic contexts (Feelgood and Hoyer 2008). Through the therapeutic support of the group of non-offending pedophilic/hebephilic men, the PPD follows a new approach to the prevention of child sexual abuse and makes possible the non-forensic review of data from the forensic context. To this end, an outpatient center was established, offering diagnosis and therapy for persons who feel attracted toward children and

K. M. Beier (✉) · H. Gieseler · H. Ulrich
G. Scherner · E. Schlinzig
Charité – Universitätsmedizin Berlin, Corporate Member of Freie Universität Berlin, Humboldt-Universität zu Berlin, and Berlin Institute of Health, Center for Human and Health Sciences, Institute of Sexology and Sexual Medicine, Berlin, Germany
e-mail: klaus.beier@charite.de

© The Author(s), under exclusive license to Springer Nature Switzerland AG 2021
K. M. Beier (ed.), *Pedophilia, Hebephilia and Sexual Offending against Children*,
https://doi.org/10.1007/978-3-030-61262-7_4

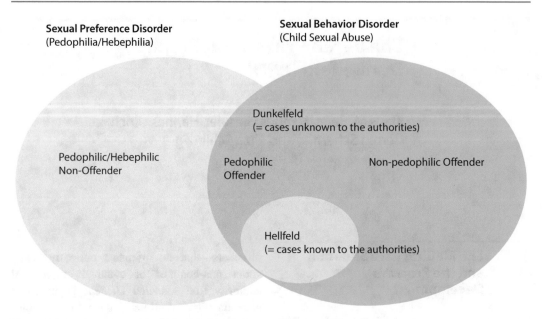

Sexual Preference Disorder
(Pedophilia/Hebephilia)

Sexual Behavior Disorder
(Child Sexual Abuse)

Dunkelfeld
(= cases unknown to the authorities)

Pedophilic/Hebephilic
Non-Offender

Pedophilic
Offender

Non-pedophilic Offender

Hellfeld
(= cases known to the authorities)

Fig. 1 Schematic representation of the differentiation of paraphilias and dissexuality

worry about committing sexual abuse against a child—for the first time or again.

The overarching goal of the PPD is the improvement of preventative measures against child sexual abuse and the use of child sexual abuse images through the extension of an offer of help to a thus-far rather unaccounted-for group: self-described pedophilic/hebephilic individuals who are aware of their problem and currently living within the general population in the community. At the beginning of the project, a specific goal was also set to develop a Germany-wide media campaign to reach the target group described above. The diagnostic and therapeutic process was to be accompanied by scientific research and data collection, in order to review assumptions about this group and evaluate therapeutic treatments. Furthermore, a program for the prevention and treatment of dissexual behavior was also developed and evaluated.

Excursus

In Germany, all those working in community-based treatment programs are subject to the requirement of confidentiality (section 203 of the Criminal Code: "Violation of Private Secrets"—imprisonment for not more than one year or a

fine), which also includes information regarding child sexual abuse (the only explicit exception is the treatment of previously convicted offenders in the context of so-called supervision of conduct, section 68a (8) of the Criminal Code).

The requirement of confidentiality also applies to possible future child sexual abuse, since it is not listed in section 138 of the Criminal Code ("Failure to Report Planned Crimes")—in contrast to, among others, serious trafficking in human beings, murder, manslaughter, or other crimes against personal liberty (in which case the failure to report would constitute a punishable offense).

However, with reference to section 34 of the Criminal Code ("Necessity as Justification"), medical confidentiality can be broken and the case reported to the police if, in the context of a community-based treatment relationship, the therapist is convinced that a patient will commit a sex offense. In this case, the clinician can invoke the fact that, upon weighing up the conflicting interests, the protected interest that is in danger (abuse of a child) substantially outweighs the one interfered with (the requirement of confidentiality). Nevertheless, under the Criminal Code, this only applies to the extent that reporting the matter "is a proportionate means to avert the danger."

That is questionable, since the person reported will deny any motivation whatsoever to commit the offense when official investigations are instituted and permanent deprivation of liberty cannot be justified on this basis. In addition, and according to the experience gained from the PPD, self-referred pedophilics who seek professional help usually want to prevent any sort of abusive behavior from happening. A conflict could only arise if different assessments were made of the risk that an impulse could no longer be controlled and the person concerned would not act on the means recommended by the therapist of averting the danger. But even in the event of such a case (which, to date, has never come up in the PPD), the participant would not reveal his inner life to the authorities if he were reported and he would no longer be accessible for interventions.

For that reason, the legal situation in Germany must be regarded as an extremely favorable starting point for preventative treatment in this field, because it enables a protective framework, which leads to potential offenders or real undetected offenders being prepared to accept help in the first place. Since, however, these offenders certainly do exist and the probability that they would commit their first offense or further sexual offenses or the use of child sexual abuse images (CSAI) is much greater if they did not accept help, it is definitely better to have the opportunity to begin an intervention than not to gain any access to this target group at all. The legal situation in Germany is especially notable when compared with other countries, where therapists working in community projects are subject to the requirement of disclosure if they become aware of acts of child sexual abuse (CSA) or the use of CSAI, or if they have reason for suspecting that their patient will commit such acts.

An ethical debate on this matter would raise the question of whether utilitarian principles (choice of the lesser evil) in view of the benefit achieved (being able to prevent offenses against sexual self-determination) permit a procedure obligated more to protecting children than a strictly normative orientation (duty to report cases on account of the interest being in danger), which is also linked to the restriction of civil liberties (lifting of requirement of confidentiality).

The ethical dilemma at hand is not about the question of whether or not a therapist reports one single individual to the authorities in order to try protecting one single child. The ethical dilemma is about the question of whether a society creates or obstructs circumstances, which allow a higher number of individuals to face their problem, granting professionals the opportunity of protecting a greater number of children.

2   Target Group

In the general population, persons with the following characteristics are the targets of the PPD:— Those who suffer from their sexual preference or sexual behaviors toward prepubescent and/or early pubescent children and wish to seek help for this

- Those who fear that they could commit child sexual abuse (again)
- Those who are not currently being prosecuted for sexual offenses against children or the use of child sexual abuse images

The target group consists of people with exclusive or non-exclusive pedophilic and/or hebephilic sexual preferences corresponding to the diagnostic criteria for pedophilia (DSM-5; APA 2013) or hebephilia (Blanchard et al. 2009). However, a background of sexual interactions with children or past use of child sexual abuse images without the simultaneous occurrence of sexual thoughts, fantasies, or impulses about/toward children is not regarded as sufficient for a /hebephilia.

The sexual orientation of the project participants toward the male and/or female sex is evaluated based on the fantasies occurring during masturbation and on persons experienced as sexually arousing. A diagnosis of exclusive pedophilia/hebephilia is made when a person reports recurring and intensive sexual thoughts, fantasies, and impulses exclusively about/toward prepubescent and/or early pubescent children and if no sexual fantasies about adults are reported. The PPD and its treatment program are directed at:

- Persons who have not committed child sexual abuse or used child sexual abuse images but fear doing so in the future (non-offending persons with pedophilia/hebephilia)
- Persons who have committed child sexual abuse or used child sexual abuse images but have remained unknown to the justice system (offenders with pedophilia/hebephilia in the *Dunkelfeld*) and fear offending again
- Individuals with pedophilia/hebephilia, who have been prosecuted in the past for child sexual abuse or the use of child sexual abuse images, but are no longer under judicial oversight and fear relapsing

The program is directed furthermore at persons with the intrinsic motivation to seek support and are not being pushed to participate by external pressure.

Requirements for participation in treatment are as follows: the diagnosis of a pedophilic and/or hebephilic sexual preference; a minimum age of 18 at the time of initial introduction; and sufficient command of German. Persons with acute (e.g., untreated) drug or alcohol problems, developmental disorders, or acute psychiatric disorders, whose treatment must be prioritized cannot be taken on into the treatment program. They may, however, get in touch with the project again after the successful treatment of their acute psychiatric symptoms, as applicable.

3   Treatment Rationale

The integrative theory of Ward and Beech (2006; see Sect. 4 in chapter "Child Sexual Abuse and the Use of Abuse Images") has resulted in a multidimensional treatment approach that takes into account that in primary preventative therapy for people with pedophilic and/or hebephilic sexual preference, sexual preference itself must be seen as an influencing factor displaying a high degree of stability (Grundmann et al. 2016; see Sect. 3 in chapter "Therapeutic Options"), and the modification of which cannot be seen as a goal of therapy—though the improvement of behavior control regarding sexual impulses toward children may.

This makes it clear that a treatment should comprise biomedicinal (pharmacological), psychological (cognitive behavioral therapy), and sexological (couples counseling that takes the sexual relationship into account)   intervention strategies. Accordingly, the Berlin Dissexuality Therapy is in its original conception (Neutze et al. 2005; Neutze et al. 2008) a therapy program that looks largely to a cognitive behavioral approach and has been expanded to include sexual medicine and pharmacological treatment options (Beier and Loewit 2011). The interventions are based on a cognitive behavioral model as well as the principles of Relapse-Prevention, Self-Regulation, and the Good Lives Model (Pithers 1990; Ward and Gannon 2006; Ward and Hudson 2000; Ward et al. 1998). BEDIT corresponds to current treatment standards of the USA and Canada, where most therapeutic institutions for sex offenders known to the authorities draw on cognitive behavioral approaches (McGrath et al. 2010). A number of adjustments to existing treatment approaches were necessary, however, to appropriately meet the conditions necessary for an outpatient institution for sexual medicine offering individual treatment of sexual preference disorders. These conditions are as follows (Beier et al. 2005).

- Both the sexual preference for a certain developmental body age and sex, as well as possible additional paraphilic arousal patterns, must be seen as relatively stable components of the individual personality. A person is not responsible for their sexual attraction but is responsible for behavior that may result from it (Beier et al. 2009). The treatment of sexual impulses toward children is thus normally connected with lifelong challenges regarding sexual self-regulation and behavior control.
- As sexual fantasies may be seen as a part of the individual self-concept, confrontation with children perceived as sexually attractive results in a lasting burden on feelings of self-worth, which can lead to the denigration of one's own person. This itself can make the development of socially adequate management strategies and control of sexual impulses all the more difficult.

- On the basis of a multidimensional understanding of sexuality (the pleasure dimension, the reproductive dimension, and the relationship dimension; Beier et al. 2005), it must be taken into account that persons with a pedophilic/hebephilic attraction also seek fulfillment within the relationship dimension (with focus on the basic biopsychosocial needs of acceptance, security, and warmth) with a child as partner. It is thus helpful for the patients to build up other relationships (friendships, etc.) to experience these emotionally stabilizing factors, even when these persons are not perceived as attractive on a sexual level.

4   Treatment Objectives

Likelihood to commit child sexual abuse (for the first time or again) is not distributed uniformly throughout a person's lifespan. Although pedophilia/hebephilia represent a significant risk factor for child sexual abuse and the use of child sexual abuse images, biological, psychological, and social factors all further influence whether or not someone will act in accordance with their sexual attraction. Factors that exist in connection with the likelihood to offend or re-offend and may be subject to influence through therapeutic interventions are described in scientific literature as dynamic risk factors (DRF). Theories of child sexual abuse or the use of child sexual abuse images has since taken the significance of dynamic risk factors into consideration (Davis 2001; Finkelhor 1994; Hall and Hirschmann 1992; Marshall and Barbaree 1990; Ward and Beech 2006; Ward and Siegert 2002; Quayle and Taylor 2003, see also Sect. 4 in chapter "Child Sexual Abuse and the Use of Child Sexual Abuse Images"). In addition, they represent important treatment goals in the context of preventative approaches for sex offenders who are known to the criminal justice system (Andrews and Bonta 2006; Marshall et al. 2006).

According to findings from research conducted in the *Hellfeld,* alongside the sexual attraction to children, four dimensions of dynamic risk factors are associated with sexual relapse and thus with influence on sexual motivation: abuse-supporting attitudes, sexual and general self-regulation deficits, and emotional or intimacy deficits (Hanson et al. 2007). A number of factors, such as deficits in victim empathy, could not be empirically attested (Mann et al. 2010). Nonetheless, they are regarded by clinical experts as core elements in the treatment of sex offenders (McGrath et al. 2010).

To what extent these empirically relevant risk factors for relapse and the derivative treatment goals can be applied to persons with pedophilia/hebephilia with a risk for first-time child abuse and offenders with pedophilia/hebephilia in the *Dunkelfeld* is still unknown (Duff and Willis 2006). In any case, the first results of the PPD's group comparisons point to the applicability of most described risk factors to persons unknown to the justice system and accordingly represent relevant treatment goals (Beier, Grundmann et al. 2015; Neutze et al. 2012).

The therapy program of BEDIT fundamentally aims at strengthening the motivation for abstaining from problematic sexual behaviors, as well as increasing the experience of self-efficacy and behavior control (including sexual fantasies and interests). The goal is to replace emotion-oriented, avoidance-oriented, and sexualized coping strategies by building up adequate management strategies, strengthening social functionality (with a focus on the relationship dimension of sexuality), reducing abuse-supporting attitudes and behaviors, fostering empathy regarding the victims of child sexual abuse, and finally, developing appropriate measures and goals for relapse prevention. The general model of therapy-relevant factors in BEDIT (Fig. 2) provides an overview of basic factors that can be used to specify individual treatment goals.

As an overview, group therapy focuses on the following treatment goals:

1. Integration of sexual preference and sexual behavior disorder into the individual self-image (realization, strengthening of awareness)
2. Acceptance of an experienced biographical stability of sexual preference

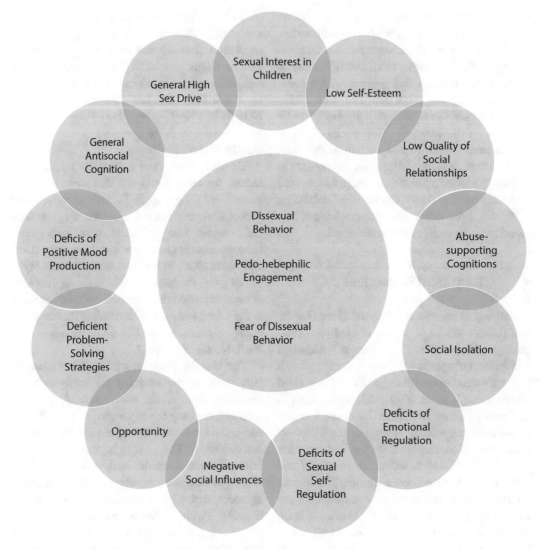

Fig. 2   General model of therapy-relevant factors in BEDIT

3. Improvement of the experience of self-efficacy and self-observation (also regarding sexual fantasies and interests) and the reduction of sexual coping mechanisms via the acquisition of alternative coping mechanisms

4. Improvement of the levels of social functioning through a focus on the relationship dimension of sexuality (basic needs for acceptance, security, and warmth, e.g., through the inclusion of partners) and/or the building up of networks that provide social support

5. Improvement in adopting other perspectives and empathy for victims of child sexual abuse and victims of child sexual abuse images

6. Complete and radical acceptance of responsibility for one's own behavior (specifically socio-sexual) in the past, present, and future

7. Formulation of one's understanding and knowledge of the connections/interactions between perception, feelings, and behavior

8. Identification of pathognomic perception failures (denial and trivialization) and correction of dysfunctional perception and

behavior patterns, as well as the reduction of abuse-supporting views and positions

9. Identification of high-risk situations, risk constellations, and stimuli that could lead to risk-likely behaviors
10. Development of a comprehensive and effective repertoire of (control and relapse-prevention) strategies to better cope with problematic day-to-day situations in general and in confrontations with children in particular
11. Information and support regarding the possibility of pharmacological interventions

5   Effects of Treatment on Risk Factors and Sexual Behavior—Initial Results

The efficacy of one year of the BEDIT treatment program was examined via a sample of participants with pedophilia/hebephilia in the PPD (Beier, Grundmann et al. 2015). Through the use of a non-randomized waiting-list control design, data were taken multiple times from the treatment group ($n = 53$) and the waiting control group ($n = 22$). In order to evaluate changes throughout the course of therapy, comparisons were run both within the groups and between the groups. It was assumed that previously identified dynamic risk factors and sexually abusive behaviors would improve considerably in the treatment group, while no changes would arise within the control group. To this end, the therapy evaluation concentrated on the sexually abusive behavior of three different groups:

- Men who displayed continued sexually abusive behavior ("persisters") regardless of whether or not they were known to the authorities
- Men who had not committed child sexual abuse or had refrained from the use of abuse images ("desisters")
- Men who, for the first time, displayed sexually abusive behavior during treatment ("beginners")

The results corresponded as a whole with the assumed changes and in the desired direction.

After treatment, the participants reported less isolation, showed fewer emotionally oriented coping strategies, fewer deficits in emotional empathy with victims, fewer abuse-supportive attitudes, fewer deficits of self-efficacy, and less preoccupation with sex. The effect size of these improvements tended toward the middle to high range. Contrary to the hypothesis, however, no significant change was shown to deficits of self-worth, cognitive empathy with victims, or sexualized coping. Evidence for the stability of the positive changes were shown in a follow-up examination one year after therapy. The data collected at the one-year mark showed no significant changes from that collected directly after the end of therapy, which supports the hypothesis of the stability of the positive changes. Additionally, a subsample of the persons who took part in the follow-up examination displayed a decrease in deficits of intimacy and cognitive empathy with victims after the completion of therapy.

This corresponds generally to existing research results on the modifiability of dynamic risk factors through therapeutic interventions for sex offenders and indicates that results from the forensic field are at least partially applicable to men with pedophilia/hebephilia living in the general population. This does not, however, apply to the evaluation of repeated behaviors of sexual assault. Regarding child sexual abuse, 20% of the sample group reported new assaultive behavior and were consequently categorized as "persisters" (0% "beginners"). As for the use of abuse images, 90% of the sample reported continued use, even when a reduction in the frequency of use and the degree of severity of the materials had been achieved. They were accordingly categorized as "persisters" (11% "beginners"). This confirms the significance of the *Dunkelfeld* population on the sexual traumatization of children (for detailed results, see Beier, Grundmann, et al. 2015; Amelung et al. 2012; Kuhle et al. 2012; Neutze et al. 2012).

On the basis of its exploratory character, small sample size, and relatively small follow-up time frame, the results of the PPD must be regarded as preliminary. Further studies with larger samples and longer follow-up time frames would be necessary to confirm its results. As a whole, however, the results underscore the significance of preventative treatment approaches.

---

6   Follow-Up Examinations

The basis for the follow-up examinations of PPD patients (Gieseler et al., forthcoming) is a systematic sampling of 56 subjects. As of the end of December 2016, 2465 interested persons had contacted the Berlin site of the prevention network "Kein Täter Werden." A clinical exploration followed with 1033 affected persons, of whom 507 were presented with an offer of therapy; 247 accepted the offer and began therapy. At that point, 45 participants were currently participating in psychoeducation or individual/group therapy; 79 had stopped therapy for different reasons; and 126 had completed a therapeutic treatment. Of these, 110 fulfilled the requirements for the study—those who had completed therapy at least one year prior. This sample was recruited via telephone or e-mail between June 2015 and August 2017. A €100 compensation was offered, to be paid out upon participation. Forty previously treated project participants could not be reached, as there was either no contact information or the information on file was no longer current. One potential subject had died. Sixty-nine previous participants could thus be contacted; 11 of these 69 did not agree to participate due to distance, or without stating a reason. Three initially agreed, but then could not be contacted again. This resulted in a sample of 56 subjects.

The data were collected by six scientific and therapeutic staff members of the Institute for Sexology and Sexual Medicine at the Charité—Universitätsmedizin Berlin, on their premises between July 2015 and August 2017, in the form of semi-structured interviews and questionnaires. It was ensured that the subjects were not questioned by their former contact therapists, so that the interviewer was as unknown to them as possible.

The participants of the follow-up examinations were on average 45.6 years old (SD = 10.6, range: 24–67 years) and had, excluding one participant, German citizenship. About 42% met the requirements for higher education and the majority (62.5%) were employed at the time. Over one-third (41.1%) of the participants were currently in relationships, with an average length of 10.2 years (SD = 9.5 years). Eight participants were currently living in a household with one or more children.

On average the subjects had participated in 14.68 months of therapy (range: 11–25 months): fifty three participants (94.6%) had been to group therapy, six participants (10.7%) received supplementary individual therapy, three (5.4%) had exclusively done individual therapy, and four (7.1%) had accepted an offer of supplementary couples counseling or couples therapy.

The length of time since the end of weekly therapy was essential to the duration of observation, which lasted between 12 and 118 months, with an average of 73.6 months. At the time of the interviews, nine of the participants made use of the follow-up care offered three to four times weekly.

In accordance with the treatment program's therapy goals, interviews with the subjects focused on problematic sexual behavior before, during, and after therapy. These focused on child sexual abuse and the consumption of abuse images.

At different points before the beginning of therapy, 28 subjects (50%) had committed one or more sexual offenses of varying severity against children or teenagers. Six (10.7%) were known to the authorities—e.g., previously in the *Hellfeld*—before the beginning of the treatment program. One subject (1.8%) committed child sexual abuse during the observation period; 55 participants (98.2%) reported no further offenses against children or teens since the end of therapy. None reported contact with the authorities because of child sexual abuse since the end of therapy.

Forty-four participants (78.6%) used abuse images of varying kinds and with varying frequency before the end of therapy. Five (8.9%) were known to the authorities (in the *Hellfeld*) before the treatment program for this reason. Twenty-eight subjects (50%) continued this behavior during the observation period. Ten participants (17.9%) had never used abuse images at any point before the interview. Eighteen participants (32.1%) reported no further use after the end of therapy. Within the group of those that did use further, the frequency of use and severity of the images were reduced in a number of cases. One subject (1.8%) only began to use during the observation period. Two subjects (3.6%) came into contact with the authorities because of the use of abusive images after the end of therapy.

An initial qualitative assessment was undertaken by selecting from the first 23 participants who reported no further problem of sexual behavior during the observation period. Above all else, this group experienced the perception, acceptance, and integration of sexual preference into their self-conceptions, as well as the feeling of not being alone in their sexual responsiveness to children, as helpful factors for behavior control. Contact with the authorities before the beginning of therapy was also shown to have had a positive effect on the regulation of the use of abuse images.

To that end, quotes from interviews with different subjects:

> Subject A: "…in the end I was also glad that I had done it, because I could say it for myself, so I know now what the problem area is, so to speak, and how I need to control it.
> Subject B: "It's part of me, it's my tendency, it's allowed to be there, this fantasy (…). It's okay."
> Subject C: "And it's nice. You learn a lot about yourself. Why you are the way the you are, and what's actually behind this sexual attraction. Like what the commonalities of normal sexuality are."
> Subject D: "Yeah, like imagining how being abused really makes a child feel, for instance. Like that you really just destroy everything, and that was really the main point, and I mean at the end of the day it's the fantasies that no one can take out of me, that as long as I can control them, in connection—or not act on them, let's say, then I can live pretty well with that, and that's what I've learned since then."

The results provide clear tendencies that preventative therapy can have a decisive impact on problematic sexual behavior. There was notably only one subject (out of 56) who reported having committed sexual abuse during the catamnesis period (the victim in question was a boy of early pubescent developmental age).

7 Discontinuation Rates

Up to this point, the question of reasons for prematurely discontinuing or quitting therapy has played a secondary role in research's assessment of psychotherapeutic offerings. Studies of therapeutic efficacy are increasingly describing and analyzing the numbers of those who have quit or who did not get into therapy in spite of pertinent indications. One goal of research is in the corresponding improvement of therapeutic services and the reduction of discontinuance of therapy. Premature discontinuation of therapy is associated with not achieving stated therapy goals, poorer results for these patients in the reduction of symptoms and improvement of quality of life (well-being), as well as higher costs for the health care system and society in general, on the economic side (cf. Archer et al. 2000; Walker et al. 1999). One of the few systematic meta-analyses (125 completed individual studies) of therapy discontinuation reported an average discontinuation rate of 47% (SD = 22.25) (Wierzbicki and Pekarik 1993). Earlier studies (such as Baekeland and Lundwall 1975) describe rates between 31% and 79%. It should be noted that the different discontinuation rates may be primarily explained by different operationalizations and definitions of therapy discontinuation (e.g., number of sessions, appraisal of the therapist, achievement of goals, absences, etc.). A newer meta-analysis of 669 completed studies showed a weighted discontinuation rate of 19.7% (Swift and Greenberg 2012). As for possible relevant factors/variables in connection with therapy discontinuation, no clear and credible results have thus far become available.

Reducing the risk of sexual assault on children is always a therapy goal in the case of persons with pedophilic/hebephilic sexual preference. Along with the general results, discontinuations of therapy are to be regarded in connection with possible risk for child sexual abuse and the use of child sexual abuse images, and they are thus of particular relevance. In the context of therapies in the forensic field with sex offenders, sociodemographic factors such as age, gender, relationship status, level of education, and employment have been analyzed in studies. As possible influencing factors in connection with therapy discontinuation, areas such as low self-esteem, loneliness, emotional coping, cognitive bias, perceived low self-efficacy, impulsivity, psychopathy, deficits of intimacy, deficits of empathy, and above-average sexual preoccupation have been discussed. Results of individual studies up to this point are inconsistent and in part contradictory. In a meta-analysis including 114 forensic studies with convicted persons who offended sexually, the authors found an average cessation rate of 27.1% and sociodemographic factors such as age, relationship status, employment, and level of education to be predictive of therapy discontinuation (Olver et al. 2011). Within the Prevention Project Dunkelfeld, the discontinuation rates in the first phase of the project from 2005 to 2012 were analyzed (Scherner, forthcoming). During this period treatment was set beginning and were conceived for a duration of one year and without psychoeducational sessions. The operationalization of treatment discontinuation was set conservatively. Participants who had begun therapy and then quit between the third session and the regular end of therapy were classified under "discontinued therapy." Plausible premature cessations of therapy related to change of residence or organizational incompatibilities with a new workplace were also classified as "discontinued therapy." Interested persons who met the acceptance criteria for the project—in whose case the indication for therapy was given—but either did not accept the offer of therapy or participated in a maximum of three sessions were classified under "declined therapy." Participants who took the offer of therapy and completed the program in its full extent were classified under "completed therapy." Taken into the analysis were fundamentally only those for whom fully evaluable datasets were available. This resulted in a total sample size of 425 participants, classified as follows: 253 "declined therapy," 60 "discontinued therapy," and 112 "completed therapy." The discontinuation rate of those who had recently begun therapy was at 35%—within a range not uncommon in psychotherapy. Because of the above-mentioned issues of a possibly untreated risk of assault, the sample was further examined for possible factors that might be associated with discontinuation of therapy. The same applied to those who did not or could not make use of an offer of therapeutic treatment. Compared to those who accepted the offer of therapy, the following factors proved themselves relevant for those classified under "declined therapy."

Persons who declined the offer of therapy tended to live outside of Berlin, in part in neighboring or more-distant German states. This result may be seen as evidence of a shortfall in corresponding care options near potential patients' places of residence. Furthermore, fewer of those who declined therapy tended to have a sexual preference structure directed exclusively toward prepubescent or early pubescent body age. This group also reported a higher experience of control over sexual impulses, a more problem-oriented coping style, fewer feelings of isolation, and fewer cognitive biases. To what extent these results indicate a possible lower degree of psychological strain or less-acute need for therapy must be regarded critically, as these persons stated a general interest in therapy and this group also contained individuals who had displayed sexually abusive behavior and/or used child sexual abuse images in the course of their life.

These results contributed to bolstered efforts to establish further therapeutic offerings in other German states, in order to establish a care infrastructure in proximity to more peoples' places of residence. Through the establishment of the network "Kein Täter Werden," which includes 11 sites working in cooperation, great advances could be aimed for.

Compared to other groups, those classified under "discontinued therapy" showed higher numbers in the areas of cognitive biases and, on the sociodemographic level, a lower formal education level than those who completed therapy. It could furthermore be shown that within the group that discontinued therapy, those who stopped within the first four months of treatment generally showed a higher degree of cognitive bias and reported lower experienced self-efficacy regarding sexual impulse control than those who discontinued in the period between 4 and 12 months after beginning therapy. Significant differences between the groups were also found. These results contributed to critical analysis and targeted modification of previous approaches in the sense of therapeutic treatment following a set time frame and manual procedure. Instead, the therapy could be tailored—including in the group setting—more to individual participants, thus reducing the discontinuation rate as much as possible (e.g., in the case of participants with strong cognitive biases, addressing these early on through motivational work and thematization and focusing treatment in light of their responsiveness). These considerations led to designing a therapy program more flexible, interactive, and customizable to the time constraints of patients, which contributed in part to this manual. To what degree a reduction of the discontinuation rate is achievable cannot be measured at this time. A decrease in the discontinuation rate can be observed, though not within a statistically significant range. To this end, a larger sample must be analyzed in the future.

8   Adaptation for Juveniles

8.1   Initial Situation and Development of the Berlin "Prevention Project for Juveniles"(PPJ)

Founded in 2014 at the Institute for Sexology and Sexual Medicine at the Charité-Universitätsmedizin Berlin, the Prevention Project for Juveniles (PPJ) represents a clinical extension of the Prevention Project Dunkelfeld (PPD). The PPD is directed exclusively at persons over the age of 18 (as described in Sect. 2). Nearly ten years of clinical experience at the Berlin site have shown, however, that the majority of adults who contacted the PPD to report pedophilic attraction had already been aware of their sexual preference as minors, with many having already abused children when they themselves were minors. Most of them would have appreciated therapeutic help, but did not know of any place to go and did not dare speak to anyone directly around them—for fear of denigration and stigmatization.

The picture drawn from clinical knowledge was confirmed by (among other sources) the police criminal statistics (*Polizeiliche Kriminalstatistik* [PKS]). According to the PKS (Bundeskriminalamt 2017), a total of 12,019 known cases of child sexual abuse (§§ 176, 176a, 176b of the German Criminal Code) were committed in 2016. Of the 9159 reported suspects, 8.4% were children (individuals under 14 years of age) and 20.9% were juveniles (individuals between 14 and 18), so that a total of 29.3% of suspects were under the age of 18. Or in the case of the criminal offense of the distribution, acquisition, possession, and production of child pornographic materials (§ 184b German Criminal Code), which numbered 5687 cases, of the 4859 suspects, 5.9% were children and 9.2% were juveniles—meaning 15.1% of suspects in total were under the age of 18 (Bundeskriminalamt 2017).

It can be assumed that, like those committed by adults, the majority of sexual offenses committed by juveniles take place in the *Dunkelfeld*. It must furthermore be taken into account that juveniles' sexual preference toward children is much easier to realize due to the smaller gap in age to the victims. Moreover, this does not tend to result in the child informing a third party about the traumatic experience, as the likelihood of victims reporting their experiences is low and only increases with age (McElvaney 2013).

Further concordances between the clinical experiences gained through the PPD and those from suspects apprehended by the judicial system are reflected in pertinent empirical literature. Studies of various conceptions report that 30–50% of offenders who sexually abuse children had already been aware, as juveniles, of their sexual interest in children (cf. Abel et al. 1987; Elliott et al. 1995; Marshall et al. 1991). In 40-50% of adult sex offenders, abnormalities in sexual development or sexually inappropriate behavior had been observed during childhood and in the juvenile years (cf. Abel et al. 1993; Longo and Groth 1983).

In their review, Worling and Langström (2006) analyzed the tenability of numerous empirically specified risk factors for (repeated) sexual offenses against children committed by juveniles. They concluded, among other things, that deviant sexual interests counted as a sure risk factor for the (repeated) commission of a sexual offense by a juvenile (Worling and Langstrom 2006). A subsequent meta-analysis by Seto and Lalumière (2010) showed that in the differentiation of juvenile criminals and juvenile persons who offend sexually, the biggest difference in the groups was the presence of atypical sexual interests ($d = 0.67$). Pullmann and colleagues (2014) both confirmed and expanded upon these results: compared to offenders who committed both sexual and non-sexual crimes, their study showed that juvenile sex offenders generally displayed more atypical sexual interests, as well as greater problems in romantic relationships (Pullman et al. 2014).

The cited empirical studies suggest that a need for treatment is already present at juvenile age. It should therefore also be assumed that the majority of sexual offenses committed by juvenile offenders—as with adult offenders—take place in the *Dunkelfeld*.

8.2 Pilot Study 2013

The presented clinical experience and corresponding empirical evidence led to a pilot study undertaken between July and December 2013, financed by the Federal Ministry for Families, Seniors, Women, and Youth (Bundesministerium für Familie, Senioren, Frauen und Jungend [BMFSFJ]). In total, 16 juveniles between the ages of 11 and 18 approached the Institute, in 14 of whom sexual particularities could be identified. Thirteen of these represented a sexual attraction to the development body age of a child. Additional comorbid paraphilias were ascertained in a number of these juveniles, including some belonging to the fetishistic and sadomasochistic spectrums. The majority had already committed offenses against children ($n = 10$, i.e., 63%) or had made use of child sexual abuse images ($n = 5$, i.e., 31%). Nearly 75% of sexually inappropriate behavior had taken place in the *Dunkelfeld* (see Beier et al. 2015c).

From this pilot study, it follows that the intended target group of the PPJ exists and that sexual particularities can already be ascertained at juvenile age, as the juveniles were ready—after the development of a trusting and nonjudgmental atmosphere— to report on these in the form of fantasies accompanying masturbation. It could furthermore be ascertained that the great majority of those who contacted the Institute had already displayed sexually abusive behavior, primarily in the *Dunkelfeld*. It also became obvious that contact between the youths and the PPJ was initiated primarily by way of an adult guardian or youth services social worker. The given aspects led to the launch of the main phase of the PPJ project on April 4, 2014, funded by the BMFSFJ (Federal Ministry for Family Affairs, Senior Citizens, Women and Youth).

The high number of psychiatric comorbidities identified in just seven juveniles during the pilot phase led to cooperation with Child and Juvenile Psychiatry, Psychotherapy, and Psychosomatics of the Vivantes Klinikum in Berlin-Friedrichshain (Kinder- und Jugendpsychiatrie, Psychotherapie und Psychosomatik des Vivantes Klinikum). The aim of this cooperation is to be able to offer inpatient and outpatient child and juvenile psychiatric or pharmacological treatment, in the event of pertinent indication. Careful and specific diagnostics and treatment designs are necessary to correctly serve the developmental aspects of a juvenile patient. The PPJ thus seeks to join sexological and child/juvenile psychiatric expertise, which is fundamental to the following treatment manual (BEDIT-A; see chapter "BEDIT-A Manual for Adolescents"), and recommends the application of this manual in a correspondingly structured setting and to a comparable clientele.

8.3 Target Group and Diagnostic Services

The goal of the PPJ is the prevention of dissexual behavior by juveniles toward children—in the sense of the initial or repeated sexual abuse of a child, as well as initial or repeated use of child sexual abuse images. As a diagnostic and therapeutic care service, the PPJ is aimed at juveniles between 12 and 18 years of age with sexually conspicuous behaviors or fantasies that point to a non-normative sexual attraction for the child body age in the sense of pedophilic preference. Principally, it employs a primary preventative approach to potential juvenile offenders who, because of sexual particularities for the child body age, are in particular danger of acting upon their fantasies and displaying sexually abusive behavior toward children. The goal is to offer "support with managing and controlling sexual impulses toward children to affected juveniles as early as possible in their development" (Beier et al. 2015c, p. 31).

Through thorough diagnostics with the individual youth and their contact persons with a sexological focus (see Beier et al. 2015c; 2016), the aim is to clarify the sexual preference structure with a focus on any paraphiliac content, in particular whether or not a sexual particularity for the child body age is involved. Previous sexually inappropriate behavior is recorded, cognitive faculties are assessed by way of an intelligence test, evidence of any present (comorbid) child or juvenile psychiatric/somatic illnesses is compiled, and individual risk factors are identified in order to propose appropriate specific therapy options.

Due to their age, juveniles are in a period of physical, psychic, and emotional development. This will be taken into account, in that—in accordance with the current classification systems of the ICD-10 (WHO 1992) and the DSM-5 (APA 2013)—a diagnosis of "pedophilia" will not be made for anyone under the age of 16. The focus in the semi-structured clinical interviews will rather be on pre-orgasmic masturbation fantasies, which will be evaluated in the context of previously experienced sexual contacts and the consumption of pornographic materials. Subsequently, this is used as an indicator of the presence of a sexual particularity for the child body age in the sense of an initial and provisional diagnostic evaluation.

8.4   Therapeutic Services

Should the diagnostics show that sexual particularities for the child body age are currently present, an offering of therapy can be presented with the voluntary agreement of the patient and the guardian, accounting for the patient's current status in the *Dunkelfeld*. The foremost purpose of the treatment is to achieve the acceptance of personal fantasies that may arise and the integration of these into one's own self-image. In addition, the development and strengthening of capabilities in dealing with sexual desires and impulses in a way that does not endanger others or the self will be aimed for. A cure in the sense of a change to sexual preference will, in accordance with the current state of empirical research, not be held as a prospect, although the therapeutic component of the PPJ may be characterized as open to other results. The patients and their close contacts will work on being able to identify and manage individual risk factors. Abuse-supporting attitudes and cognitive biases will be analyzed and reflected upon together. Along with this, the strengthening of social skills and the resulting improvement in relational abilities can come into focus. The whole therapy is offered free of charge and under therapeutic confidentiality.

8.5   Procedure in Borderline Cases

In the event of evidence of any danger to a child's well-being, a structured procedure was developed within the PPJ in accordance with the Law on Cooperation and Information in Child Welfare (specific German Child Protection Law, Article 1, §4(1)).

In the case of a borderline situation articulated by the juvenile himself or the contact system, a tiered series of measures are to be turned to. The procedure works from the assumption that as per the acceptance criteria to the project, the juvenile is a voluntary participant, meaning that a readiness to cooperate on the part of the patient or the welfare system can be assumed. The point of departure is the recognition of a borderline situation on the part of the therapist. The borderline situation is first discussed between the therapist and the patient, in particular when one's estimation of risk deviates from the other's. An awareness of the problem is to be worked on with the patient in order to work toward solutions together. Should the juvenile show an understanding of the situation, solution strategies are to be developed and implemented. Should he not display a credible and unequivocal readiness to cooperate, it must be made clear to them that their guardian will be informed. Parallel to this, a test for indications necessitating medicinal measures should be undertaken, in particular aiming at suppression of sexual impulses. Should the guardians show credible understanding and readiness to cooperate, concrete measures toward minimization of risk (in accordance with the specific German Child Protection Law, Article 1, § 4(1)) should be taken, and an inpatient stay in a child/juvenile psychiatric clinic can be considered, as applicable. In the absence of readiness to cooperate on the part of the guardians, the responsible child protective services agency should be informed, about which the guardian must also be made aware of. Should an explanation of the mandatory report to child protective services not increase the guardians' readiness to cooperate, a report of child endangerment should be made to child protective services, in accordance with spe-cific German Child Protection Law, Article 1 § 4(2). The therapist then communicates the assessment of the borderline situation to a relevantly experienced social worker from child protective services. The communication of the situation, as well as transmission of data about the case, is pseudonymized and thus presents no conflict with the confidentiality agreement. Should substantial evidence of child endangerment be ascertained by child protective services, following § 8a SGB VIII (Schutzauftrag bei Kindeswohlgefährdung [Protection Mandate in the Case of Child Endangerment]), a consultation of specialists on the assessment of danger will be initiated by child protective services. This institution will decide about further procedure and involve itself with additional authorities (e.g., family court and police) as necessary. For more details on risk management within the PPD, see also Sect. 5 in chapter "Therapeutic Options", which contains another section on high-risk situations   (See Sect. 5.2 in chapter "Therapeutic Options").

BEDIT Manual for Adults

Working Group of the Prevention Project
Dunkelfeld

1 Fundamental Premises of the BEDIT Group Therapy

The BEDIT manual consists of 13 modules and was originally intended for a 12-month group therapy in a closed group setting (fixed composition of participants, fixed beginning, and conclusion of the therapy) with weekly sessions (altogether approx. 45–50) each lasting two hours. Each session is led by two therapists and is carried out with a minimum of five and maximum of ten participants per group. Some locations within the prevention network, however, opt to conduct sessions in a semi-open group setting (flexible beginning and end of the therapy with mandatory participation and participants can be in different stages of treatment) or in an individual setting. In these cases, the manual is adapted accordingly.

The BEDIT manual provides a general orientation for the treatment of people with pedophilia and hebephilia in the *Dunkelfeld* and should not be understood as a standardized procedure. The therapeutic approach and the suggested interventions must be adjusted to the specific setting, the composition of the group, as well as the needs of individual patients. Therefore, it is necessary to develop an individualized model of the disorder and, where appropriate, of the dissexuality together with each patient at the beginning of the treatment in order to determine specific and approach-oriented goals. Furthermore, the interventions can be tailored not only to the needs of the patients but also with respect to the professional background of the therapists. The worksheets are to be understood as suggestions for interventions which can be adapted or extended according to the needs of the participants and the objectives of the therapists.

The changes to semi-open groups are mainly for practical reasons, because in this way individuals can be cared for more easily and the waiting time for admission to the groups can be shortened. An additional advantage to the semi-open group setting is that group members who have already been participating in the therapy for a longer period of time are confronted with the social challenge of opening up to the new group members and integrating them into their system (Sect. 2). They also have the opportunity to reflect on their own progress by comparing their situation at the beginning of the therapy with what they have achieved or changed since. New group members can get an impression of how they can benefit from the therapy by looking at the positive examples of those who have been

Working Group of the Prevention Project Dunkelfeld
Charité – Universitätsmedizin Berlin, Corporate Member of Freie Universität Berlin, Humboldt-Universität zu Berlin, and Berlin Institute of Health, Center for Human and Health Sciences, Institute of Sexology and Sexual Medicine, Berlin, Germany
e-mail: klaus.beier@charite.de

participating for a longer time. The concept of semi-open groups does not require the group to start anew with each new member. Rather, the current needs of the participants (e.g., regarding problematic behavior or risk factors) and their individual progress in treatment (e.g., which modules have been completed successfully and which risk factors have not yet been treated) determine the content of the sessions and the aims of the therapy modules. The essential content of the modules is also repeated during the course of the therapy sessions so that the patients can work on the same material at different stages of the therapeutic process, which serves to reinforce the learning process. The semi-open group setting requires a high degree of flexibility and discipline on the part of the therapists. The therapists have to consider the individual needs of the group members because not all interventions can meet everyone's needs at the same time. Regarding the therapeutic goals within each module, the therapists must also keep an overview of the therapeutic progress of the individual group members.

In semi-open group settings, the group is a functioning system, in which a person's progress is determined by the duration of their participation in therapy, and departing group members are replaced by the admission and integration of new group members. For example, some group members start the therapy with a high level of awareness and already have effective methods of sexual impulse control at their disposal. They can benefit from a reduced number of group sessions and end the therapy after eight or nine months. For other group members, however, it is advantageous to increase the recommended number of 45 group sessions in order to deal with certain topics more intensively and thus have the opportunity to repeat and reinforce. Consequently, semi-open groups provide better opportunities for addressing the individual needs of the group members.

With regard to the composition of parallel groups, the PPD, following the RNR principle, endeavors to compose the groups according to the risk status and needs of the participants. Thus, group composition can be based on past offenses,

for example, by establishing groups that focus on child sexual abuse, or non-offenders and others that focus on abuse images. This grouping is based on the assumption that men who have committed sexual abuse in the past have an increased life-long risk of engaging again in abusive behavior that involves physical contact. Some participants, for example, committed a single act of sexual assault many years ago and currently use abuse images for masturbation on a daily basis. In this case, the placement in a group that focuses on direct sexually abusive behavior would probably not correspond to the needs and risk situations of this participant. The above-mentioned algorithm used for group-assignment is based on past misconduct and therefore provides only one assignment option for each participant. It appears to be important to make the group-assignment process transparent for the respective participants involved by discussing their needs and goals. Furthermore, all therapists working with this manual are encouraged to develop their own modus operandi.

2   Structure and Interactivity of the Therapy Manual

The 13 modules of the BEDIT manual, together with the visual material and the worksheets, constitute a framework for the contents, processes, and goals of the therapy. The primary goal is to maintain or increase self-control over sexual behavior, especially in regard to direct and indirect abuse. The single modules in this manual complement and build upon each other because they address different risk dimensions which are then integrated into the final modules on future planning and protective measures. The different modules can be applied to specific therapy issues, i.e., they can be used sequentially or independently in the context of specific interventions and therapy priorities. As a result, the degree of structuring and sequencing can be adapted to the individual needs of each group (Allam et al. 1997).

It is recommended to start this manual with Module 1 "Psychoeducation" and then use it as a kind of toolbox, selecting treatment options and single modules or module sets according to the needs of the group members and the group as a whole. Most of the modules are linked to each other, which encourages an open and interactive approach to the relevant content and the practical implementation of the methods learned. Furthermore, the structure of the manual makes it possible to work on specific contents in one module and in so doing already prepare for another module. The structure of the manual facilitates a high degree of flexibility so that the focus can be placed explicitly on the participants and on the repetition and reinforcement of important treatment goals during the therapy process.

Within the PPD, Module 1 "Psychoeducation" is offered at regular intervals of two to four months and is intended for persons on the waiting list for group therapy. The module is conducted in separate psychoeducation groups. This allows a reduction of the waiting time for patients, as well as a flexible and low-threshold initiation of the intervention even before the patients are assigned to the running semi-open groups. In addition, therapists and new participants can get to know each other in this way even before the group therapy begins. Furthermore, it is expected that one of the group therapists and the new group member will meet for a one-on-one consultation after the psychoeducation session to discuss the patient's expectations of group therapy, his motivation, and personal therapy goals before entering the semi-open group.

3 Practical Implementation in the Sessions

Beginning and End of the Session

Each group session (with the exception of the first one) starts with a short session introduction ("Flash Feedback") and ends with a short closing round, for which about five to ten minutes should be scheduled. For the opening of the session, each participant is asked to give an outline in a few sentences of the issues with the highest priority for him at that moment (difficulties or successes, thoughts or moods, problematic sexual behavior with regard to children, or the use of abuse images). Let the group decide who should begin, and then continue with the others in a clockwise or counterclockwise fashion. Let the participants decide what they want to share with the group. Neither the therapists nor the other group members should interrupt the presentations. However, an agreement should be made within the group as to whether the participants are allowed to ask clarification questions or other kinds of questions. This way of opening the session should serve to focus everyone's attention so that they may begin the group session. It also gives each participant the opportunity to confide in the group and to be heard. Individual topics that are raised by the participants at the opening of the session can be taken up again in the subsequent group session.

The procedure for closing the session is similar to that of the introductory phase. Each participant should explain in a few sentences what he has experienced in the session, what messages he will take with him, and what new insights he has gained. Participants have the opportunity to make final comments on the preceding discussions, to give positive feedback to other group members, or to support them in other ways. Neither the other group members nor the therapists should interrupt the individual synopses. After all group members have expressed themselves, the therapists will briefly describe their impressions of the session, group-work, and group cohesion. The therapists can also encourage the participants to highlight particularly important aspects of the discussion or give the participants a final take-home message.

Therapy Goals

At the beginning of each module, the therapeutic goals are to be specified, as they will serve as reference points during the sessions. The structure of a session in a semi-open group setting is determined by both the personal concerns of the group members, as well as by the modules and the specific therapeutic goals. Therapists typically are aware of the progress of the individual group members before they start a session. Therefore, it can be helpful to prepare content and worksheets pertaining to the module. Ultimately, however, it

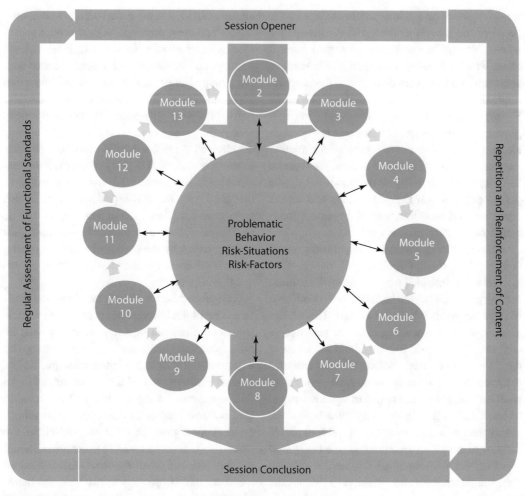

Fig. 1 Model of sequential and interactive embedding of modules within the BEDIT

is up to the group (under the guidance and support of the therapist) to decide what to focus on in a session. It requires flexibility on the part of the therapist to broaden or shift the focus regarding current issues and goals. The therapists are not necessarily obligated to follow all the objectives of the module description. A model for embedding modules in a sequential and interactive fashion within the BEDIT therapy is described in Fig. 1.

Material, Preparation, Homework

A flipchart and markers in different colors or an interactive whiteboard is necessary for the organization of a group session. When preparing specific topics for the session, there should always

be enough worksheets available. Regularly assigning homework between meetings is helpful so that the participants can continue to work on relevant topics between sessions. The worksheets can be found in the back of this manual and are labeled with the name of the corresponding module, as well as the name of the particular worksheet. They are in some cases adapted from other manuals or simply newly developed within the PPD process. They can of course be modified as needed.

Time Allocation for the Meetings

As an example of how to determine the duration of a group session, we suggest dividing it into two blocks of about 50 minutes, each with a break of about 10 minutes. This arrangement however is only intended as a suggestion and can be managed flexibly according to the needs of the group and the therapists. However, it is important to discuss and agree on the time frame and structure of the sessions in advance. The time limits for the sessions facilitate better planning for both therapists and patients and prevent unstructured situations.

Excursus – The Role of Transference

Although the BEDIT takes a cognitive behavioral approach, it has proven beneficial to reflect on the role of transference in the therapeutic process.

According to the orientation of this manual, an individual's sexual preference is a structural component of his or her personality. For this reason, individuals with pedophilic tendencies often exhibit low self-esteem, which leads to the devaluation of their own person and prevents the development of socially adequate coping strategies in dealing with their own sexual impulses. This has an impact on the role of transference, which according to Freud (1910) is always a hindrance. Freud postulates that transference is a spontaneously arising factor in every human relationship, as well as the true driving force of the patient. Its effect is all the more strong, the less aware he is of its existence. The patient's fantasy is most likely accompanied by the fear of encountering rejection (aversion and punishment) due to his sexual preference structure. Therefore, it is possible that he may project these feelings onto the therapist and expect rejection. The source of this fear may be his low self-esteem, which can be associated with pedophilic sexual preference, as well as its stigmatization (Faistbauer 2011). Therapists should respond to this by taking a clear position that accepts the person with his sexual preference as such but that clearly and unequivocally rejects sexual

abuse. This differentiation can support the patient and help him to integrate his own sexual preference structure into his personal self-perception.

4   Concepts of Cognitive Behavioral Therapy

In order to achieve the above-mentioned therapeutic goals, the following four basic methods are employed:

- Cognitive restructuring
- Model learning
- Positive reinforcement,
- Role-play

4.1   Cognitive Restructuring

One of the main methods of cognitive behavioral therapy is the restructuring of cognitive distortions or dysfunctional expectations. The following steps are recommended:

1. A fundamental clarification of the role of cognitive distortion in the emergence and persistence of maladaptive and deviant behavior
2. Providing corrective information (psychoeducation)
3. Recognizing one's own cognitive distortions
4. Engaging in an in-depth investigation of specific cognitive distortions and placing these under scrutiny

This approach can be used in both group and individual sessions. In the context of cognitive restructuring, the Socratic dialogue is particularly suitable for questioning existing attitudes among the participants that favor risk behavior. In the context of the Socratic dialogue, the therapist assumes a naive attitude and questions the participant's existing attitudes with the help of various disputation techniques. The therapist's attitude should not be hostile or critical but, rather, neutral and disinterested. This attitude helps the group members reflect upon themselves, which can help them facilitate changes in certain thoughts and assumptions. Questions that contain assumptions, that aim at confrontation, or that predetermine possible answers (closed questions) should be avoided.

The following are some examples of Socratic questions (for example, see Beck 1995):

- Which facts support your thoughts and assumptions? What connection can you see between your (specific) behavior and the thoughts which preceded it? (Revealing the problem)
- What could be a different way of viewing the situation? (Development of alternative perspectives)
- What are realistic consequences? (Review of the different possible consequences)
- What effects might occur from abandoning this viewpoint and thinking differently? (Evaluation of the consequences)

4.2   Model Learning

The therapist can serve as a role model by taking responsibility for his own behavior, respecting the rights and integrity of others, and acting honestly and sincerely within interpersonal relationships. For this kind of model-learning to take place, the therapist's demeanor and behavior must be clear and unambiguous.

Conditions for a model's effectiveness:

- Respect for others in communication and behavior
- Respect for the rights and feelings of other group members
- No placing of blame onto others for one's own problems and difficulties
- Admission of mistakes and acceptance of criticism
- Acceptance of praise
- Adherence to agreements
- No expression of unsolicited advice
- No denigration of oneself or others
- Forgiveness of the mistakes of others

4.3   Positive Reinforcement

In the given context, the concept of reinforcement includes any form of verbal and nonverbal recognition or reward. For effective reinforcement, three conditions must be met:

- Direct (verbal or nonverbal) reaction to or immediate comment on the statements of a group member; nonverbal reinforcement through eye contact, nodding, or smiling.
- Explanation and justification of the reaction.
- The expression of reinforcement must be distinguishable from the generally open and interested demeanor of the therapist; otherwise, it won't be recognized as such.

4.4   Role-Play

The technique of role-play developed out of the approach of psychodrama (Moreno 1943). As a primarily experience-based and problem-detecting method, it was further developed by Kelly (1955) into fixed type of role-play therapy. In contemporary cognitive behavioral therapy, role-play is mainly used in training certain behavioral patterns (Wolpe 1958; Lazarus 1966; Kanfer and Phillips 1975). Role-playing techniques are of particular importance in group therapy where they may promote social learning in a protected therapeutic setting (Grawe 1980).

In this manual, these different role-playing techniques can be distinguished:

- Diagnostic role-play as an effective method for making problematic behavior more approachable. This facilitates a deeper understanding than what is achievable through the
- purely subjective descriptions of the patient. The therapist encourages the participant to re-enact the interpersonal encounter or conflict situation that was previously recounted by him with the participation of the other group members. In this way, the original situation can be repeated and the other group members can directly respond to the thoughts, emotions, and behavioral patterns associated with it.

- With role-play as a behavioral experiment, the patient adopts different positions in order to try out different behavioral patterns. The therapist encourages the patient to try out new ways of behaving beyond their typical habits, thus encouraging behavioral changes. This change in perspective paves the way for changes in attitude and increases flexibility in thinking and acting.
- The technique of role-reversal enables the patient to experience the effects of his own behavior on others. By assuming the role or position of others, the patient learns about different attitudes, opinions, and emotions. At the same time, he develops flexibility and empathy. Research results indicate the effectiveness of this technique in changing attitudes (Kanfer et al. 2000).
- Role-play for the development of coping strategies is a method of hypothetical problem-solving in which critical situations of the past, present, and future are simulated and coping skills are adopted. This takes place in a framework in which the person is less invested than in the original situation. The rehearsal of new behavioral patterns systematically reinforces what has been previously learned and simplifies its transfer into everyday behavior. In this manner, many small role-playing sequences with increasing difficulty may be performed and critical situations can be anticipated and simulated. The aim is to establish clear principles for future situations in order to increase the patient's sense of self-control.

Participating in role-play for the first time is a demanding task for most patients. The transition from a conversation to an active game therefore requires an appropriate introduction and a clear description of the goals and the process. The preparatory time should be between 10 and 15 minutes. Good preparation ensures adequate execution, reduces the probability of failure, and increases the patients' self-efficacy. For a detailed description of the preparation and procedure for role-play, see Fliegel 1996.

5 Advices for the Method of Application of the Therapeutic Approach

5.1 General Advices for the Method of Application

The preferred form for implementing the therapeutic approach, as it is practiced within the framework of the PPD (*Präventionsprojekt Dunkelfeld*), is the treatment of adults in groups (group therapy). This has pragmatic reasons, on the one hand, such as a significantly better cost-benefit ratio with group therapy as compared to multiple individual therapies, not to mention a reduced time commitment for therapists. On the other hand, professional considerations, especially in regard to the patient population targeted by the therapeutic approach, speak for the application of group therapy. Even for the experienced therapist, it can be helpful to continually recall the specific operating factors and mechanisms of group therapy, which is why they are again briefly summarized in Table 1.

Of course, the therapeutic approach can also be used for individual therapy, e.g., if there are any contraindications for the application of group therapy. The relevant reports on therapy experiences are also available (Faistbauer 2011; Konrad et al. 2018). In these cases, however, certain adaptations and deviations from the procedure of the manual have proven to be helpful. It is advantageous, for example, to replace the role-play in the first sessions with imaginative exercises. If in a later phase of therapy a favorable therapeutic partnership has been established, role-play may also take place in the individual therapy sessions. Exercises for the adoption of new perspectives should be given special priority. Homework can be used to a much greater extent.

For both methods of application (group and individual therapies), the theme of transparent and continuous clarification of goals and values has proven to be central. According to the concept worked out by Bordin (1979), a relationship between therapist and client can be regarded as especially favorable if there is a consensus

Table 1 Specific impact and mechanisms of group therapy

Universality of suffering	Participants realize that other people have similar feelings, thoughts, and problems
Altruism	Participants strengthen their self-concept by offering help to other group members
Hope for cure	Through the success of other participants, an optimistic attitude toward one's own possibilities for change can develop
Providing information	Participants receive information and advice from therapists or other group members
Corrective recapitulation of primary family relations	Participants can re-enact critical family dynamics with others in a corrective fashion
Development of techniques for interpersonal interactions	The group offers its members a framework in which adaptive and effective communication can be experienced and learned
Imitative behavior	Participants expand their personal skills and abilities by observing other group members and exploring new behaviors
Group cohesion	Group members experience feelings of trust, belonging and togetherness
Existential experiences	Participants take responsibility for their life decisions
Catharsis	Participants are given free rein to express intense feelings about past or present experiences
Interpersonal learning – input	Participants gain an impression of their interpersonal impact through group feedback
Interpersonal learning – output	Participants create an environment that allows other members to interact in a more adaptive way
Self-understanding	Participants gain insight into the psychological motivations underlying their behavior and emotional reactions
Openness	Openness means that the participants can discuss intimate, private, or personal matters in the group
Trust	Trust in the group develops when the members feel they have achieved something in the group and can count on the support of the others. Only participants who have trust in the group will speak openly about themselves
Working behavior	Willingness of the participants to engage in something new and to cooperate, even if they themselves are not always the focus of the therapeutic group work
Receive and accept feedback	Participants can learn how they affect others
Feedback	Feedback in a group means crossing the private boundaries of others. Therefore, criticism as well as praise should be constructive and helpful for the person being criticized, as well as expressed in a way that would be acceptable to the person who is criticizing
Support	A person can be supported by the group in dealing with problematic issues. For example, it may be helpful if other group members describe their experiences in comparable situations

(Adapted from Fiedler 1996; Yalom and Leszcz 2005)

between the two concerning the therapeutic aims and the approach used to achieve them.

- To help participants understand why a change is worthwhile for them, it is important to keep a constant focus on their motivations for participating in therapy.
- The participant should be informed about what the therapy entails, what possibilities and changes it could bring with it, and what formal process the therapy adheres to. A high degree of transparency and information-sharing facilitates the involvement of the participants in the therapeutic process and increases their independence and active participation.
- Furthermore, the underlying problem should be worked out cooperatively, and its origins, resulting behavior, the conditions that sustain it, and possible solutions should also be reflected upon (Hautzinger 2000). A transparent clarification process, especially in the group context, ensures

that the therapists and participants will identify the same problems and develop common goals in response to them. Each participant will have his own conception of his problems, where they come from, and what success from therapy might look like. The therapists also have their own agenda, an overriding therapeutic goal ("not to become a perpetrator"), which cannot and should not be deviated from. A critical and informative clarification at the beginning of treatment diminishes faulty or obstructive perceptions of patients and thus strengthens the coordination of (realistic) therapy goals (Ellis and Hoellen 1997).

5.2 Special Advice for Group Therapy

Avoidance of Overly Conflictual Group Dynamics

In psychoanalytically based therapy procedures (e.g., depth psychology-based and psychoanalytic psychotherapies), conflictual developments in group dynamics can play an important role and are often intentional. In problem-, method-, and goal-oriented behavioral therapies (as well as in the therapeutic approach described here), however, developments that are too conflictual often prove to be counterproductive. Clinical experience has shown that group cohesion suffers from overly dynamic conflicts between the participants and that they are then less willing to open up and openly address taboo subjects, such as their own sexual fantasies, their own sexual behavior, as well as their everyday interpersonal interactions in the group.

The focus of the therapy program lies specifically in the analysis and management of problems in everyday life outside the therapy group and not (at least not primarily) in the analysis of ongoing problematic interactions within the group. The following procedures can reduce the development of conflictual group dynamics (see also Fiedler 1996):

- The therapists promote disorder-related and goal-oriented approaches.
- The therapists provide concrete help and feasible instructions for making changes in everyday life, which enable the participants to make immediate changes regarding their problems.
- If possible, the feedback in the group should refer to problems outside the group and to a specific situation in everyday life (constructive suggestions for implementation).
- Therapeutic goals and procedures should always be made transparent, and the group work should be precisely structured.
- Conflicts between the participants in a group are to be immediately clarified and made transparent.

Use of the Group Constellation for Therapeutic Purposes

The procedure described above can also lead to the situation that therapists (and other members of the group) refer only to the descriptions and problems of one person. In our therapeutic approach, the mere accumulation of therapist-participant dyads or, exaggeratedly stated, multiple parallel individual therapies in a single group enable essential and decidedly desirable success factors of group therapy to be overlooked. The use of these success factors (Table 1) does not contradict the concepts of behavioral therapy. If a participant describes a problem that seems only to affect himself, the other group members and the therapists will always experience it as well. Such a situation always offers a multitude of possibilities to use the social energy for the benefit of all members:

- Highlighting shared experiences of group members
- Drawing attention to the relationships between the group members
- Using a group mode of speech ("the group" instead of "me" or "you")

- Transferring direct questions addressed to the therapist to the group
- The therapist makes nonverbal active participation clear (through eye contact, nodding, etc.)

5.3   Role of the Therapist

Another advantage of the group setting is that the therapists have the other participants as assistants. The therapist has the obligation to take care of the formal and content-related structure, as well as to immediately resolve potential disturbances. Beyond the creation of this clearly structured framework and the offering of a content-related concept, the therapists should not work alone but, instead, enable the members of the group to engage themselves. They should take advantage of the given structure and fill it with content. The primary function of the therapist is to help the participants to help themselves. If therapists feel exhausted after a group session, they might have worked too actively during the session.

Modules for Adults

Working Group of the Prevention Project
Dunkelfeld

1 Module 1: Psychoeducation

1.1 Goals

- Communicating the process and structure of BEDIT
- Communicating knowledge about sexuality, sexual preference, and dissexual behavior
- Communicating defined psychological risk factors for sexually abusive behavior
- Making emotional relief and anxiety-reduction possible (understanding, exchanging experiences, contact with other affected persons)
- Supporting therapeutic interventions by facilitating a positive therapist-patient relationship and a corresponding higher therapeutic compliance
- Communicating information on supplementary pharmacological treatment options
- Supporting intraindividual processes of defining realistic therapy goals and expectations regarding the treatment

Working Group of the Prevention Project Dunkelfeld
Charité – Universitätsmedizin Berlin, Corporate
Member of Freie Universität Berlin, Humboldt-
Universität zu Berlin, and Berlin Institute of Health,
Center for Human and Health Sciences, Institute of
Sexology and Sexual Medicine, Berlin, Germany
e-mail: klaus.beier@charite.de

1.2 Rationale

Talking about sexuality, especially one's own sexuality—not to mention one's own problematic sexuality—is difficult for most people and can trigger feelings of anxiety, shame, or guilt. Many don't have the words and concepts. The first module accordingly serves to communicate fundamental information on concepts relevant to treatment and to develop through this a common language and shared basic knowledge. This is of particular importance, as participants may display widely differing degrees of familiarity with the topics of sexuality, sexual preference, potential risk factors for sexually abusive behavior (e.g., child sexual abuse or the use of CSAI), and treatment options. The module should thus precede and prepare the content of the actual therapy.

1.3 Content

The module is broken up into five thematic blocks. A structured procedure is advisable for the first module, as all five topics should be discussed in the group. The individual themes are only introduced here and will be explored more deeply in the course of the therapy. To promote a more group-centered and less therapist-centered process of psychoeducation, the recommended interventions aim to strengthen group dynamics.

Group members should have the opportunity to meet one another, break down inhibitions and prejudices, and build up relationships of trust.

1. Organizational aspects and BEDIT's general conditions for therapy: In the first session the therapists and the participants introduce themselves and organizational aspects are clarified.
2. Sexuality: In this session, general information about one's sexual preference structure is communicated.
3. Dissexuality and problematic sexual behavior: This session serves as an introduction to the concept of dissexuality.
4. Risk factors for sexually abusive behavior: This session elucidates concepts of empirically proven factors that can increase the risk of problematic sexual behavior toward children.
5. Pharmacological treatment options: In this session, medicinal treatment options for the reduction of an elevated sex drive or a strong sexual preoccupation are introduced.

1.4   Interventions

1. *Organizational aspects and BEDIT's general conditions for therapy*
   > Therapists can serve as models at this point by laying out a wide range of possible sexual preference and modes of behavior. Through this they can create a safe and nonjudgmental framework that allows participants to share and discuss topics that might elicit feelings of shame or guilt.
   - Introduction of participants and therapists
     - The therapists introduce themselves and encourage the participants to give a short personal introduction consisting, for instance, of the following information: age, vocation or current occupation, social background, relationship status, children of their own, motivations and goals for participation.
   - Overview of the topics to be covered in this session

- Explain the fundamental requirement of confidentiality and its conditions to the patients.
- Clarify the legal framework (§ 203 German criminal code) and the meaning of confidentiality for the therapeutic relationship.
- Clarify the therapeutic options in the event of self-endangerment or endangerment of others (in particular the endangerment of children).
- Introduce different treatment settings (e.g., group therapy vs. individual therapy, open/running groups vs. closed groups, offense-specific vs. nonspecific groups, etc.) and lay out their respective advantages and disadvantages.
- With the participants, develop possible strategies for dealing with concerns, e.g., rules within the group and treatment contracts (Worksheet Agreement for Group Work [Participants], WS Agreement for Group Work [Therapist]).

2. Sexuality
   - *Expression of Sexuality:* sexual activities/ sexual behavior: have the participants consider different kinds of sexual activities and types of sexual behavior, and write them out on a flip chart. Talk about different autoerotic and partner-oriented sexual interactions and discuss different standards of evaluation (interindividual differences, morals, relevance to criminal codes, social conventions).
     - Refer to the *Three Forms of Sexual Activities:* genital sexual interaction with a partner (e.g., vaginal, oral, or anal intercourse and digital penetration), extra-genital sexual activities with a partner (e.g., kissing, petting, cuddling, fondling), and masturbation (stimulation of one's own genitals for sexual arousal).
     - Focus on the different expressions of intimacy (e.g., kissing, petting, cuddling, stroking, intimate talk) and introduce paraphilic interests (fetishism,

voyeurism, sadism, coprophilia, necrophilia, etc.).

- *Dimensions of Sexuality:* collect different motivations for sexual interactions on a flip chart and organize these into the three (functional) dimensions of sexuality:
  - The *Dimension of Desire* includes all possible ways of experiencing and intensifying pleasure and sexual arousal through sexual stimulation. The importance of this dimension begins with the ability to experience physical pleasure and arousal, which is most likely already possible in the intrauterine phase and early childhood (the so-called infantile masturbation), and generally remains significant throughout one's entire lifespan.
  - The *Dimension of Reproduction* emphasizes the role of sexuality in reproduction. With the onset of puberty, this dimension fluctuates between overemphasis, on the one hand, and complete meaninglessness, on the other. Gender differences must be kept in mind, as even men of an advanced age are generally able to father children, while the reproductive capabilities of women cease with menopause.
  - The *Dimension of Attachment* emphasizes the importance of sexuality in fulfilling the fundamental biopsychosocial needs for acceptance, intimacy, warmth, and security through sexual communication in a partnership (Beier and Loewit 2011). This social-communicative dimension manifests itself even in the earliest phases of life (infancy) in the sense of non-genital-centric preforms of infantile sexuality. It reaches a strong form early in life and bears further influence on an individual's life, but generally remains unreflected upon.
- *Sexual Preference*: explain the assumption that sexual preference is mostly expressed on the level of sexual fantasies and can be represented along three axes (chapter "Pedophilia and Hebephilia"):
  - *Three Axes of Sexual Preference*: sexual attraction to a gender (male, female, or both), responsiveness to a certain body age (prepubescent, early pubescent, or post-pubescent), and responsiveness to desired practices with a preferred partner (sexually preferred interactions/modes of interaction).
- *Three Levels of Sexuality:* sexual behavior, sexual fantasies (particularly those experienced during autoerotic activity), and individual sexual self-concept
  > *The focus on sexual fantasies instead of sexual behavior is based on the understanding that individual sexual preference is reflected in fantasies (more so than in sexual behavior).*

3. *Dissexuality and Problematic Sexual Behavior*
   - Definition of sexual acts: all acts that are sexually motivated, that is, acts that serve toward sexual arousal or sexual pastimes and/or that precede or prepare for sexual activity.
   - Definition of dissexuality: socially dysfunctional sexual behavior that injures the integrity and individuality of another person, regardless of whether or not this behavior is being investigated.
   - Discuss and question the participants' individual concepts of dissexual behavior. Try to go beyond the legal criteria for CSA (child sexual abuse and the use of abuse images). For this, the following worksheets can be used: WS *Dissexuality and Child Sexual Abuse* and WS *Categories for Describing CSAI.*
   - Discuss the question of who commits child sexual abuse (men, women, teenagers, persons of all ages and social backgrounds) and differentiate between various motivations or reasons for sexual abuse of children (e.g., as a replacement for sexual contact with adults that is actually desired, against the backdrop of psychological disorders or sexual developmental disorders, or because of a pedophilic/hebephilic preference).

> *Because of a series of myths about consent, it is an important topic in therapy. Be aware that the discussion can become very difficult when participants reflect on situations which they considered to be consensual (e.g., in perceived equitable relationships to adolescents).*

Excursus

Sexual Behavior

Every sexual act that emerges from individual sexual interest in a person is sexual behavior. Sexual behavior can consist of the following:

* Watching the child for whom they have an inclination when it is aware or not aware of it ("peeping")
* Making sexual remarks or comments
* Exposing oneself (to demonstratively expose the partially- or fully-unclothed body), with or without masturbation
* The production of pornographic materials (photos, videos, or audio recordings) of a child, or showing pornographic materials in the presence of a child
* Encouraging a child to perform sexual acts with their own body (e.g., masturbation)
* Initiating bodily contact, such as grabbing, rubbing, or kissing
* Penetration of the vagina, anus, or mouth with the penis, tongue, finger, or any object

Consensual Sexual Behavior

* The other person is fully informed about the content, execution, and possible consequences, and understands these.
* The other person is able to consent, i.e., physically and mentally capable of making their own decision (possible examples for discussion: A child wants to drive a car. A ten-year old child who has had sex education in school exposes themselves and wants to be touched in their genital area. What do you do?).
* The other person agrees freely and without pressure.

Sexual Abuse

Discussion in the group:

* How do participants define sexual abuse? Where does sexual abuse begin?
* Do the participants consider the use of CSAI to be sexual abuse?

Discussion of the following questions:

* What does it mean when a child neither verbally nor physically says no?
* What does it mean when a minor consents to certain behavior? Who is responsible for the sexual act?
* Are children responsible for sexual abuse (e.g., through the way they dress, their behavior, or their lifestyle)?

4. *Risk Factors for Committing Child Sexual Abuse*

> *Therapists should consider empirically proven risk factors, such as strong sexual preoccupation, abuse-supportive attitudes, conflicts in intimate relationships, and weak problem-solving skills* (Sect. 4 in chapter "Child Sexual Abuse and the Use of Abuse Images").

* Have the group members divide themselves into two groups based on the focus of their problematic sexual behavior. Each group is then asked to determine, discuss, and write down factors associated with their problematic sexual behavior. Each group then presents their ideas on a flip chart to the whole group.
* Discuss the results and organize the risk factors into respective risk dimensions (e.g., sexual and general self-control, socio-affective deficits, offense-supportive attitudes, sexual tendencies, and situational factors).
* Explain the central strategy of the therapeutic approach in first identifying the (empirically supported and individually relevant) risk factors in order to change these in the next step, thereby reducing the risk of sexual abuse.
* Protective factors should also be identified and strengthened during the course of ther-

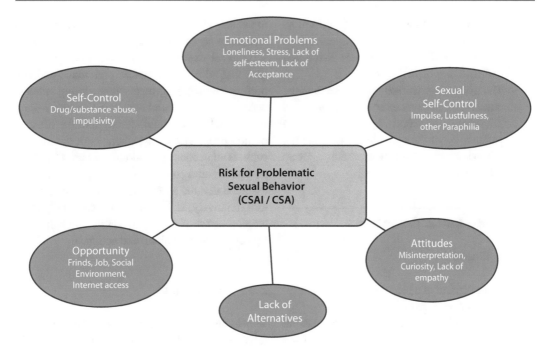

Fig. 1 Risk for problematic sexual behavior

apy. Be sure to point out that the individual models of risk and protective factors will be continually reviewed and modified throughout therapy.

Example: Result of group work by participants (Fig. 1)

5. *Medicinal Treatment Options*
   > *Medications can affect individuals in different ways or lead to different side effects. Physical activity, such as endurance sports and outdoor sports, can influence the effects/side effects of a medication on a person.*

In this session, different medications are discussed as treatment options for improving sexual behavior control and influencing sexual experiencing.

• With the participants, collect and discuss the advantages and disadvantages of the use of medications with the aim of reducing sexual desire and sexual impulses. Keep in mind that the same aspect may be seen as an advantage by one participant and a disadvantage by another.

– Possible advantages: reduction of stress, reduction of the use of abuse images and masturbation, more calmness in contact situations with children, feelings of relief and freedom, sexuality is felt to be less of a compulsion, more trust in oneself and security not to commit CSA, fewer sexual fantasies.
– Possible disadvantages: reduced masturbation, reduced erectile function, fewer orgasms, reduced interest in sexuality (e.g., with a partner), reduced sexual interest in children, life is less exciting without sexuality, uncomfortable side effects of the medication, such as enlargement of the breast (gynecomastia), fatigue, weight gain, etc.
– Discuss the role of testosterone and chemical processes in the male body (Worksheet *Regulation of Testosterone Balance in Men*).
– Inform participants about areas of indication and effects/side effects of relevant pharmacological options, beginning with the antiandrogens (gonadotropin-releasing hormone [GnRH]-analogues and cyproterone acetate) as specific medication for the reduction of sexual impulses and then onto

selective serotonin reuptake inhibitors (SSRIs) as less-specific medications (Worksheet *Medications for the Reduction of Sexual Impulses*).

– The following worksheet can be handed out: *Patient Reports after Pharmacological Treatment* (a report by previous PPD patients about their medicinal treatments). Discuss the worksheet with group members.

2   Module 2: Acceptance

2.1   Goals

• Communication of a biopsychosocial etiological conception of sexual preference.
• Communication of knowledge about sexual preference as a stable constituent part of the personality.
• Communication of the therapeutic concept of acceptance and providing support for its implementation.
• Communication of the notion that, in this therapy, change means the building up of behavior control in order to directly and indirectly prevent child sexual abuse. In this context, change does not mean changing one's sexual preference.

2.2   Rationale

The current state of empirical and clinical knowledge does not offer a definitive etiological theory of the development of pedophilic/hebephilic sexual preference. An integrative model that looks to biological (e.g., genetic factors, premature birth, handedness, neurological structures), psychological (e.g., shyness, anxiety, self-consciousness, "immaturity"), and social factors (e.g., aversive childhood experiences or abandonment, mistreatment or [sexual] abuse, lack of contact to people of the same age) and their interactions can be regarded as currently favored among available explanatory models. The hypothesis of an integrated model of this sort can be seen as a first step

in dealing with one's own sexual preference from a place of acceptance.

Clinical experiences and empirical data suggest that both sexual gender preference and age preference manifest themselves during adolescence—or young adulthood, at the latest—and remain (relatively) stable throughout the lifespan of most people. Looking to therapeutic approaches such as dialectical behavioral therapy (DBT) or acceptance and commitment therapy (ACT), it is assumed that the acceptance of sexual preference as a (relatively) stable—and thus constantly challenging—part of one's personality can help open up new ways of thinking and acting.

2.3   Contents

The hypothesis that sexual preference remains relatively stable throughout one's life implies that the therapeutic process should concentrate more on acceptance than changeability. Participants should be supported in accepting their sexual preference as a constant part of their personality so that a constructive examination of their sexuality, and in particular their sexual behavior, can be made possible. Rather than attempting to change the sexual preference per se, group members should be encouraged to accept their sexual preference, take responsibility for it, and change/control their problematic behavior.

As people cannot choose their sexual preference, it should be regarded as fate rather than a choice. This therapy aims to support group members in accepting this fate. "Acceptance" is not meant in this context as a passive putting-up with, but rather the acceptance of, oneself and one's own emotions. For many participants, this is a long and difficult process. At the same time, however, this often means the beginning of a change toward preventing abuse and to a greater satisfaction with life.

2.4   Interventions

• Gather etiological concepts from group members about their sexual responsiveness toward prepubescent or early pubescent children. Clarify the biopsychosocial approach as a possible explanation for pedophilia/hebephilia through graphic representations of each of the factors and their associations on a flip chart.

- Let the participants reflect on the history of their sexual preference within the group and collect their ideas:
  - Since when have you been aware of your sexual interest in minors?
  - Do you hope that your sexual preference will change?
  - Have you ever actively tried to change your sexual preference?
- Differentiate between management strategies for dealing with urgent sexual impulses and attempts to alter sexual preference structure.
- Summarize: Sexual preference is a (relatively) stable part of the personality.
- Compile together aspects that participants associate with their pedophilic/hebephilic sexual preference and record the positive (e.g., happiness, lust/desire, enjoyment, and sexual fantasies) and negative (e.g., shame, self-doubt, fear of committing abuse, and media representations of the topic of child abuse) associations on a flip chart.
- Elaborate on the danger of internalizing the hostile perceptions of people who condemn person with pedophilic and/or hebephilic preference as violent criminals. This kind of internalization can lead participants to self-denigration.
- Work out the way that pedophilic and/or hebephilic preference is a part of the participants' personalities, but that the personality structure also consists of other components, such as the actual behavior that determines the way a person is perceived in a social context. In deciding to work on themselves, thus questioning their previous strategies and ways of behaving, the participants have made a responsible decision on the way toward changing.
- Give an introduction to the concept of acceptance. Acceptance of one's own sexual responsiveness serves as the basis for change. Only a

sufficiently stable foundation can lead to meaningful change in a person.

- Discuss the concept of acceptance with group members. You can use the following guidelines to explain the approach:
  - Acceptance does not mean finding something good.
  - Acceptance is the acknowledgment of reality.
  - Acceptance means not fighting something any longer.
  - Acceptance is the decision to face the present moment.
  - Acceptance is the only way to reduce pain when one realizes that things cannot be changed.
  - The acceptance of an existing reality requires a conscious decision.
  - The steps toward more responsibility must be continually renewed. Sometimes it is necessary to repeat them within the space of a few minutes.
  - Acceptance means giving up the wish to change a given reality.
- To foster an active engagement with the theme of acceptance, have the group members answer the following questions:
  - What might be stopping you from accepting your sexual preference?
  - What could help you accept your sexual preference?
  - Should you accept your sexual preference, what could the possible consequences for your experience and behavior be?

Explain the following therapeutic principles:

- Attempts to change one's sexual preference are going to fail. Therapy should support the acceptance of one's sexual preference.
- The acceptance of one's sexual preference makes dealing with it easier and thus helps to change and better control one's behavior.
- Better behavior control and acceptance of that which is contributed both directly and indirectly to stopping sexual abuse of children and gaining better self-esteem and more satisfaction.

Excursus

Example to Introduce the Concept of Acceptance

To introduce the concept of acceptance, you can tell the following story of a broken down car in the desert (perhaps as an imagination exercise): You are totally alone on a trip in the desert, and your car breaks down. Sand in front of you, sand behind you; sand to your left, sand to your right. Nothing but sand. You are desperate. You are afraid. All you have is two bottles of water. No one knows of your trip. You become enraged, pound on the steering wheel. You scream, get out of the car, kick it, and run about looking for an explanation. But you don't know enough about cars to understand the problem.

At the end of it, you're worn out and tired, and your car is still just sitting there broken down in the middle of the desert.

The conclusion might be that one must first accept a situation (that you can't change anything about the broken down car) before one can deal consciously with the problem and start searching for solutions.

(Example taken from Hayes et al. 1999)

Excursus

Further Example to Introduce the Concept of Acceptance

Imagine you are a bus driver on your way to a specific place. The road you are driving down is windy and full of potholes, and sometimes you cannot really even see where it is taking you. On the way, unfriendly passengers get in—some from the first stop, while some get on later. One passenger is perhaps named Loneliness, another Pedophilia or Self-Denigration. The passengers are loud and demanding. They interrupt your concentration on the road, give you advice, and try to convince

you to turn right or left. Others doubt you and say that you will fail at whatever you do. After a while you realize that you've been so occupied with calming and looking after your passengers that you haven't even been looking at the street. Maybe you've turned the wrong way or missed an important road sign. Maybe you stop the bus, turn around, and reprimand your passengers instead of concentrating on the street in front of you. You don't advance and instead just busy yourself with things that have nothing to do with your goal. You have the choice: you can either keep fighting with the passengers and flounder, or you let them go on, put your hands on the wheel, and concentrate on the street so you can get to where you want to go. You may have to take them all with you and might not be able to get rid of them, but it is your choice as to whether you concentrate on the road in front of you or the noise of your passengers.

3 Module 3: Motivation

3.1 Goals

- Praising of patients' efforts to work on their behavior and recognition of their ambivalent motives and doubts
- Working out the patients' status quo regarding their strengths and resources, current behavior, self-perception and perception by others, benefits and interests, and aspects of sexuality
- Communication of the concept of motivation as a dynamic construct with different steps
- Supporting the patients in identifying their expectations and working out concrete, individual goals for therapy
- As a whole, encouraging the patients to continually analyze the state of their own motivation and supporting the development of this motivation toward change and behavior control

3.2 Rationale

To minimize the risk of sexual abuse and strengthen protective factors and resources, participants have to change familiar patterns and modes of behavior. Changes often bring with them uncomfortable consequences that can activate avoidance schemes. In the worst case, this could lead to the discontinuation of therapy. For this reason, therapists must support the participants in reducing avoidance behaviors. As lack of motivation and insufficient therapeutic progress feed one another, the motivation for change must be continually assessed and fostered. In particular, the patient-centered approach of Motivational Interviewing (Miller and Rollnick 2013), upon which our therapeutic approach to this topic is oriented, follows the hypothesis that a therapist who leads or claims too strongly may damage a patient's autonomy, which can lead to resistance to change. People are more likely to motivate themselves to change than to be motivated by others. It is furthermore presumed that patients who enter therapy are ambivalent regarding their own motivations for change, and not resistant to change. It is thus important to identify already-present motivations for change and to strengthen these aspects. At the same time, reasons that run contra to change should be understood and acknowledged. This means however that at no point should the therapist deviate from their fundamental position and directive: The prime goal of therapy remains the prevention of immediate and indirect child sexual abuse.

3.3 Contents

One cannot assume that motivation for change is a given. They should rather be regarded as a dynamic construct defined by short-term, medium-term, and long-term influences. It is likely that slumps in motivation will occur throughout the therapeutic process. Prochaska and DiClimente's (1984) transtheoretical model of behavior change offers a helpful orientation to deal with these situations by dividing the process of change into five stages:

- Stage 1—Precontemplation: Persons at this stage have no intention to cease their problem behavior in the near future or are not (yet) conscious of the necessity of change. In this phase, the communication of information should come to the foreground. These persons should be encouraged to learn more about the advantages of behavioral change. They should be made aware of their behavior's (negative) consequences for themselves and others.
- Stage 2—Contemplation: Participants at this stage have the intention to cease their problem behavior (e.g., dissexual modes of behavior) and recognize the advantages that a change would bring. At the same time they also see many disadvantages. These persons should concentrate on what it could mean to change their problematic behavior and should learn from others who have changed their behavior (e.g., stopping the use of CSAI).
- Stage 3—Preparation: Persons at this stage are ready to act and take small steps that promise to end their problematic behavior. These persons should be encouraged to seek support within the group and to think about how they might feel once they have actually ceased their problematic behavior.
- Stage 4—Action: Persons at this stage have changed their behavior and must work hard to maintain this change. These participants must learn to strengthen their self-obligation toward change and stave off the impulse to fall back into old behavior patterns. It is advantageous for them to develop techniques to stay focused on their intention, e.g., through replacing problematic behavioral modes with positive activities, through rewarding steps toward change, or through the avoidance of situations that could tempt them to fall back into old behavior patterns.
- Stage 5—Maintenance: Persons at this stage have successfully changed their behavior for months. It is now important to recognize situations that could lead them to fall back into old behavior patterns. During this stage, it is recommended that they seek support from people close to them and dedicate themselves to healthy activities that reduce stress, instead

of reaching back to old management strategies.

- A relapse into problematic behavior is often accompanied by insufficient expectations of self-efficacy (e.g., "I won't manage it anyway; why should I even try?"). People who describe a relapse should look to the conditions of the relapse situation as a source of information. The experience of self-efficacy should be reinforced, partial successes emphasized, and the plan of how to get back to positive management abilities taken up anew.

3.4   Interventions

- Hand out WS *My Current Self* as homework, with the aim of ascertaining the status quo that can act as the basis for a change in problematic behavior.
- Give an introduction to the aspects of motivation in other areas of life. Ask the participants if they have ever tried to get on a diet or give up smoking or alcohol.
- Collect participants' experiences of successes or failures and segue into the existence of ambivalent motives and feelings that can influence one's willingness to change.
- With reference to participants' current statuses, work out the different stages of motivation as suggested by Prochaska and DiClimente in the five-stage model.
- Compile the advantages and disadvantages of changing the problematic sexual behavior on a flip chart. Keep in mind that therapists should acknowledge reasons both for and against change. Confirm the existence of both sides and acknowledge that decisions in either direction (maintaining the familiar behavior or changing the behavior) have their price.
- Hand out the WS *My Therapy Goals and Expectations* and let the participants answer the questions.
- Support the participants in their efforts to find realistic goals and expectations. Segue into the aspects of acceptance and changeability.

4   Module 4: Perception

4.1   Goals

- Introduction to the basic principles of perception and information processing
- Communication of the differences between perception, interpretation, emotion, and experience
- Communication of the differences between external perception and self-perception
- Development of an awareness of problematic perceptions, attitudes, and cognitive distortions regarding interactions and sexual behavior with children
- Strengthening participants' capacity for self-control through reflection on perception and interpretations and their interrelationship with emotions and behavior
- Supporting participants in their immersion into introspective and reflective processes

4.2   Rationale

Perception is never neutral. It is always influenced by our experiences, memories, schemata, and personality. Situations are not merely perceived but, rather, also interpreted, which leads to specific thoughts (cognitions), emotions, physical reactions, and behavioral impulses. As a part of our personality, sexual preference also determines our perception: We desire what we see when we see what we desire. The mechanisms of our perception of interactions with persons who correspond to our sexual preference are fundamentally identical in all humans. For pedophilic/hebephilic men, this means that (analogous to teleiophilic men) they long for emotional and sexual contact with children who are sexually attractive to them. They may have the tendency, however, to interpret interactional behavior from children as an expression of sexual interest. This is principally the case when children display natural sexual curiosity and a propensity for experimentation. Perception is thus distorted in this context by sexual preference. This tendency is particularly pronounced in cases of infatuation. It is important to address these distortions ("seeing things through rose-colored glasses") in therapy and to discuss different, alternative points of view in the perception of situations ("seeing things clearly"). In so doing, participants' individual problematic perceptions should be identified, reflected upon, and modified.

4.3   Contents

The examination of the discrete components of perception should enable the patients to differentiate between different perspectives and understand the influence of sexual preference on information processing. During therapy, the risk of distorted perception and judgment of situations involving interaction between adults and children should be explained, for example, through neutral situations that could be interpreted as sexual. It can happen that sexual wishes and the sexual desire of the patient may be perceived as being actively initiated or encouraged by the child, thereby delegating responsibility away from the adult. The patient must understand that perceptions and interpretations of sexual aspects of interactions between adults and children are solely his and that children do not seek sexual stimulation, arousal, or pleasure in interactions with adults. Participants should acquire an awareness that they are the ones who sexualize situations and that the responsibility lies with them to understand, reflect upon, and reassess their own individual mechanisms in order to control their behavior.

> *Elucidate the connection between perception, judgment, impulse, and behavior and emphasize the difference between an impulse (for a behavior) and the actual behavior itself.*

Excursus
Offense-Supportive Cognitions

Offense-supportive cognitions (e.g., cognitive distortions) are a form of offense-supportive attitudes. They are empirically shown to be a risk factor for reoffending in terms of child sexual abuse. These are beliefs or convictions that justify or excuse sexual abuse. Cognitive distortions relate more to the direct perception of information than information processing and interpretation. A pedophilic individual who sees a child that they feel sexually attracted by will automatically be confronted by their problems. This confrontation provokes internal and external conflicts (self vs. surroundings) and induces inner tensions that lead to a psychological imbalance. The resulting interpretations and information processing lead to self-exculpation and restoration of psychic balance through the reduction of cognitive dissonance. This often culminates in downplaying and denial, and leads to the delegation of responsibility, to overlooking of possible traumatization of victims, or to an inability to take on other perspectives.

There is a connection, or even an alternating dependence, between problematic perceptions and cognitive distortions. This is quite difficult to differentiate. Their differentiation is nonetheless important for therapeutic progress, and the therapists should take note that problematic perceptions and cognitive distortions are strongly influenced by the sexual preference of the participant. Additionally, it is useful to explain how problematic perceptions and cognitive distortions generally result more from internal and external conflicts than from deliberate and conscious decisions.

Distorted perceptions and cognitions can lead to lasting problematic attitudes, which can in turn be regarded as the result of the lasting internal and external conflicts that participants are confronted with regarding their sexual preference. They can cause basic attitudes and positions that hinder therapeutic work. The motivation to change can be called into question in these cases. Problematic attitudes might be, for example, "Children want sexual experiences with adults," "Sexual relationships between children and adults were common in ancient Greece," or "I don't have a problem, it's society that's denying me my right to have sex with children."

Excursus

Accounts of Children Initiating Sexual Contact

It can happen that participants recount situations in which children seem to have initiated sexual contact. Possibly they refer to children who behave in a sexually provocative manner to seduce adults, or of children who intentionally touch adults sexually, or of children who even ask to be touched themselves. It may indeed be the case that children behaved in ways that correspond to these descriptions. As a rule, a sexual motivation in the adult sense cannot be attributed to these behaviors. In absolutely exceptional cases, however, children may act in this manner because they have experienced this behavior as normal, because sexual contact seems to them like the only way to be close to someone, or because they do in fact want to test out their own sexual effect on others without having considered the next steps or consequences. In many cases, the situation has not been scrutinized by the patient because of his sexual preference but, rather—corresponding completely to his own desires and needs—is perceived as intentional sexual behavior on the part of the child ("selective perspectives"). Therapists should listen carefully to these descriptions, call the behavior and underlying motivations of the children into question, and emphasize the adult's non-negotiable responsibility to abstain from sexual contact with children. Writing off such descriptions as nonsense can engender reactance.

4.4   Interventions

- Collect from the group possible components out of which perception might consist (such as sensations, thoughts, judgments, and feelings).
- Ask the patients to think of a specific situation with a child in order to work out the components of perception. Gradually introduce the WS *Behavioral Analysis*.
- Collect and discuss different possibilities of the perception and judgment of stimuli by comparing participants' different interpretations of a single situation (Fig. 2). Concentrate on the role of sexual preference and its effect on the process (e.g., how a situation involving a little girl would have a different effect on a pedophilic who is attracted to girls versus a pedophilic who is attracted to boys). You can use the WS *Imagination Exercise for Self-Observation* (1) + (2) to clarify the principles of perception.
- Use the WS *Influencing Perception* to work out the connection between thoughts, feelings, impulses, and behavior, and practice possibilities for influencing sexual arousal and impulses with the participants.
- Discuss the role played by intentional and unintentional attention in the interrelationship of perception, judgment, and impulses in behavior and the alterability of perspectives.

>*Take care that participants differentiate between sexual behavior with themselves and sexual behavior with others.*

Make sure that all participants unequivocally understand the concept of consensual sexual activities.

- Apply the general understanding of information processing to sexual impulses and behaviors. Discuss the following questions:
  – What is sexual behavior?
  – What is consensual sexual interaction?
  – What is dissexual behavior?
  – What is sexual abuse?

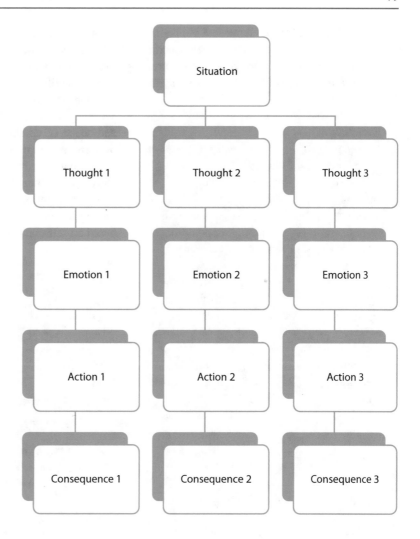

Fig. 2 Flowchart illustrating different perceptions and judgments of a single initial situation

- Work out and explain the following:
  - In the absence of consent or the ability to consent, sexual contact is defined as abuse not only in the case of children but also of adults.
  - Children are not under any circumstances responsible. To make this position clear, you can use the following analogies:

    A young boy says to his father, "Let's box! Not a play fight, a real one!" The father says, "Okay," and then punches the child in the chin. The child is knocked out. The father then says, "But he wanted it that way. He even asked for it!"

    An eight-year old girl says to her uncle, "Let's play husband and wife. Give me a kiss!" To the girl's horror, the uncle French kisses her and touches her chest.

> *Questions must be answered explicitly (e.g., "Children are not able to consent to sexual contact because of their physical and developmental state").*

- Focus should be placed on the triad of perception-judgment-impulse regarding the behavior and perspective of others. Participants should be put in a position where it is possible for them to reflect and apply the themes discussed to their personal problematic situations (WS *Dissexuality and Child Sex Abuse;* WS *Categories for Describing Abuse Images of Children;* WS *Myths About Child Sex Abuse*).
- Expand participants' capabilities for self-observation by applying the themes worked on by the group to individual situations in the everyday lives of participants (e.g., situations

with children and sexual fantasies). As home-work, ask the patients to analyze their specific situations and learn more about inner pro-cesses with the help of WS *Behavior Analysis.*

Excursus
Influencing Perception and Impulse Control
  Perception is a process that not only necessarily entails thoughts, judgments, and emotions of a person but is also cor-rectable and can thus be changed. Participants often describe situations that they experienced as sexually arousing. They recount, for instance, that they met a child and could think of nothing else for hours afterward. Behavior analysis often reveals in these situations a concentration on sexual thoughts and feelings, as well as an insufficient experience of self-efficacy ("I couldn't help myself, I just had to stand there and look."). At the same time, patients report situations in which they do not fol-low the first signs of sexual arousal and concentrate for a variety of reasons on something else (e.g., out of fear that some-one might discover them and because of other compelling activities). It can be help-ful in this case for the therapists to work out underlying mechanisms of perception and support patients in solidifying their expec-tations of self-efficacy in order to stabilize already-present attempts at impulse con-trol. Recommendations for helpful inter-ventions can be found in WS *Influencing Perception.*

5   Module 5: Emotions

5.1   Goals

- Communication of concepts and knowledge about the main categories of emotions
- Communication of knowledge about the inter-connectedness of emotions, cognitions, and actions

- Communication of the importance of emo-tions in social interactions
- Supporting participants in perceiving emo-tions, identifying emotions, and expressing emotions in another way
- Working on the ability to evaluate the quality and scope of emotions in order to decide if they are helpful or a hindrance to the achiev-ing of goals
- Developing strategies for the regulation of unwanted emotions
- Laying the groundwork of a prevention plan based on self-control

Excursus
Discussion   on   Consensual   Sexual Interactions and Dissexual Behavior
  Participants' experiences could be help-ful as the basis for a discussion on consen-sual sexual interactions. Alternatively, the following examples can help to clarify the concept of consensual sexual activity.

- A 10-year-old child who had sex educa-tion in school exposes himself nude and asks to be touched in his genital area. A 24-year old woman with a mental dis-ability and with the mental developmen-tal state of an 8-year-old asks a man to have sexual intercourse with her. A 16-year-old girl who has a relationship with a 30-year old man wants to have sexual intercourse with him. A 16-year-old boy has a relationship with a 30-year-old woman and wants to have sexual intercourse with her (While legal under German law, this might not be the case in other jurisdictions).
- What do you do?
- Ask yourself the following questions: Is it legal? Is it friendly/consensual? Is it respectful? Is there a choice? Is it on equal terms?
- You can also discuss the following questions:
- What about when there is no verbal refusal and no physical resistance? What

about when the underage person consents? Are children partially responsible for sexual abuse (e.g., in the way they dress or behave, or because of their lifestyle)?

Excursus

Example of a Behavioral Analysis and the Questioning of Interpretations

Patient	It was my sister's birthday and we were celebrating in the garden, when my nephew asked me to come to his room so he could show me his new video game. We sat at the computer, played the new game, and were fooling around. My nephew started to tickle me, and I had an erection. He kept tickling me, so I took his hand and placed it on my penis. He didn't say anything, so I undid my pants and showed him how he should masturbate me. We didn't talk about it later, but he went back to the others in the garden.
Therapist	Let's look at the situation more closely. You told us that your nephew brought you to his room. What did you think when he asked you to come with him?
Patient	I was happy.
Therapist	Why? What did it mean for you that he asked you?
Patient	He clearly liked me and wanted to be alone with me.
Therapist	Why do you think he wanted to be alone with you?
Patient	I don't know.
Therapist	What did you think would happen in his room?
Patient	I dunno, I thought we could get closer, have some time for ourselves, talk more intimately…
Therapist	Did you think of touching him or hope that sexual activity might take place?
Patient	Not directly. I was just excited to be alone with him.
Therapist	What did you think when he started to tickle you?
Patient	I mean that he wanted to get closer to me.
Therapist	You had an erection. How did that feel?
Patient	I was excited, my heart was beating, I was sexually aroused. I wanted him to touch me, but I was afraid he'd stop tickling me…
Therapist	But he didn't stop. What did that mean for you?
Patient	Hmm, I think he had noticed my erection, but he didn't stop touching me. So I thought he was curious or that he liked it, even.
Therapist	When you put his hand on your penis he didn't say anything. Why do you think that was the case?
Patient	I thought he was into what I was doing. I mean otherwise he would have said something.
Therapist	Why do you think he wanted to go back to the others after what happened?
Patient	I'm not sure. Maybe he was ashamed of what happened or was afraid someone would come looking for us.
Therapist	How did you feel?
Patient	I was still excited and couldn't believe what had just happened. I was just happy.
Therapist	And later? How did you feel in the following days? And how do you feel now?
Patient	I'm not sure. I know that it probably shouldn't have happened—that's not allowed. But on the other hand he agreed to it, and I didn't use force or make him do it.
Therapist	You said you hoped to be alone with him and to be more intimate with

Table 1 Perception and interpretation

Situation	Thoughts	Emotions and physical reactions	Impulse for my behavior	Actual behavior	Consequences (long term and short term)
Fooling around with the nephew	He likes me; he wants to be alone with me; I want more intimacy; he likes to touch me; he notices my erection; he wants to touch my penis	Happy, excited, sexually aroused, erection, heart beating	I cause him to touch me	I cause him to touch me	Short term: excited, happy. Long term: uncertain, anxious

	him. Do you think your nephew wanted to be alone with you?
Patient	I mean he said he wanted to show me his new game.
Therapist	Do you think that was a pretense? Do you think he wanted something else?
Patient	I thought it could have been more.
Therapist	And did you think he also wanted more?
Patient	Maybe.
Therapist	How did you come to that conclusion? Does he have to feel the same way you do?
Patient	No, probably not.
Therapist	Could it be that he really just wanted to show you his game because he likes you and wanted to play it with you?
Patient	Yeah, could be.
Therapist	When you had the erection he didn't stop tickling you. Why do you think that is?
Patient	He wanted to…
Therapist	Did he…? Are there maybe other explanations?
Patient	Maybe he didn't notice it? At first I thought maybe not, but then I put his hand on my penis and he agreed.
Therapist	You say he agreed. What did you observe and what did he do?
Patient	Nothing. He did what I showed him.
Therapist	Do you only do things that you really want to do, or have you ever done something you didn't want to do, but didn't say anything?
Patient	Yeah I have. Do you think he didn't like it?
Therapist	It's very likely that he was uncertain, maybe afraid, and just didn't know

how he should express his feelings. There are different explanations for his behavior. Children often have difficulties asserting their boundaries around adults, particularly with someone they like and respect.

• *Assignments for Therapists*
    – Divide up the above story into perception and interpretation (see behavioral analysis for this example: Table 1).
    – Question the assumptions and interpretations of the patient.
    – Take on other perspectives.

5.2   Rationale

In everyday communication and interaction, emotions are often described in general and imprecise ways. Common descriptions like "bad" or "unwell" can encompass a multitude of emotions such as anxiety, anger, aversion, or shame, while positive descriptions such as "fine" or "good" can describe happiness, pleasure, or love. For many people, this imprecision in language also affects self-observation. The therapeutic focal point of identifying and verbalizing one's own emotional states is an important part of our therapeutic approach for two reasons.

Firstly, for pedophilic/hebephilic persons, imprecise description of emotional states often confounds emotions bound up with sexual motivation with other emotions. Patients often tend to describe their feelings of attraction to a child or even sexual desire with a variety of attributes, for instance, harmless interest, selfless care, respite from negative emotions, aesthetic sense, or disquiet. When a relationship to a child becomes sexualized, this development is often described as having "come out of nowhere." It is difficult for many patients to pin down the connection between their emotions, their needs, and the actions and consequences that follow. Reflective sensation, precise description, and the acceptance of feelings of passion or love are thus preconditions of successfully controlling problematic modes of sexual behavior.

Secondly, imprecision in the sensation and expression of emotional needs in social interaction hinders efforts to build and maintain age-appropriate social relationships. This inability can increase stress levels in everyday life. The inability to correctly identify which emotional needs are injured in frustrating situations decreases the possibilities for successful management. In becoming familiar with their emotions and needs and learning to communicate them, patients can be helped in the development and maintenance of fulfilling social relationships and functional management strategies.

As a final product, familiarity with one's own emotional needs and knowledge of their consequences will enable patients to assess their perceived emotions as helpful or a hindrance to their goals. Strategies of emotion control help patients to distance themselves from emotions that compromise their goals.

5.3 Contents

In collecting emotions, the patients will find a variety of different expressions for feelings. The focus of BEDIT falls on the categories of fear, anger, disgust, sadness, joy, shame, lust, and love, which have proven themselves helpful in clinical praxis. To facilitate communication about feelings, it is useful to organize descriptions into the main categories. The terms "doubt," "worry," "dread," and "panic," for instance, could be ordered into the category of "fear." "Horny," "hot," "passionate," etc., could be placed in the category of "lust."

The conscious naming and verbal communication of feelings are unfamiliar to many patients and could prove to be a fundamental challenge. Patients often bring up elusive emotions such as

"indifferent," "uncomfortable," or "surprised." Supplementary signs of emotional states can help them pave the way for differentiated feeling. These signs include physical feelings (heart rate, blushing, getting flushed, sweating), posture (upright, stiff, relaxed, tensed), vocal pitch (quiet, still, loud, shrill), verbalizations (swearing, excusing oneself, hemming and hawing), behaviors or behavioral impulses (fleeing, fighting, hugging, crying), and thoughts ("That's great/terrible/…";"…wait until I get my hands on you!"; "She's so sweet!").

Patients will often experience themselves as helpless, both in controlling their sexual feelings toward children and in controlling their sexual frustration. As a first step, it has proven helpful to break down clear changes in emotional states in everyday situations in order to impart a feeling of self-efficacy regarding emotional control. When this point has been reached, the feeling of self-efficacy can be strengthened. Strategies for this are similar to those in other contexts. A basic strategy for management of unwanted emotions consists of allowing the moment of the first impulse to just pass. Distancing oneself from unwanted emotions can be achieved through a reality check, through reflecting on the motion, or through self-instruction. Withstanding unwanted emotions can additionally be made easier through the imagination of a secure place, shifting of attention, contrary action, or the provocation of another strong feeling.

> *Healthy perspectives on emotions can help participants reveal their feelings and speak about them.*

> *It can be difficult for participants to speak about, define, and categorize their emotions. Examples of participants' everyday situations and emotions can be helpful in the beginning stages.*

5.4 Interventions

• Collect descriptions of emotional states from the patients and let them order them into the main categories. Discuss the fine differences between the emotional states and points of crossover between categories.

- Have the patients document their emotions. Discuss the advantages and disadvantages of a broadening of one's knowledge about their own emotional needs and reaction patterns in stressful situations. Practice during a session filling out the column for the behavioral analysis regarding a real or fictitious situation (see the below example). Together with the patients, practice orienting oneself to the structure of the behavioral analysis.

Examples of emotional states				
Angry	Sad	Happy	Anxious	Excited
Upset	Despondent	Glad	Dreading	Aroused
Livid	Distressed	Satisfied	Nervous	Ecstatic
Sore	Depressed	Optimistic	Scared	Nervous
Enraged	Dejected	Delighted	Afraid	Energetic
Glowering				

>> *For example: A woman says to her husband, who arrives home very late at night without having called, "Where were you all night?"*

- What happened? What led to the situation above?
- What did you think in this situation? How did you judge this situation?
- What did you feel? What physical feelings manifested themselves?
- What behavioral impulse did you have? Was there only one impulse or multiple ones?
- What did you do? What were your intentions?
- What consequences did your actions have?

Ask the patients to concentrate on emotions in social interactions with a special focus on frustrating experiences and situations involving children. Work out patterns of emotional reactions to social stress and contact situations with children. Do these patterns correspond to the self-perception of the patients? What consequences do the patients take from potential discrepancies? (WS *Behavioral Analysis*; WS *Feelings in Situations with Children*)

Example
Situation
An acquaintance from the neighborhood, who is a single father, calls you on a Friday evening

after a hectic week. He would like to get away for the weekend with a woman he is interested in.

This is only possible if you agree to look after his 8-year-old son, whom you find sexually attractive, for 2 days. He asks if you are willing to do so.
Thoughts
This can't be true: He wants to go have a good time and the child has to suffer?

- The boy is being left behind. I'll look after him.
- I like it when he's around.

Emotions and Physical Sensations
Anger, empathy, suspense, excitement, the thrill of anticipation
Behavioral Impulse
I'd like to tell him he's being really selfish. I'd like to spend the weekend alone because I'm worn out. I'd like the opportunity to be able to spend some time with his son.
Behavior
I call back and agree to look after his son. I wish him a fun weekend and discuss the details of my looking after his son.
Consequences
I'm in the company of a child.
I'm not alone for the weekend. I have to take my needs and my fantasies in stride. I'm knowingly putting myself in a risky situation.

- Have the patients analyze individual emotions. This can be done in the group or alone. The emotions can be examples or taken from the patients' notes in their behavioral analyses. Discuss the "helpful signs" of emotions and how these can help patients correctly identify emotional states (WS *Perception of Emotions*).
- Collect patients' attitudes and beliefs about dealing with emotions. Discuss the consequences of these kinds of attitudes. How do these attitudes influence a patient's readiness to communicate their emotions? How do these attitudes influence the patient's image of other people?
- Talk about the function of emotions: Why do humans need emotions? What would it

be like if the participants had no emotions? Do different emotions fulfill different functions in life? Put special focus on the social environment. Discuss the relevance of emotions for initiating or preventing action. Discuss the consequences of different emotions for specific situations (WS *Behavioral Analysis*).

Example
Possible Attitudes When Dealing with Emotions

- Showing emotions means showing weakness.
- Emotions come and go for no reason.
- Some emotions are wrong.
- I am the only person who can know how I'm feeling.
- Others know better than I do how I'm feeling.
- People who show their emotions lose their self-control.
- After a good feeling, things can only get worse.
- Showing emotions makes us vulnerable.
- It's better to ignore uncomfortable emotions.
- Only women can talk about their emotions.
- Emotions are addictive.

- Work on strategies to modulate emotions. In one sitting, provoke an emotion, e.g., with a short, emotional film, an image, or an imagination exercise. Have the patients analyze the elicited emotion with a worksheet or in groups. Have the patients then evaluate their emotional state again. Did their emotions change? Did the degree of their emotional arousal change? How could the patients use this change in emotions in their everyday lives? Repeat the exercise. Use palpable sensations (e.g., mints, candies, and fizzing beverage powder) to induce a change in emotional state (WS *Regulation of Emotions Through Strong Physical Sensation*, WS *Influencing Perception*, WS *Imagination Exercise for Self-Observation* [1] + [2]).

Excursus
Healthy Perspectives on Emotions

- Emotions are neither good nor bad, neither right nor wrong. Feelings are just there. It is not helpful to judge (one's own) emotions.
- Emotions are not the same as behavior. There is a difference between feeling an emotion and acting because of this emotion.
- Emotions do not remain forever. Whatever you are feeling will eventually change, and another emotion will replace the previous one.
- When a strong emotion comes up, you don't have to let action follow what you are feeling. You only need to recognize and feel.
- Emotions are not facts. Sometimes they feel as if they were, as emotions can sometimes be very intense.
- You can't get rid of emotions; they fulfill essential survival functions. Be ready to accept your emotions as they are.

6 Module 6: Sexual Fantasies and Sexual Acts

6.1 Goals

- Participants becoming experts on their own sexual fantasies and sexual acts
- Practice perception of one's own sexual fantasies and acts
- Differentiating between internal and external boundaries that influence sexual behavior
- Determining the resources that each of the group members has to control sexual impulses
- Communication of knowledge about mechanisms such as downplaying, denial, and rationalization of sexual fantasies and acts

- Reduction of participants' anxiety in describing their own sexual fantasies and acts
- Internalization of the concept of dissexuality in general, as well as reflection on one's own (potentially) problematic sexually motivated behaviors (e.g., the use of CSAI)

6.2   Rationale

Sexual fantasies and sexual acts are an important source of information to help describe the sexual preference structure. Detailed reflection on sexual fantasies and acts can shed light on important characteristics of one's own inner processes, needs, and sexual preference. Describing one's own sexuality to third parties can also reveal central cognitive tendencies such as downplaying, justification, and rationalization. These cognitive tendencies provide insight into a participant's fundamental assumptions about himself and the world around him and can call attention to (potential) problematic attitudes.

6.3   Content

- *Dissexuality and Problematic Sexual Behavior*

  > *There is no informed consent with sexual behaviors in the relationship between adults and children.*
  The concept of dissexuality will be explained in the following theoretical section.
  Any activity can generally be understood as a sexual act when they are sexually motivated or partially sexually motivated, that is, when they serve as sexual arousal, sexually arousing conduct, and/or the preparation for direct sexual activity. Sexual acts can be described as dissexual when they injure the integrity and individuality of another person, particularly when the person in question is incapable of consent. Sexual abuse is defined here as every sexual behavior toward a person that takes place without their explicit consent or with persons who fundamentally cannot consent. Every use of sexually explicit images of such sexual behavior is defined here as indirect

sexual abuse. Dissexuality is a clinical (nonlegal) construct and is as such very relevant for therapeutic praxis. Because of the high risk of harm to one's own person or to others, however, there is overlap with legally relevant sexual behavior.

> *For example, I have sexual feelings when I look at a child in a public bus. When the child looks at me, I see their gaze as confirmation that they know my intentions and want the same thing I do. When I go to get off the bus, I pass by the child and touch their back in passing to increase my sexual arousal.*

Along with the legal criteria for (direct and indirect) child sexual abuse (child sexual abuse and the use of abuse images), it is important to discuss and question the participants' concepts of (their own) dissexual behavior toward children. It is additionally helpful to discuss who commits child sexual abuse (men, women, persons of different social backgrounds and age groups) and to differentiate between various motivations and reasons for child sexual abuse (e.g., as a replacement for sexual contact with a consenting adult partner, against the background of a mental disability or sexual-developmental problem, because of a pedophilic/hebephilic sexual preference).

- *The Vicious Cycle of Child Sexual Abuse*

Judicially sanctioned child sexual abuse and the use of abuse images often exhibit an escalating progression playing out in phases: a preparation phase, an action phase, and a follow-up phase. Cases of repeated abuse or the use of abuse images may additionally follow a cyclical pattern, wherein the follow-up phase immediately bridges over into the preparation phase (Fig. 3).

A participant can identify his own preparation phase, and thus the accompanying-individual risk factors for child sexual abuse, ahead of time. The more attuned the ability to recognize these risk factors in the preparation phase, the more possibilities for behavior control are available. An early awareness of the preparation phase increases the timeframe in which the participant can counteract. One of the goals of this therapy is thus to improve impulse control through a more developed awareness of one's own sexual desire

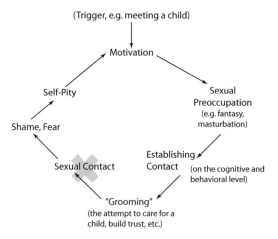

(Trigger, e.g. meeting a child)

Motivation

Self-Pity

Sexual
Preoccupation
(e.g. fantasy,
masturbation)

Shame, Fear

Establishing
Sexual Contact   Contact   (on the cognitive and
behavioral level)

"Grooming"
(the attempt to care for a
child, build trust, etc.)

Fig. 3 Example of a vicious cycle of sexual abuse

and one's own needs in order to break the cycle depicted, or to halt it in time.

To this end, it is vital to speak explicitly about past sexually abusive behavior or use of abuse images. German therapeutic confidentiality laws, which make possible the necessary confidential framework for engaging with past dissexual behavior not necessarily known to authorities, should be brought up again in this context (Sect. 5.1 in chapter "Therapeutic Options"). A detailed analysis of the course of events surrounding the behavior and associated conditions, perceptions, thoughts, feelings, and sequence of actions offers participants and the group various opportunities and learning experiences to help stop future abuse. The patients should understand, for instance, that a sexual assault represents intentional behavior and requires a certain degree of planning (in opposition to patients' frequent perception that abuse "just happened.") that the patients may not always be conscious of. It should also be recognized that certain steps that may have taken place over a longer period of time or decisions between different behaviors may eventually lead, or have led, to the abusive act. This recognition is central to taking responsibility for one's own decisions and problematic modes of behavior—both past and future. When patients can recognize the development of their individual risks early on, they are also in the position to employ helpful strategies and countermeasures to protect themselves and others.

Example of a Vicious Cycle of Sexual Abuse (Fig. 3)

Excursus
Principles for the Exploration of Sexual Experiences in Fantasies and Modes of Behavior

- Support and facilitate the participants' reflections.
- Avoid interpretations.
- Pose open-ended questions (how, what, why, etc.).
- Dig deeper into individual experiences and facilitate the reconstruction of the problematic behavior through the recollection of details (atmosphere, colors, other people, weather, temperature, etc.).
- Repeat the participants' thoughts in your own words and answers.
- Use present tense to make the descriptions as authentic as possible.
- Take care to look at the scene from the perspective of each of the patients.
- Make sure to keep the intensity of contact between therapist and patient in mind.

Bodily Sensations

During the exploration of sexual experiences in fantasies and behavior, keep the following five areas in mind: (1) behavior, (2) thoughts, (3) feelings, (4) physical sensations, and (5) sensory perceptions.

Analyze these areas before, during, and after sexual experiences. This can help toward a better recognition of mechanisms such as denial, downplaying, and justification, and lays down the basis for a future individual prevention plan.

Some aspects may make the description of sexual experiences in fantasies and behavior more difficult (e.g., fear, sadness, feelings of shame, strategic reasons, low introspective capability, memory gaps, repression, and discrepancy to one's own ideal self).

Should emotional reactions such as anger, sadness, or shame occur during descriptions, ask the patient about his feelings and thoughts. If the participant claims to have not experienced or not remember any sexual fantasies, there are different possibilities for initiating this discussion:

- Tell me about the fantasies you had last time you masturbated.
- What are your thoughts like when you see a child you find sexually attractive? What do you like about this child? What would you like to do with him/her?
- What sexual thoughts and fantasies have you had recently (e.g., as teenager, adolescent, and young adult)? Begin with the thoughts and fantasies that you can remember.

- *Participants as Experts on Their Own Sexuality and Sexual Preference*

Sexual preference can be described on three axes (sexual orientation toward gender, sexual orientation toward a body age, and sexually-preferred practices), human sexuality on three levels (sexual behavior, sexual fantasies, and sexual self-concept), and sexual behavior in three forms of sexual activity (masturbation, extragenital, and genital) [see chapter "Pedophilia and Hebephilia" and Module 1]. To sensitize participants to sexual attraction to a certain body age, of particular relevance is the differentiation between sexual interest in prepubescent children (pedophilia) and early pubescent children (hebephilia), as well as between exclusive attraction (pedophilia, hebephilia, pedo-hebephilia) and nonexclusive attraction (pedo-teleiophilia, hebe-teleiophilia, pedo-hebe-teleiophilia) to a specific body age or body schemata. The completion of the following module should leave participants with their own diagnosis and extensive knowledge of their sexual-preference structure. They should become aware in the process of the possible discrepancies between self-concept, fantasies, and socio-sexual behavior.

> *It can happen that participants become sexually aroused during descriptions of explicit sexual fantasies or behaviors. This should be addressed by the therapists and depathologized as a natural reaction. Sexual arousal that occurs can be used in the framework of exercises for emotional regulation, wherein the participants experience being able to actively increase or decrease their sexual arousal with the help of various instructions (e.g., intensification of sexual thoughts vs. concentration on nonsexual content, such as math problems) (WS **Influencing Perception**).*

6.4   Interventions

- *Dissexuality and Problematic Sexual Acts*
    - Have the group members give examples of sexual acts (alone, with others, etc.) and with which partners sexual acts can take place (men, women, children, teenagers, adults, older people, animals, corpses, objects, etc.). Collect the results on a flip chart. Discuss, and mark which interactions with which partners could be regarded as consensual. Discuss the criteria for consent (see Module 1, WS *Dissexuality and Child Sexual Abuse*).
    - Explain and discuss the concept of dissexuality (see Module 1) and the model of the age of consent. Every group member should think of a real or invented sexual situation in which a nonconsensual sexual interaction could have taken place. Differentiate in the description of the situation between "My Expectations" and "The Other Person's Expectations" to help sensitize group members to the concept of nonconsensual sexual behavior, specifically against minors.
- *The Cycle of Sexual Abuse*
    - Discuss in the group if sexual contact with others happens unexpectedly or if there are specific intensifying conditions (emotional, cognitive, situational) in which acts of abuse take place.
    - Use behavioral analysis to recognize individual risk factors and analyze with the

group members the individual steps or phases of sexual abuse (chain of events), as well as the elements of the vicious cycle of (repeated) sexual contact. Help participants who have committed real sexual abuse of children or used abuse images in the past, together with the other patients, to reconstruct how the abuse happened, as well as all the steps and decisions that eventually led to the abuse.

– Support the group in understanding that sexual contact with children follows patterns that are individual, yet also repetitive and recognizable. Be sure that patients understand that sexual contact does not happen "out of nowhere" or "for no reason," but is rather the product of a chain of events.

• *Participants as Experts on Their Own Sexuality and Sexual Preference*
  – Discuss with the participants why it makes sense to have a nuanced knowledge of one's own sexual behavior and sexual fantasies.
  – Collect participants' ideas on a flip chart and make sure that the participants are aware of the following aspects:
    To become an expert on one's own sexual fantasies and behaviors means protection from unwanted surprises and helps to reduce fears—especially about oneself and one's own behavior.
    Knowledge means more competence and self-confidence.
    To know one's own desires and needs increases one's accountability: I can only change that which I know.
  – Give the participants WS *Sexual Preference Mannequin* and WS *Guidelines for Describing Sexual Experiences in Fantasy and Behavior* as homework. Explain the different levels of sexuality. The homework can then be discussed in the group. By the end, participants should be able to name their own sexual-preference structure.

7 Module 7: Empathy and Adopting Other Perspectives

7.1 Goals

• Fostering the ability to put oneself in someone else's shoes and to understand their feelings and perspectives
• Application of this ability to real and/or imagined sexual contact and to the perspective of children (thoughts, feelings, consequences of victimization)
• Application of these abilities to the use of abuse images, the perspective of children (thoughts, feelings, consequences of victimization), and the fact that images on the Internet may be freely accessed by anyone ("once it's on the Internet it's on the Internet forever").

7.2 Rationale

Empathy is defined as the ability to perceive the emotions of others and to understand and share in their feelings, desires, ideas, and actions. Through strengthening empathy, the ability to show understanding and concern is improved. Considering that the ability to adopt another's perspective and empathy also influence sexual motivation, most therapy programs for convicted sex offenders contain units on empathy with victims. Improved impulse control and reduced aggression levels are crucial for a greater degree of empathy. Even in patients who have never had sexual contact with children, increased empathy can further strengthen impulse control, thus fostering the development of behavioral control.

According to scientific research, sex offenders—particularly pedophilic sex offenders—show an adequate degree of empathy for victims of other sex offenders, but not for their own victims. This can be interpreted as the result of cognitive distortions (see Module 4, "Perception"). Empathy is generally regarded as an ability learned within sociocultural contexts. It can, however, be impaired by cognitive distortions, negative emotions, and/or sexual arousal.

7.3 Content

> *Participants who have used abuse images of children but have never had direct sexual contact with children may possibly have greater difficulty in adopting the perspective of children.*

Patients will be confronted with feelings, thoughts, and sensations experienced by victims of sexual abuse or that could be experienced by potential future victims. This applies too to victims of abuse images: in this case, discussion will turn to feelings, thoughts, and sensations experienced by the victim of child sexual abuse committed for the production of images and/or those that emerge from a victim's sexual abuse being made public and remaining available to others.

7.4 Interventions

>*Patients can be asked to share their own experiences or imagine situations (For example, someone abused your trust; someone filmed you in the shower and posted the video on the Internet; therapists secretly recorded you during a sessions and played the recording for others. How would you feel?)*

- Give examples of empathy in everyday life (e.g., a child that falls and hurts himself while playing). Ask the participants for typical reactions and reasons for these reactions. Explain that emotional reactions and behavioral impulses are based on empathy and concern.
- Collect features of empathy and considering another's perspective and let the group work out important aspects, such as (1) the ability to change perspectives; (2) walking in someone else's shoes and understanding their thoughts and feelings; (3) understanding how one's own behavior affects others.
- Have the participants explain the importance of empathy for therapy: (1) understanding and

acknowledgment of how children think and feel enable the participants to resist sexual impulses and thus behave toward children in non-harmful ways or without crossing boundaries; (2) empathy can be a great asset in interpersonal relationships.

- Work on letters from victims of child sexual abuse and abuse images (WS *Letter from a Victim*). For example, have a participant read the letter aloud. Ask the participant to share the feelings and thoughts this elicits with the group.
  - What could victims feel directly after being sexually abused? What are some possible short-term consequences?
  - How could victims feel weeks/months/ years later? What are some possible long-term consequences?
  - Are there differences between short-term and long-term ramifications?
  - Are there group members who can identify with the letter, either as offender or as victim?

> *Before any role-play, rules and boundaries—especially regarding touching the other participants—must be discussed and set.*

- Have the group members write letters to victims of their own actual behavior or their sexual fantasies (WS *Letter to My Victim(s)*, WS *Letter from My Victim to Me*).
  - The discussion should focus on the relationship between abusive behavior toward children (child sexual abuse and abuse images) and a lack of empathy. Further discussions should focus on the question of how the ability to have empathetic concern can affect actual abusive behavior. Discuss the relevance of empathy for the motivation to carry out or refrain from an act.
- Use role-play to strengthen participants' victim empathy for (potential) victims of child sexual abuse. Patients are asked here to stage their own real or fantasized sexual contact with children from the perspective of the child.

Excursus
Recommendations for Establishing Rules and Boundaries in Role-Play

1. Before getting started, have the group reflect on possible fears. Collate and discuss them.
2. Emphasize that all fantasies are okay for the purposes of masturbation, but that it is important to develop a feeling for how the children being fantasized about might feel or think if these fantasies were to be lived out.
3. Patients should not portray themselves, as this makes it difficult to take on the perspective of the victim.
4. Establish that touching is only allowed when this has been agreed upon and defined in advance ("When I touch the outer side of your upper thigh with my hand, that is supposed to represent the moment when you pushed your penis up against the child's body.")
5. The use of physical violence is not permitted.
6. Should one of the therapists or one of the participants say "stop," all action must be stopped immediately. Participants may take a break at any time.

8 Module 8: Biography and Schemata

8.1 Goals

- Conveying the impact of self-perception and the perception by important people in one's life on one's current life situation and current behavior
- Reflecting on individual learning history, sexual development (i.e., sexuality, self-image), and social and intimate relationships in the context of individual sexual preference
- Contributing to a better understanding of individual problems, problematic behaviors,

strengths, weaknesses, and resources, as well as individual sexual preference
- Developing a better understanding of one's own thinking, attitudes, and emotions
- Working out resources based on the participant's individual learning history
- Building the foundation for a prevention plan and protective measures based on behavioral control

8.2 Rationale

Analyzing a person's biography and learning history make it possible to recognize connections between past, present, and future experiences and behavior, as well as one's current self-image. Basic individual patterns of behavior, perception, and development can be revealed and put to use for therapy. Working with the biography and current self-image of a patient is part of many therapeutic approaches. With persons with pedophilia, it may be helpful to discuss individual etiological explanation for the own sexual preference. However, as it is not possible to determine and treat the causes of sexual preference, this therapeutic approach places its emphasis on developing self-control. The biographical work therefore serves to uncover schemata that obstruct the fulfillment of fundamental psychological needs and thereby influence future behavior. Schemata are acquired in childhood and are sustained over the course of one's later life and contain a broad pattern of memories, emotions, perceptions, and feelings that determine behavior. They can be maladaptive and dysfunctional. Reflecting upon individual life history and drawing connections between lived experiences and current self-image generally reveal significant patterns that are relevant for the therapeutic process.

8.3 Content

> *Therapists should keep in mind that the patients are likely to focus on events in their lives that they believe to be etiologically connected with their*

sexual preference (e.g., their own experiences of being sexually abused).

The analysis of the connection between self-image and biography can bring many interesting aspects to light, but not all subjects have proven to be equally relevant for the therapeutic process. As part of the therapy within the BEDIT framework, the following issues should be given priority: the concept of an intimate relationship/partnership; the way in which people enter into, develop, and form relationships; the concepts of sexuality and intimacy; making reference to problematic situations in life and the desire for change; strengths and resources; comparing one's own viewpoints with those of key figures in one's life.

Biographic work can take up a lot of time. If patients are going into too much detail, you should refocus them on relevant subjects. For example, they could start by writing out a detailed personal history for themselves, and then mark out important and therapy-relevant experience, events, and milestones on a timeline.

8.4 Interventions

- Have the participants reflect on their current self-image and the influence it has on their behavior, perception, and emotions, as well as their personal well-being. Focus on the influence of their sexual preference and on their actual behavior (WS *My Current Self*).
- In the group, discuss ideas about how biographic work could be used, which broader themes their life course should include, how the life course should be discussed (constructive criticism), and which focus could be relevant for therapy. Then, each group member should write a detailed life course for himself at home. In the next step, the group members should narrow down the therapy-relevant experiences and events and prepare a timeline that will serve as a basis for the discussion in the group (WS *Sexual Development*).
- Together with the group members, work out individual patterns, schemata, and concepts as they pertain to the central themes and questions, and discuss possible influences on the sexual perception of the participants and on their feelings and their behavior in connection with their sexual preference. Compile instances of self-experienced or committed violations of personal intimate and sexual boundaries.

Excursus
Therapy-Relevant Subjects for Life Histories

- Concept of partnership
  - Think back: How would you describe your previous partnerships?
  - Think (back) about your parents' partnership: How important was/is this as your model?
  - Which (socio-sexual) experiences in your youth have influenced your perspectives today?
  - What do partnerships mean for you today? Do people even need partnerships? What do they need them for?
- Forms of partnership
  - Why do you have relationships?
  - What have you learned about forming relationships with other people over the course of your life?
  - What kinds of patterns do people display when they meet and get to know each other?
  - What does one have to do to get to meet and get to know people or to be liked by people?
  - How do you usually deal with criticism? How do you usually deal with acceptance? How do you feel about this?
  - How do you present yourself? Are you happy with this?
  - How do you deal with conflicts? Are you happy with this?
- Concept of sexuality
  - Why do you/people in general have sex?

- What is the difference between masturbation and sex with another person?
- What is the difference between sex with an adult and sex with a child?
- What is your sexual orientation like? Since when have you had this orientation?
- Concept of intimacy
  - Which conclusions do you draw from your life experiences in regard to trusting other people?
  - Where have you experienced acceptance, closeness, security?
  - How do you experience physical affection and hugging? How would you feel if you were forced to give this up?
  - How do you react if someone tries to be physically affectionate with you? Could you try to explain your reaction based on life experiences and conflicts in your past?
- General questions for participants for analyzing a life history
  - Which of your behaviors would you like to change due to the repeated difficulties and problems they have caused?
  - Which behaviors would you like to keep? What are your strengths?
  - Which insights were new to you?
  - Which subjects or themes were important to you?
  - Which patterns in your relationships to adults (partners, friends) could you recognize?
  - Who has given you recognition, acceptance, and security? Who treated you with disapproval and rejection?
  - Which situations lead/have led to physical reactions such as sweating outbreaks, stomach aches, headaches, neck pain, and heart issues now and in the past?

- In what situations, or on which occasions, do you usually react by withdrawing?
- In what situations, or on which occasions, do you usually react with anger or rage?
- How do you deal with criticism?
- How do you deal with praise and recognition?
- Which of the difficulties and problems mentioned here are the important people in your life informed about? What is keeping you from telling them about them?

9 Module 9: Management and Problem-Solving

9.1 Goals

- Assessment of management strategies based on their short-term and long-term effects
- Communication of the concept of functional and dysfunctional management strategies
- Identification and strengthening of individual functional management strategies

9.2 Rationale

Scientific research on people who have committed sexual abuse show that impaired abilities in the management of everyday tasks is connected to reoffending. People who had committed sexual offenses were found to have dysfunctional, maladaptive management strategies for emotional stress—such as sexual strategies—that may contribute to the risk of reoffending. Patients often describe in therapy that boredom, increased stress levels, or emotional loneliness preceded the use of abuse images and/or sexual acts with children. Development and training of management strategies for the long-term reduction of averse, stressful states thus represent a meaningful goal in the reduc-

tion of risks for abuse. The successful management of external and internal stressors and
situations is significant for participants' long-
term psychological well-being.

9.3   Content

Patients are often plagued by a variety of external
and internal stress factors (stressors) that they
feel they are no match for. External stressors consist of challenges such as unpleasant bureaucratic
tasks, work-related demands, or interpersonal
conflicts. Internal stressors consist of uncontrollable negative emotions, deviant sexual fantasies
and impulses, and sexual behavioral impulses
that   are   experienced   as   uncontrollable.
Pedophilic/hebephilic persons frequently turn to
denial, avoidance, and emotion-oriented strategies such as self-incrimination or self-pity. These
strategies may lead to short-term relief but provide no long-term solutions to the problem.
Strategies for long-term relief from emotional or
situational stress encompass the solution to the
problem, the division of a given task into smaller
tasks, utilization of social support, acceptance of
external or internal conditions that cannot be
changed, and intervention based on one's own
needs or a reassessment to regain control of a
situation perceived as uncontrollable.

9.4   Interventions

- Collect examples for problem and stressful
  situations from participants' past experiences.
  What did you do to make situations like these
  more tolerable? How did you react to difficulties? Develop a definition of management,
  understood as thoughts or acts that can be
  used in dealing with internal or external stressors (WS *Behavioral Analysis*).
- Consider short-term and long-term consequences of the measures taken. Explain how
  temporary relief can be helpful in reinforcing
  oneself during stressful situations, but problems nonetheless require long-term solutions.

In general, the ability to call up short-term and
long-term strategies represents an important
resource. Collect strategies in the group that
could lead to long-term solutions to problems
and those that lead to temporary relief (WS
Types of Management Strategies, WS
Evaluation of Consequences).

- Have the participants identify patterns of management in specific situations. Are there situations that can be solved without great effort?
  Are there situations in which you normally do
  not use strategies that nonetheless contribute
  to solving a problem? (WS *Behavioral
  Analysis*)
- Have the participants consider context. Have
  there been internal or external factors that
  contributed to your ability to develop problem-
  solving strategies in a specific situation? (WS
  Behavioral Analysis)
- Have the participants develop a problem-
  solving strategy for a situation currently occu-
  pying them. Pay attention to both the patients'
  resources as well as situational and internal
  factors. Divide up strategies into small, man-
  ageable steps, and have the patients evaluate
  their implementation (WS *Development of a
  Solution to a Problem*).

10   Module 10: Social
Relationships

10.1   Goals

- Identification of important partners in social
  interaction and the communication of the
  importance of emotional relationships
- Communication of knowledge on typical individual patterns in social interactions
- Identification and analysis of problem modes
  of behavior in social interaction with trusted
  people/contact persons (close friends and/or
  partners) and the development of alternatives
  for problem behavior
- Strengthening participants' experience of self-
  efficacy in interactions with emotionally significant persons

10.2 Rationale

Functional social relationships with contact persons are an important factor for both mental and emotional well-being, as well as for physical health. Persons who lack certain social competencies can have great difficulty in building a social network of supportive friends and acquaintances, which can lead to social isolation, loneliness, or emotional problems. Many people are taught neither general nor additional social skills. This can mean a challenge for, or even a burden on, the ability to function socially, as well as communication and problem-solving in relationships with family members, partners, and close friends.

10.3 Content

Clinical experience of the PPD has shown that social isolation and a lack of close relationships with acquaintances, friends, and family members are common problems among patients. Some patients have reported trying to shield themselves from unpleasant questions about relationships or sexuality by avoiding intimate social contacts. The main goal of this module is therefore to encourage participants in improving their social skills and competencies in order to overcome social isolation. The module aims for the psychic stabilization of patients in order to strengthen their ability to control sexual impulses. At the core of this module is the construction or further development of an individual social network generally, as well as the maintenance of intimate social relationships in particular. With the help of behavioral analysis, resources and deficits in social interactions should be identified and treated, as a lack of intimacy in social relationships represents a risk factor for the sexual abuse of children.

10.4 Interventions

- *Emotions and Social Interactions*
  - Have each member of the group create an overview of their social relationships and organize them on a scale from "very comfortable" to "very problematic" (WS *My Social Network*).

  Group members should then discuss the following questions:

  Who in your life has provided you with recognition, acceptance, and emotional security?

  Who has showed you refusal and repudiation?

  How would you describe your current situation as it relates to these aspects?

  What does your ranking of your social relationships look like?
  - Have group members identify recurring problem situations that are burdens on close and intimate relationships. Are there recurring patterns? Is there a connection between the quality of the relationships and the difficulties that persons in the relationships have to deal with?
- *Behavioral Analysis*
  - Every group member should concentrate on a specific problem in their social relationships that they would like to change or improve, or about which they would like a greater degree of clarity.
  - Each participant should recall a typical situation with a certain contact person in which this problem manifested itself. Therapists can use WS Behavioral Analysis to help achieve a better understanding for personal experiences and modes of behavior in typical social situations (thoughts, feelings, physical sensations, behavioral impulses, actual behavior). The short-term and long-term consequences of each situation's described behaviors should then be discussed.
  - Group members' understanding can be deepened via a further analysis at home of stressful situations with the help of the worksheet. Discuss their results in the next session.
  - Together with the participants, develop ideas for alternative modes of behavior.

Excursus

Social Competencies

Because of limited social competencies, patients can display a lack of social relationships. It can therefore be helpful to discuss this in therapy. Concentrate on knowledge about the mechanics of feedback, strengthen awareness of personal boundaries, communicate concepts of successful communication, etc. It may be helpful to identify problems and resources in the social realm and accordingly refer to the mechanics of feedback (e.g., making contact, expression of positive/negative feelings, and dealing with rejection/criticism). Therapists should be knowledgeable about social competencies and communication and should make use of therapy manuals as needed.

11   Module 11: Intimacy and Trust

11.1   Goals

- Communication of the concept of intimacy
- Communication of the connection between a lack of intimacy and loneliness
- Communication of the effects of insufficient intimacy and emotional loneliness on quality of life
- Reflection on the relevance of intimacy and emotional closeness and distance on interpersonal relationships
- Communication of basic rules of friendly and social communication
- Strengthening of participants' competencies in the communication of feelings
- Communication of knowledge on the origin and meaning of sexual dysfunction
- Insight into the ramifications of pedophilic/hebephilic sexual preference on the structure and development of relationships (desires, needs, fantasies)

11.2   Rationale

Acceptance, acknowledgment, security, and safety are the basic needs of humans. They can be fulfilled in interpersonal relationships, in particular in intimate relationships. A greater degree of intimacy in relationships leads in turn to increased overall personal satisfaction and emotional well-being. Intimacy is defined as the familiarity with or nearness to another person. While sexual relationships stand out in their high degree of intimacy, they can simultaneously lack intimacy; accordingly, intimacy is not the same thing as a sexual relationship. As sexuality can be regarded as an important factor for communication and the intensification of intimacy in interpersonal relationships, it must be kept in mind that a pedophilic/hebephilic sexual preference can make it much more difficult, or even impossible, to experience and utilize sexuality as an expression of intimacy with a partner. At the same time, sexuality plays no role in most intimate relationships (e.g., friendship and parenthood) and is therefore not a necessary condition for the initiation and maintenance of these kinds of relationships.

11.3   Content

A low level of experienced intimacy (e.g., few to no trusting relationships) is connected to increased emotional loneliness. It follows that pedophilic/hebephilic men lacking in or deprived of intimate relationships experience a higher degree of emotional loneliness. A weak feeling of belonging to the adult world, the impression of being stuck in one's own development, and the emotional identification with children can result in intensifying relationships with children to satisfy individual needs for intimacy, nearness, and sexuality. Initiation and intensification of trusting and intimate relationships with adults can, by contrast, lead to a reduction of feelings of loneliness, improved satisfaction with life, psychological stability, and increased impulse control regarding sexual abuse.

Excursus

Partnership and Pedophilic/Hebephilic Preference

Depending on the exclusivity of an individual's sexual preference, participants may have opportunities to experience sexuality in intimate relationships with other adult partners. Someone responsive in the same degree to both adults and children (i.e., non-exclusive pedophilia) can lead an intimate and sexually fulfilling relationship with an adult partner, whereby a portion of their sexual fantasies remains unfulfilled. Someone who is exclusively responsive to children, on the other hand, has no possibility of realizing their sexual fantasies and desires without committing child sexual abuse. They may have relationships to adults, but which remain sexually only partially satisfying and/or may be accompanied by sexual dysfunction. Therapists should look out for this and acknowledge feelings of sadness, despair, anger, or feelings of injustice that may arise. It can be helpful to turn to the Good Lives Approach and work from its focus on resources, future perspectives, and fulfilling activities.

11.4   Interventions

> *Emphasize that while the term intimacy is often used synonymously with sexuality, this is an insufficient reduction. Sexuality is in particular suitable for the expression of intimacy, but it is not necessary to feel intimacy with someone. At the same time, there can also be sexual contact that is not perceived as particularly intimate.*

• Discuss the term intimacy and its meaning for each of the participants. Collect characteristics of intimate relationships, such as the following:
  – Feelings of security, trust, and emotional closeness
  – Communality and shared experiences (e.g., free time together)

> *Extra attention should be paid to the age of the persons in the relationships listed by participants. If they should report social (and intimate) relationships to children who are not their own, these must be scrutinized.*

  – Care for one or more other person(s)
  – Experience of affirmation, esteem, and acknowledgment
  – (Mutual) support in crisis situations
  – Feelings of an intimate connection
  – Functional verbal and nonverbal communication
  – Self-disclosure (e.g., revealing insecurities)
  – (Shared) resolution of problems and conflicts
  – Optional: consensual sexuality

• Identify with whom participants lead intimate relationships and to whom they have authentic, close connections (currently or in the past). Analyze the individual meanings of intimate relationships with adults. You may use WS *My Social Network* to help ascertain the level of intimacy for the listed relationships.

• Discuss the advantages (e.g., the feeling of leading a fulfilling life, positive contact to others, improved mental and physical health, increased resistance to stress, less aggressiveness, and greater self-awareness) and disadvantages (e.g., the risk of being hurt, exhaustion of individual initiative and effort, necessity of compromise, and necessary self-disclosure) of intimate relationships with adults.

• Point to possible problems that can arise in intimate relationships with children such as the following:
  – The relationship is always and in every dimension asymmetrical.
  – Because of their cognitive, mental, and emotional development, children can never fully grasp the problems of adults.
  – Children live in their own emotional and cognitive world. This cannot be congruent with the world of adults.
  – In contrast to relationships with adults, sexuality in relationships with children is never an option for the expression of intimacy.

Excursus

Expression of Emotions in Intimate Relationships

Therapists may discover deficits in the expression of feelings in participants' existing intimate relationships. To address these deficits, it can be helpful to turn to Module 5, "Emotions," to discuss the verbal and nonverbal expression of fundamental emotions such as sympathy, fear, or shame. Compassion, for instance, can be expressed by taking relevant aspects into account (e.g., eye contact, smiling, nodding, spending time together, fulfilling needs and wishes, positive feedback, verbal support, paraphrasing, showing interest, and communication of one's own feelings). It can additionally be helpful to use current observable behaviors of participants in the group context (e.g., lack of reaction to the statements of another group member and lack of eye contact): these can be mirrored, discussed, and, for example, addressed in a role-play to allow a person to experience the effects of these kinds of behaviors himself.

12 Module 12: Planning for the Future

12.1 Goals

- Development of new, approach-oriented life goals, taking into account intermediary goals and cost-benefit analyses
- Reduction of dysfunctional management mechanisms and the building up of functional alternatives for management
- Clarification of existing cognitive dissonance between the desired self-image and problem sexual behavior
- Development of strategies that will support a long-term change on the basis of one's own resources

12.2 Rationale

The Good Lives Model and other resource-oriented approaches are based upon the hypothesis that risk-oriented and avoidance-oriented approaches are necessary, but insufficient for a comprehensive treatment program. They work from the position that pedophilic patients, like all people, strive to lead a good and fulfilling life ("Good Life"). Part of this striving for a good life is the attempt to achieve important goals in life. For the development of goals for the future, the practicality of the applied strategies and available resources must be examined. In order to aim for real and sustainable change, strategies should be task-oriented and focused. Regarding the development of goals (e.g., to lose weight), it must be kept in mind that approach-oriented goals (e.g., to eat more fruit) are easier to achieve than avoidance-oriented goals (e.g., to stop eating chocolate). It can therefore be sensible to reformulate the avoidance-oriented goal—to not commit further sexual abuse—as an approach-oriented goal (for instance, "I want to live a satisfying life without harming others."). Intermediary goals should be additionally worked out, as these make expectations for self-efficacy easier to achieve, which in turn increases motivation for pursuing the greater goal.

In connection with this, it is important to address the topic of reward and the concept of long-term and short-term costs and benefits. For the effective achievement of goals, it may make sense to forego immediate reward and instead push on, using intentional goal-oriented behavior, toward a later positive result.

12.3 Content

Participants often concentrate on avoidance-oriented goals. In this module, patients will be supported in their attempts to weigh costs and benefits (e.g., short-term and long-term consequences of their goals). Goals will furthermore be analyzed based on their actual and longer-term applicability. Participants will learn to designate intermediary goals that can be achieved in the near future. The importance of intermediary goals as milestones on the way to primary therapy goals, as well as the disadvantages of unrealistic goals or exclusive concentration on primary goals, will be discussed in the group.

> *It must be emphatically communicated that although participants may desire sexually intimate relationships with children, these can never be consensual and are therefore always abusive.*

12.4   Interventions

- Together with the participants, develop individual plans for the future. You can orient discussion based on the following questions: What will I be doing in the future (work, lifestyle, living conditions, behavior)? How will I spend my free time (social relationships, hobbies, etc.)? What problems will I be confronted with and how will I deal with them (e.g., anger, depressive moods, alcohol, working together with others)? Where will I be (places, situations)? How will I feel (moods, emotions)? How and what will I think regarding my need for sexual gratification? What will this need look like (regarding moods, emotions, behavior, thoughts)? What will be important to me in the future (values, attitudes, lifestyle, relationships, work, etc.)? What will I be proud of, what will I have achieved? What personal resources and strengths will I make use of to get there? (WS *My Future Self*)
- Introduce the concept of approach-oriented and avoidance-oriented goals and discuss the consequences of patients' behavior within the group (passive behavior vs. active behavior). Practice reformulating avoidance-oriented goals into approach-oriented ones using participants' examples. Consider the required resources (strengths, effort, capabilities, thoughts, feelings, etc.) that are necessary to increase the likelihood for a sense of achievement.
- Explain the concept of short-term and long-term costs and benefits of behavior. The topic

of immediate reward (both its positive and negative aspects) should be addressed in connection with this (WS *Evaluation of the Costs and Benefits of Goals*).

- > *Patients often report that their previous attempts to reach their goals have failed. This can be explained by goals that are too ambitious or a negative perception of self-efficacy. Therapists should address previous failures, elicit the reasons, and work on alterations to patients' goals.*
- Discuss with participants the function and necessity of intermediary goals in the step-by-step construction of a stable and positive lifestyle. Dysfunctional coping styles and cognitions should be addressed via reflection on the current situation and communication of how current coping styles, thoughts, and emotions can influence the success of an attempt to change ("It's too hard, I'll never make it," "If this doesn't work soon, I give up," "I feel powerless when I think about my problematic sexual behavior," "Why do things like this always happen to me?" etc.).
- With the group, take a closer look at how the elaborated and realistic goals of the patients could contribute to a reduction in problematic sexual behavior, more self-control, positive self-management, and a good life (in the sense of the Good Lives Model). Discuss this.

Excursus
Immediate Reward and Problematic Sexual Behavior

Problematic sexual behavior often goes hand in hand with immediate reward that makes abstention difficult. The weighing of short-term and long-term costs and benefits can be addressed in this context. The use of abuse images of children (e.g., in stressful situations) leads in the short term to sexual arousal, excitement, and the reduction of negative feelings. Long-term consequences, however, might include feelings of shame and guilt, bad conscience, self-doubt, depression, or even legal ramifications.

Nonetheless, the replacement of problematic behavior with new modes of behavior can be made more difficult by a variety of aspects: new modes of behavior are often initially bound up with costs (e.g., they might be time-consuming and unfamiliar) and the short-term consequences of new behaviors may be less fulfilling than the problematic behaviors. Additionally, it can take time before advantages emerge from the new behavior (i.e., comparably to learning a new instrument). Old behavior can, on the other hand, be activated more easily, particularly in challenging or difficult situations that accompany emotional stress.

13   Module 13: Protective Measures

13.1   Goals

- Communication of an understanding that child sexual abuse and the use of CSAI are the results of a chain of events, thoughts, emotions, and actions that are controlled and executed by the patient.
- Communication of an understanding of the controllability of different risk situations in that participants come to understand their individual cycles of problematic behavior. Explain that it is possible to interrupt the cycle at different points and that it is easier and less risky to do this at an early phase.
- Collection of participants' individual risk factors, warning signs, and high-risk situations relevant to committing sexual abuse.
- Develop a hierarchy of individual risk factors and warning signs in the chronology of an individual's vicious cycle of problematic sexual behaviors and regarding potential offending.
- Development of intervention strategies for risk situations at the different levels within the cycle of problematic sexual behaviors.

13.2   Rationale

This module is based on the concept of relapse prevention. Participants should attain an understanding of which events, thoughts, emotions, and actions have cleared the way for sexual abuse or for the use of CSAI in their lives thus far. The communication of this concept should give the patients a sense of how the development of risk situations for problematic behavior and child sexual abuse can be controlled and influenced. Based on behavioral analyses, biographical work, and schemata analyses, the patient can identify decisive steps that lead to risk situations. With reference to social competencies and functional problem-solving strategies, participants will identify measures that can be taken to manage the development of problems. As risk-supportive circumstances are often accompanied by destabilization, these abilities can help improve the patient's general quality of life.

13.3   Content

BEDIT differentiates between risk factors and warning signs for child sexual abuse. By this terminology, risk factors describe conditions that increase the likelihood of committing child sexual abuse. Among these, for example, are the initiations of an intimate relationship with a child, interpersonal conflicts, situations of being alone with a child, or other opportunities to act sexually with a child unbeknownst to others. Warning signs, on the other hand, are external or internal indicators that point to imminent child sexual abuse. Internal indicators cannot be perceived by others, e.g., thinking about sexually abusive behavior, feelings of rejection, the assumption of a right to sexual satisfaction, or other thoughts and emotions that are generally related to these processes. External indicators are those that can be perceived by others, e.g., social retreat, regular visits to a playground, or other preparatory activities.

The patient should be prepared to deal with risk factors in the future. Warning signs should be taken as an occasion to react to problem developments, though there is quite often a connection between risk factors and warning signs. Visits to a public swimming pool, for instance, could represent a risk factor for pursuing dissexual activities. A successful strategy in this case could be switching to a different sport or activity, for example, in order to reduce the impact of this risk factor. At the same time, frequent visits to a public swimming pool could also represent a warning sign, even when the visits are not considered as problematic behavior per se, but rather when they transpire in such a way that they could lead to a higher likelihood of making contact with children, e.g., during a time when swimming lessons are being held or during family swim periods.

The maintenance of self-control over sexual impulses toward children may represent a serious challenge for participants. This is particularly true when other forms of sexual activity appear to be unacceptable to patients and when sexual satisfaction within the bounds of social norms may only be achieved via masturbation to their preferred fantasies.

Managing this challenge of their own volition may supersede the patient's resources. Friends or family members who are informed about the patient's sexual problems can represent a source of great relief in these situations. A confidant might be a person who can speak openly with the participant about their identified risk factors and warning signs and is therefore capable of authentic social support. In any case, a partner's, family member's, or friend's knowledge of the patient's deviant sexual interests may be perceived as a great burden.

A comprehensive plan for relapse prevention should contain the following aspects:

- Knowledge of individual risk factors and warning signs, as well as strategies to manage risk factors and warning signs
- Individual differentiation between potentially risky and harmless contact situations with children, as well as risky situations regarding the use of child sexual abuse images
- Identification of confidants and clarification of their role within the prevention plan

> *The differentiation between risk factors and warning signs can be difficult for participants, as these are often interrelated. A participant may describe a risk factor as a warning sign. When one looks at the cycle of problematic behavior and the successive situations within this cycle, what is a warning sign in one situation can become a risk factor in the next situation.*

Excursus
Examples of Warning Signs and Risk Factors

- *First Situation:* I was given notice a week ago.
  - Thoughts: It doesn't matter to me. Let me be. I'm good for nothing.
  - Emotion: I'm angry, distraught, depressed (risk factor: depressive mood; self-denigration).
  - Behavior: I haven't answered the phone in two weeks (risk factor: social retreat).
- *Second Situation:* I see Kevin (age 10), my neighbor's son, playing in the garden (risk factor: watching children).
  - Thoughts: He looks really sweet and shy. He looks at me; he's interested in me. (warning sign: cognitive distortion; "he wants something from me").
  - Emotion: Happiness, excitement.
  - Behavior: I go into the garden, call over the fence, and invite the boy to come swim in the pool with me (warning sign: making contact with a child).
- *Third Situation:* Kevin comes into my garden and shows me his new fire truck (risk factor: socially uncontrolled situation in the sense of an *opportunity*: the child is in my garden; warning sign: I invited him over).
  - Thoughts: He wants to play with me, he likes me. Maybe I can convince him to get undressed and go swimming (warning sign: sexual fantasy).

- Emotion: Happiness, excitement, sexual arousal (warning sign: physical reaction).
- Behavior: Being nice to the boy, playing with him, and swimming with him in the pool (warning sign: piquing the child's interest, strengthening the connection).
- *Fourth Situation:* Kevin takes his clothes off and swims nude (warning sign: the child is now naked in a socially uncontrolled situation).
  - Thoughts: He looks so sweet. He has no reservations to take his clothes off; maybe he wants me to watch him (warning sign: "rose-colored glasses").
  - Emotion: Sexual arousal, joy, excitement (warning sign: sexual arousal).
  - Behavior: Drying the boy off and applying sunscreen to him (warning sign: initiation of pretended non-problematic physical contact).

13.4 Interventions

- Discuss the paths that lead to child sexual abuse and/or the use of child sexual abuse images. Clarify that these paths can manifest themselves hours, days, or months before the actual problematic behavior develops. Keep in mind the individual offense cycle (see Module 6, "Sexual Fantasies and Sexual Behaviors").
- Discuss the concepts of risk factors and warning signs with the help of examples. Support the patients in coming to understand warning signs and risk factors by way of past situations and experiences, attitudes, and values.
- Develop a concept for a comprehensive plan that could stop future child sexual abuse. Account for risk factors and warning signs, management strategies, as well as both potentially risky and non-problematic contact situations with children (WS *Warning Signs*)

- > *Discuss the guidelines of a successful prevention plan with the group*
- Collect individual risk factors from the participants. Consider external situations, thoughts, and modes of behavior. Have there been certain constellations in the patient's life in which risk factors came up more often than usual, e.g., certain events in their life or conflicts? Have the patients compile a list of their individual risk factors (WS Risk Factors).
- Collect individual warning signs from the participants. Have them discuss feelings, thoughts, and modes of behavior that were indicators for a chain of actions that led to sexually abusive behavior. Develop a hierarchy of individual steps. Point out that earlier steps in the chain of actions are easier to interrupt (WS Warning Signs).
- Develop strategies for the management of warning signs and risk factors. Differentiate between strategies for groups of warning signs and risk factors, on the one hand, and individual situations, on the other. Give an example during the session (WS Strategies for Dealing with Risk Factors and Warning Signs).
- Support patients in finding a confidant. Are there family members, close friends, or professionals to whom patients can safely disclose their pedophilic/hebephilic sexual interest? Have the patients share their experiences. Patients should be encouraged to make a list of confidants (Who can support me?).
- Stage a role-play that simulates a pedophilic or hebephilic person outing himself as such to a confidant.
- Compile management strategies for risk factors and warning signs into a comprehensive protection plan. Discuss participants' individual protection plans in the sessions, paying careful attention to their practicality and degree of goal orientation. To assess the strategies, stage a role-play on modes of behavior in risk situations (see Excursus: "Guidelines for a Prevention Plan").

> *Examples of guiding questions: How have patients communicated their sexual interest? How have their confidants reacted? In what*

ways have the patients found the confidant help-
ful for avoiding future child sexual abuse?
Discuss the potential burdens that come with
outing oneself.

Excursus

Guidelines for a Protection Plan

The following plan contains steps for the effective management of risk situations and dealing with warning signs.

Answer the following questions for each of the risk factors and warning signs.

1. How would you organize your life to ensure that risk situations do not occur again?
2. How do you get yourself to deal with this situation in a constructive way?
3. What would your future self say, do, and feel?

Formulate your strategies in as much detail and as clearly as possible. For example, if loneliness is a risk factor for you, you can manage this through expanding your circle of friends. It will not be enough, however, to just say: "I'm going to find more friends." Think of how exactly you plan to do that. Try to break up your goal into smaller steps, for instance, by joining a club or finding a hobby.

You can refer to WS *Development of a Solution to a Problem* for help. Be sure to include potential obstacles and how these can be managed.

Consider: Your plan will only help you if you put it into action. Try to turn the strategies you have developed into actions. With practice, putting it into action will be easier.

Excursus

Confidants

Confidants can be an enormous support in the management of stressful situations and provide security. Confidants might include close friends, family members, or other contact persons, but also professional counselors and therapists. These persons should be aware of the patient's pedophilic or hebephilic sexual interest, as well as the patient's goal not to initiate problematic contact with children and to abstain from the use of abuse images. The better the confidant is informed about the participant and their life, the better position he or she will be in to support them. To be able to provide the best support, the confidant should additionally be ready to accept the patient—including their abnormal sexual interest. Through positive communication, the confidant can support the patient in achieving their goals. However, the responsibility for abstaining from problematic sexual behavior is only with the patient.

BEDIT-A Manual for Adolescents

Working Group of the Prevention Project for Juveniles

The manual of the *Berlin Dissexuality Therapy for Adolescents (BEDIT-A)* serves as a guidebook with a modular structure for the treatment of patients between 12 and 18 years of age who have sexual particularities for the child body age. The manual is designed for an individualized therapy setting, but can also be transferred to a group therapy setting. The overall therapeutic goal is for high-risk patients to learn behavioral control in order to prevent the first or repeated acts of CSA, or the first or repeated use of CSAI. The implementation of the manual requires psychotherapeutic, cognitive-behavioral, and sexual-pharmacological competency and requires child and adolescent psychiatric expertise regarding the specified pharmacological treatment options. Psychotherapists who are interested in using the manual should have the appropriate experience and training competency, as well as a basic understanding of risk factors, regarding CSA and the use of CSAI with adolescents.

The manual was developed within the framework of the Prevention Project for Juveniles (PPJ) at the Institute for Sexual Science and Sexual Medicine at the Berlin Charité and was tested for its applicability in this context. The basis of the BEDIT-A is the manual The Berlin Dissexuality Therapy Programme (BEDIT; Berlin Institute for Sexual Science and Sexual Medicine 2013) along with additional approaches regarding the treatment of adolescent sex offenders and the current empirical literature. The development and expansion of the PPJ, and with it the present manual, would not have been possible without the support of the Federal Ministry for Family Affairs, Senior Citizens, Women and Youth since July 2013. The creation of the BEDIT-A would not have been feasible without the extensive preliminary work in connection with the establishment of the PPD and its therapy services for adults.

The present manual consists of three parts. The first part contains basic information on the general parameters, as well as recommendations for the utilization of the manual. The second part consists of the single modules of the manual for therapeutic work with the adolescent target group, which is supplemented with information for working with caregivers, dealing with comorbid psychiatric disorders, as well as drug treatment options. Finally, the third part of the appendix contains recommendations for specific interventions in the form of worksheets and information materials.

Working Group of the Prevention Project for Juveniles
Charité – Universitätsmedizin Berlin, Corporate Member of Freie Universität Berlin, Humboldt-Universität zu Berlin, and Berlin Institute of Health, Center for Human and Health Sciences, Institute of Sexology and Sexual Medicine, Berlin, Germany
e-mail: klaus.beier@charite.de

© The Author(s), under exclusive license to Springer Nature Switzerland AG 2021
K. M. Beier (ed.), *Pedophilia, Hebephilia and Sexual Offending against Children*,
https://doi.org/10.1007/978-3-030-61262-7_7

1   General Conditions

The target group of this manual is 12- to 18-year-old adolescents who have a sexual responsiveness to children and who voluntarily agree to receive therapeutic treatment in order to develop control of their behavior. The aim of the therapy is to reduce the risk of CSA and/or the use of CSAI by performing therapeutic work on dynamic as well as static risk factors. The BEDIT-A has so far only been tested in therapeutic practice with patients from the legal *"Dunkelfeld"* (with regard to CSA and/or the use of CSAI). Experience with potential participants from the legal *"Hellfeld"* is not yet existing. According to BEDIT-A, exclusion criteria for therapy are psychiatric illnesses that are in need of acute treatment, e.g., psychoses from the schizophrenic spectrum or currently relevant addictive disorders. In the case of learning or mental disabilities, it should also be examined to what extent the content of the treatment can be applied or if it may possibly have to be adapted to the cognitive performance of the individual.

With respect to establishing and maintaining a sustainable therapeutic relationship and taking into account sexual-pharmacological areas of emphasis, cognitive-behavioral basic assumptions and elements, insights from research on juveniles who sexually offended, as well as the consideration of child and adolescent psychiatric comorbidities, the following therapeutic goals are to be achieved:

- Education and fear-mitigation for patients and their caregivers
- Offering of supportive relationships to patients and their caregivers
- Acceptance of one's own sexual preference and integration into one's own self-perception
- Acquiring strategies to control sexual desires and urges directed at children
- Reduction of specific risk factors for CSA/the use of CSAI
- Treatment of relevant child and adolescent psychiatric comorbidities in accordance with related guidelines

- Integrating the social environment in order to prevent relapse

An attitude free of value-judgement is fundamental to therapeutic work with people with sexual preference particularities, since potential social exclusion usually represents the greatest and often most well-founded fear of those affected. The decisive therapeutic focus is the open-ended integration of currently occurring fantasies, so that the affected persons succeed in gradually integrating their own sexual preference, in the sense of an active condition, into their own self-image in order to ensure the development of behavioral control in the future. The latter corresponds to the goal of recognizing and reducing individual social, psychological, and emotional risk factors in order to minimize the risk of committing CSA or using CSAI in the long term. A cure in the sense of an eradication of the sexual impulses and fantasies related to the prepubescent and/or early pubescent body age cannot – according to the current empirical state of knowledge – be expected (see Beier et al. 2016a, b; Seto 2008, 2009).

2   Instructions for Use and General Conditions

The BEDIT-A consists of 9 modules for use in individual therapy with the adolescent target group, although the modules can also be adapted for use in a group therapy context. The structure of BEDIT-A is divided into an initial psychoeducation (Module 1), which is fundamental for the following treatment. Subsequently, individual risk factors will be addressed. Depending on particular needs and necessities, the frequency of the interviews with the primary caregivers may vary. If indicated, a parallel drug treatment can be initiated under the guidance of child and adolescent psychiatric expertise. This should never be done unaccompanied, but always as an embedded part of the psychotherapeutic process.

Table 1 gives an overview of the therapy modules included in BEDIT-A. It shows that the implementation of BEDIT-A is divided into con-

Table 1 Modular structure of the BEDIT-A

Constitutive modules	Facultative modules
1. Psychoeducation	4. Behavior control
2. Cognitions, emotions, and behavior	5. Social skills and intimacy
3. Fantasies and behavior	8. Treatment of comorbid disorders
6. Relapse prevention	9. Drug treatment options
7. Working with caregivers	

stitutive and facultative modules. The former should be carried out with each patient independently of the individual specific problem. It is recommended to start with the obligatory module *Psychoeducation*. Facultative modules, as well as some particular subsections of single modules, should be applied according to individual needs. It is crucial to use the manual flexibly, adapted to the individual needs and risk situation of the patient. The single modules complement each other and are designed to build on one another. The linkage of the modules to one another enables the patient to revisit certain contents repeatedly in order to process and reinforce important treatment goals. In addition to psychoeducational content as a basic foundation, the modules also deal with individual risk factors that affect the probability of an assault. A reduction of these risk factors is aimed for therapeutically. The module *Relapse Prevention* should be placed at the end of the therapeutic process in order to integrate both the content worked through during therapy as well as future planning strategies.

At the same time, situational conditions, especially those relating to the accessibility of victims or the possibility of assaults, should be therapeutically influenced. In the case of intrafamily abuse, for example, the separation of victim and perpetrator should be sought, e.g., through accommodation in a youth welfare facility. It is decisive here to include the entire system, i.e., the patient himself, but also the direct (e.g., parents) or indirect (e.g., youth welfare office) caregivers.

3 Structure of the Manual

Almost all primary modules as well as their submodules are divided into three sections: theory, goals, and interventions. In the theory section, the corresponding theoretical concepts and the current state of empirical knowledge are presented. In the goals section, the therapeutic goals defined within each module that are to be worked towards are discussed. The interventions section provides recommendations for concrete implementation. In the manual there are different materials and procedures which structure the therapeutic work and serve to support the implementation of the contents to be conveyed. The following terms (abbreviations) are used as references:

- *Psychoeducation*: Transfer of knowledge by the therapist
- *Discussion*: Joint development of substantive conclusions, guided by the therapist
- *Information sheets* (*IS*): Information sheets summarize theoretical content for the patient
- *Worksheets* (*WS*): Worksheets contain tasks for the therapy session or for homework
- *Flipchart*: Indicating which contents should be visualized for better comprehensibility

The corresponding work and information materials are referenced in the relevant place in the manual. These can be adapted to one's own therapeutic needs and style. The modules Working with Caregivers (Module 7), Treatment of Comorbid Disorders (Module 8), and Medicinal Treatment Options (Module 9) differ from the structure shown here, as all three modules can be of general relevance during the entire course of treatment. For the use of the manual a flipchart or, alternatively, a whiteboard and the appropriate pens in different colors are necessary. The sessions should be prepared in a way that corresponds to the selection of the work/information sheets, etc. Homework is mandatory for the patient and should be assigned at regular intervals. If the patient repeatedly does not do the homework, this should be discussed.

4   Organizational and Structural Framework

4.1   Individual Therapy Setting

In the individual therapy setting, a weekly cycle of 50 minutes for approx. one to one and a half years is planned with the regular involvement of the caregivers (frequency depending on necessity). Table 2 illustrates the recommended structure for the sessions. If it is necessary to deviate from the recommended schedule (e.g., bi-weekly double lessons due to long commutes), the time-table shown in Table 2 must be adjusted accordingly. Each session is to be based on the individual problem complex of the patient, thus forgoing the use of a strict time schedule. However, the main part of the therapy session should be primarily focused on the treatment of the central topic of the session.

Flash Feedback Opening and Closing of the Session

Each therapy session begins and ends with a short assessment of the patient's mood (*Flash Feedback*). At the beginning, the patient should give an overview of the issues that currently concern him in a few sentences, e.g., problems or successes since the last session, current thoughts or worries, current mood. As a therapist, ask questions, and structure these narratives if neces-

sary. The "Flash Feedback activity" at the start should serve, on the one hand, to concentrate one's attention in order to be able engage in the therapeutic session. On the other hand, it provides the opportunity to discuss any topics that are currently significant.

Flexibility is crucial! Young patients in particular can find it difficult to ignore everyday events – give them enough space without losing sight of the actual topic of the session. Stay with the patients regarding their current experiences and behavior. It may also be possible to use situations from everyday life to introduce the current topic of the session. At the end of the session, the patient should describe in two to three sentences what he has worked out for himself during the session, what he has taken away with him in terms of content, and if anything occupies him. Otherwise, give him space to assess his mood. If necessary, you as a therapist can then describe your impression of the session – it may be appropriate to praise the patient or to give feedback in cases of problematic behavior in the therapeutic context. If necessary, formulate *take-home messages* together with the patient, and give suggestions for the time outside of therapy, e.g., with regard to the application of the content or behavior addressed in the sessions.

Thermometer Method and Traffic Light Model

An essential component of each lesson is the *Traffic Light Model* or the *Thermometer Method*, used for individual risk assessment. The *Thermometer Method* is easy to learn and use for juvenile patients. At the beginning of each lesson, the patient estimates the current behavioral relevance and intensity of his sexual fantasies about children since the last therapy session by means of a thermometer on a scale of 0–100%, as shown in Fig. 1.

For each patient a flipchart sheet with a thermometer is prepared at the beginning of the therapy, in which each session is recorded (for an example, see Fig. 2). The preparation can also be done together. The patient's assessment should be reflected on together with therapist. During the course of the therapy, a curve of the behav-

Table 2 Basic structure of each therapy session

Procedure	Content
1.	*Flash feedback*: Current mood/current state of well-being? Relevant events during the week?
2.	Progression of (dis)sexual impulses in fantasy and behavior during the last week: Thermometer/traffic light Were there any actual risk situations? Were there sexual assaults (CSA), including the use of CSAI?
3.	Summary of the previous lesson's content and, if necessary, discussion of homework
4.	Working through the topic of the session and, if necessary, preliminary discussion of the homework or imminent risk situations
5.	*Flash feedback*: Current mood/current state of mind?

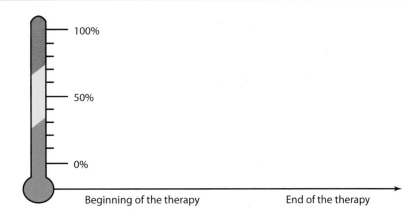

Fig. 1 Illustration of the thermometer method. (Note: For print-related reasons, the illustration is in black and white. The color gradient from green to yellow to red can be seen in the corresponding pdf)

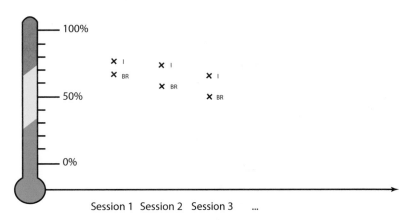

Fig. 2 An example of a progression of the behavioral relevance (BR) and intensity (I) of sexual fantasies with the thermometer method. (Note: For printing reasons the illustration is in black and white. The color gradient from green to yellow to red can be seen in the corresponding pdf)

ioral relevance of dissexual fantasies is then generated, which should be consulted again and again for analysis. In addition, the question of committing CSA or using CSAI should always be explicitly addressed, since these may not be voluntarily reported on their own, e.g., due to reasons of shame. The percentages are used for orientation and are supported by a color-coding scheme. With an increase in behavioral relevance or intensity, there is a corresponding increase in risk. On the one hand, the patients should learn to develop a sensitivity to themselves and their sexual fantasies by continuously observing themselves and reflecting on this with the help of the therapist. On the other hand, they should learn to assess their own risk and to perceive even small nuances in the variation of individual risk. Depending on the individual assessment, various strategies can be developed which can be evaluated for applicability in everyday life.

Even more simplified, the behavioral relevance or intensity of sexual fantasies involving children can be represented by means of the *Traffic Light Method*, if the percentage calculation model is not easily applicable for the patient (general illustration in Fig. 3 and as an example in Fig. 4).

Summary of Previous Content and, If Necessary, Discussion of the Homework

Depending on the cognitive abilities of the patient, the content of the therapy sessions should be repeated with differing degrees of intensity. For this purpose, it is advisable to have the patient briefly repeat the contents of the last session at the beginning of each lesson and, if necessary, to discuss the homework assigned. The therapist should pay attention to the extent to which the contents discussed have been understood and whether there is a need for further work.

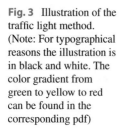

Fig. 3 Illustration of the traffic light method. (Note: For typographical reasons the illustration is in black and white. The color gradient from green to yellow to red can be found in the corresponding pdf)

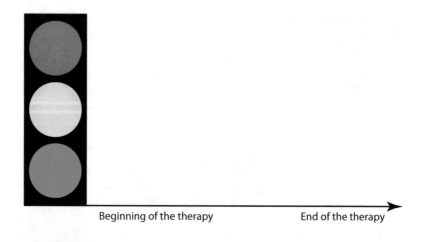

Beginning of the therapy   End of the therapy

Fig. 4 An example of a progression of the behavioral relevance (BR) and intensity (I) of sexual fantasies with the traffic light method. (Note: For typographical reasons the illustration is in black and white. The color gradient from green to yellow to red can be found in the corresponding pdf)

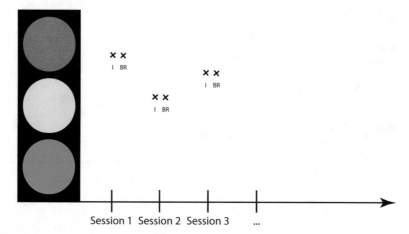

Session 1 Session 2 Session 3   ...

Working Through the Topic of the Session

Each session's topic depends on the current state of therapy. At the beginning of each module, the therapeutic goals should be discussed together with the patient, serving as guidelines. The structure of individual sessions should be adapted to the current topic, and it is up to the therapist to determine the focus.

Flexibility applies here as well. The therapist is not necessarily obliged to carry out all the details of a module. Rather, the focus should be on the individual needs and cognitive abilities of the patient, and, if necessary, some contents may have to be repeated, while others can be briefly summarized. Keep track on a regular basis of your patient's understanding of material, e.g., by asking content-related questions or by having him summarize the session.

Current Masturbation Fantasies

As described in the introduction, because adolescents are in the middle of a cognitive, emotional, and social developmental phase that affects the entire human experience and behavior, and thus also sexuality, the manual recommends recording the patient's current masturbation fantasies at regular intervals. The three-axis model according to Beier et al. (2005) (Module 1–2) can be used for this purpose (Sect. 1.2 in chapter "Modules for Adolescents"). Current sexually arousing fantasies should be regularly reflected upon with the patient, among other things with regard to possible changes and expected consistency. This contributes to the process of integrating and accepting one's own sexual preference structure and may also help reveal potential risk factors, e.g., if a child in the patient's immediate environment appears with increasing frequency in the fantasies.

4.2 Group Therapy Setting

The BEDIT-A is, as explained in the introduction, designed for an individual therapy setting. However, there are no explicit reasons against using it within a group therapy setting. Regarding basic aspects of group therapy work with individuals with a sexual preference for prepubescent and/or early pubescent body age, please refer to Sect. 1 in chapter "BEDIT Manual for Adults". Group therapy offers a number of advantages, predominantly of an economic nature (Warschburger 2006). Group members can also give each other feedback and offer emotional support; problems can be discussed from different standpoints, and solutions can be developed in a collaborative process. Groups serve as a practical training ground, group members act as role models for each other, and the transfer of therapeutic knowledge into everyday life tends to be facilitated by a reduced dependence on therapists. Nevertheless, the limited time resources for working with single patients, as well as potential negative effects from peer interventions (Warschburger 2006), have to be taken into account, the effects of which are particularly noticeable when working with adolescents who have sexual particularities that may be associated with a potentially increased risk to others. Last, but not least, a group therapy with adolescents with a sexual preference for the prepubescent and/or early pubescent body age requires a high degree of openness and trust on the part of the patient. Participation in a group therapy should be discussed explicitly in advance, and the concerns of the individual should be addressed. Even if the advantages of mutual experience and the sharing of one's own emotional burden with individuals with the same fate are to be emphasized in their significance compared to the individual therapy setting, dysfunctional group-dynamic processes must be decisively counteracted. Therefore, small groups with a maximum of four to five patients each (correspondingly less in cases where existing comorbidities such as ADHD [Attention Deficit Hyperactivity Disorder] are present) with two therapists are recommended in order to be able to continually address individual problem situations. Depending on the cognitive capacities of the group, a group session (including a break) should last between 90 and 120 minutes. At the same time, regular individual therapy sessions and accompanying consultations with caregivers should provide space for addressing individual problems.

4.3 Therapeutic Relationship

>>"There's no such thing as good therapy without a good therapeutic relationship." (Borg-Laufs and Hungerige 2005)

An essential component in therapeutic work in general, but especially when working with predominantly (initially) externally motivated adolescents, is the development of a sustainable therapeutic relationship. A functioning therapeutic relationship is also proven to be decisive for the successful treatment of sex offenders (Marshall et al. 2002, 2003). The adolescent should be provided with a corrective and safe bonding experience. Ideally, this is achieved by the therapist establishing a basis of contact and trust, but also by encouraging self-reflection in a safe space. The therapist acts as a role model for developing a positive relationship and bonding experience.

According to Grawe (2000), there are four basic human needs, which individuals strive to satisfy to varying degrees and which are also important in therapeutic relationships:

- Control and Orientation
- Pleasure
- Attachment
- Self-esteem

It is the task of the therapist to work out the individual basic needs of the patient (e.g., by means of plan analyses; see, e.g., Zarbock 2014) in order to continuously evaluate during the therapeutic process which basic needs of the patient remain unfulfilled, so that they may be actively satisfied within the structure of a cooperative relationship. While the concept according to Grawe (2000) is generally valid for therapeutic work with individuals of all ages, according to

Borg-Laufs (2009), general principles for therapeutic work with children and adolescents are: respond to preferences, stay oriented toward abilities and needs, arouse curiosity and fun, design achievable steps, celebrate success (even the smallest), leave room for repetition, introduce small changes, stimulate self-activation, and inquire to seek solutions.

With adolescent patients with regard to relationship-building, one should pay particular attention to the following points (following Borg-Laufs 2009):

- Do not take anything personally.
- Maximum transparency: the therapeutic activities must be comprehensible to the young person.
- Respectful behavior.
- Involvement of the young person in therapeutic decisions.
- Concrete statements, pay attention to the comprehensibility of one's language.
- Flexibility! Current problems and concerns should be recognized and taken into account.
- Ask open questions.
- Actively engage young people's resources (e.g., display photos, listen to music etc.).
- Neutrality.
- Cooperative reinterpreting to increase the capacity to take on new perspectives.
- Maintain sensitivity when dealing with secrets.
- Safeguard the autonomy of the young person.
- Reliability.
- Set reasonable limits.
- Cautious yet open discussion of obstacles.

Apart from the modularized therapy content, the nonspecific effects of general psychotherapy according to Grawe (2000) should also be considered during the entire therapy process, since these not only support the reinforcement of a sustainable therapeutic relationship, but also promote a positive therapeutic outcome:

- *Activation of resources*: The aim is to recognize the individual resources of the patient and to use them actively in order to achieve therapeutic goals.

- *Problem-updating*: If possible, the patient's problems should be dealt with directly in the setting in which they occur, in order to make them immediately perceptible. This effect factor should be handled with extreme caution in view of the potentially harmful effects on others that the sexual preference of these patients can have!
- *Active help in overcoming problems*: The patient should be offered goal-oriented and sensible interventions.
- *Motivational clarification*: The aim is to support the patient in becoming aware of his or her own wishes, goals, and values, but also of disturbance determinants.

Adolescents who are sexually attracted to children are aware of society's attitude toward people with a sexual interest in the prepubescent and/or early pubescent body age. They too must expect therapists to react with negative behavior, e.g., in the form of rejection, mistrust, or reproaches. They may therefore find it particularly difficult to get into contact with therapists or to open up to them. In addition, there is the fear that therapists might pass on what they have been entrusted with to parents or other caregivers.

The therapeutic relationship with the adolescent patient is easy to endanger and should always be assessed for its resilience. It should be noted, among other things, that patients often react to a primarily confrontational therapeutic style with resistance, denying their problems or showing little or decreasing cooperation. For example, they pretend not to have a problem or accept the therapist's point of view without developing an inner insight; in some cases, they may even terminate their cooperation and discontinue the therapy (Beech & Fordham 1997; Kear-Colwell & Pollock 1997; Marshall et al. 2003). It is crucial in the therapeutic process not to give the patient the feeling that he is condemned by the therapist for his non-normative sexual preference. The differentiation between behavior and fantasy should be conveyed according to an authentic therapeutic approach. Successful therapists function as prosocial role models who have a clear style of communication, encourage their patients to change, induce motivation, listen to their patients, offer solutions to problems, increase efforts in a positive way, and identify and enhance resources (Borg-Laufs 2009). In summary and in conclusion, helpful therapeutic qualities are those which promote motivation, as well as interpersonal skills such as empathy, respect, and a meaningful level of directness, warmth, authenticity, and confidence (Marshall et al. 2002, 2003).

4.4 Confidentiality

The issue of confidentiality is of particular relevance when working with adolescent patients and should be discussed in detail with patients and their caregivers. It is the job of a therapist to ensure that both parties have understood and accepted the scope and limits of confidentiality. Above all, the boundary area between the desire for a safe space for the patient and the therapist's duty to inform the persons who have custody over the patient must be discussed in detail. In particular, it must be ensured that the patient understands the circumstances under which confidentiality must be broken.

In principle, the following guideline applies: The patient is the focus of the therapy and therefore has the right to decide whether personal information should be passed on to the person who has custody over him. Adolescents generally react very sensitively when it comes to keeping their "secrets." Therefore, the therapist has to be very careful that the adolescent patient does not perceive the therapist as an agent of the parents. At the same time, it has to be made clear to the patient that the therapist is not his unconditional ally.

An attitude and approach with maximal transparency in both directions is helpful. With the adolescent patient, any upcoming sessions with parents should be discussed in advance. The decision whether he wants to take part in parental meetings should be left to him. It should be discussed with him in advance which topics should be addressed in the course of the parental talks and which aspects should not be communicated. The therapist should clarify with the patient beforehand which subjects he is obliged to inform the parents about. At the same time, it should also

be clarified with the patient that, in an analogous fashion, subjects from the parental meetings will not be passed on to him.

An additional aspect of confidentiality, which has to be discussed with the patient and the caregivers from the start, is the procedure in borderline cases (Sect. 8.5 in chapter "The Berlin Prevention Project Dunkelfeld (PPD)"). In general, it should be noted that in Germany, the prevailing confidentiality obligation for physicians and psychologists (§ 203 Violation of Private Secrets, German Criminal Code) protects the information from patients about previous offenses. The "legal situation prevailing in Germany thus [offers] an extremely favorable starting point for the successful implementation of preventive therapeutic measures to hinder (renewed) child sexual abuse and the (repeated) use of images of abuse" (Beier et al. 2015c, p. 34). The mandatory report law, which prevails above all in Anglo-American regions, is an obstacle to primary preventive treatment services. At the same time, in the event of an imminent threat to the well-being of a child, one should take recourse to the authority anchored within the German Child Protection Act if the necessary conditions have been met.

Above all it is of decisive importance, however, that the procedure for dealing with the adolescent patient's behavior that endangers himself or others is discussed with the patient and the primary caregivers at the beginning of the therapy. The principle of maximum transparency between all parties involved applies here. The therapist should inform all parties at all times about the necessity of any upcoming proceedings. If, for example, the acute endangerment of a child's well-being should arise from the adolescent, the parents as the primary guardians have to be informed, which – even if it goes against the will of the adolescent – has to be discussed with him initially. Should the application of the Child Protection Act be necessary, both the patient and those who have custody must also be informed about this process. In general, in the event of renewed CSA or the use of CSAI during the therapeutic process, the therapeutic connection should be fundamentally questioned and, if necessary, appropriate individual consequences should be determined.

4.5   The First Session

Before the modularized work of BEDIT-A can be initiated, the organizational and formal parameters should be discussed with the patient. It is important to take enough time for this and to respond to the wishes and needs of the patient appropriately.

The following formal general parameters should be discussed with the patient at the outset:

- Beginning, end, and duration of a therapy session
- Scheduled dates
- Rules regarding cancellation of appointments
- Duration of therapy
- Time-schedule
- Confidentiality

The following substantive requirements must be discussed with the patient:

- Motivation
- Transparency
- Reliability
- No verbal and/or physical aggression
- Compliance with the structure (e.g., punctuality)

The agreements reached must be documented in writing with the patient (→ WS *Therapy Contract Patient*; → WS *Therapy Contract Therapist*). Both the therapist and the patient confirm their acceptance of the formal and substantive requirements, providing the patient with a copy of both agreements. Before entering into specific therapeutic work, it is important to formulate and document realistic goals with the patient. The basic precondition for this is that expectations and fears regarding the therapeutic process are initially clarified.

Discussion: The following aspects should be discussed in detail with the patient:

- What do you understand by the term "therapy"?
- Have you ever had any experience with therapy? If so, what positive and negative experiences did you have? What positive and negative expectations do you have?
- What do you expect from the therapy? What do you wish for?
- What fears and worries do you have?
- Which issues are particularly important to you?

Afterward, the primary therapy goals should be discussed:

- Acceptance of one's own – current – sexual preference
- Learning how to deal with one's own – current – sexual preference
- No engaging in acts of sexual assault on children (CSA)
- No use of child abuse images (CSAI or "child pornography")

It should be clearly and unambiguously discussed with the patient that direct or indirect sexual assaults on children during the therapeutic process will not be tolerated. Following the explanation of the general therapy goals, an initial broad overview of the topics of the therapy should be presented. It is recommended to use a therapy folder, which should be prepared by the therapist and the patient together, that the patient can use to file all work material. The folder should be brought by the patient to every therapy session. Finally, the patient should take time to think about his individual problem areas and concrete goals (→ WS *Therapy Goals and Problem Areas*). Therapy goals and problem areas can be worked on together or given as homework. It is necessary to evaluate how realistic the goals are: Is the achievement of the desired therapeutic goals realistic for the individual patient? This has to be examined in a joint discussion with the patient. The goals should be continuously evaluated in the therapeutic process and assessed in terms of their (partial) achievement. For this, a copy will remain in the patient file.

Modules for Adolescents

Working Group of the Prevention Project for Juveniles

Guide to Implementing the Interventions

The material and approaches used in the manual within the context of the interventions are intended to provide structure to the therapeutic work and serve as aids for getting the content across. The following concepts (and abbreviations) will be used:

- **Psychoeducation:** Knowledge imparted by the therapist.
- **Discussion:** Working through the material together to draw conclusions based on the content, led by the therapist.
- **Information Sheets (IS):** Information sheets summarize theoretical content for the patient.
- **Worksheets (WS):** Worksheets contain assignments for the therapy session or homework.
- **Flipchart:** Flipchart indicates which content should be visualized for better comprehension.

Working Group of the Prevention Project for Juveniles
Charité – Universitätsmedizin Berlin, Corporate Member of Freie Universität Berlin, Humboldt-Universität zu Berlin, and Berlin Institute of Health, Center for Human and Health Sciences, Institute of Sexology and Sexual Medicine, Berlin, Germany
e-mail: klaus.beier@charite.de

1 Module 1 – Psychoeducation

Pedophilia is fate, not a choice! This is an important realization that can ease the burden and increase acceptance of a non-normative preference for those affected. Research on the etiology of pedophilia remains thinly differentiated. One can generally assume that it involves an interplay of biopsychosocial developmental factors. In other words, biological predispositions, experiences in one's primary relationships, sexually traumatic experiences in childhood, personality traits, etc., act in combination with one another. In order for therapy to have a helpful effect on people with sexual particularities for the prepubescent body age, it is important to begin by taking a psychoeducational approach to introduce ideas, to bring in concepts as well as differentiate them from one another, to familiarize oneself with the current legal situation, and to develop a concept of the individual's own preference structure.

The overriding **goals** of the **psychoeducation** module are:

- Knowing the legal situation regarding acts of sexual assault according to your country
- Learning to understand general and personal sexual preference structure
- Arriving at acceptance of one's sexual preference.

1.1   Module 1-1: Psychoeducation – Sexuality and Dissexuality

Theory

Adolescence comes with specific developmental tasks that must be dealt with in order to achieve functional psychological development (cf. Fuhrer 2013; Table 1).

It is through confrontations with psychological, physical, and social changes that the adolescent develops into an adult. Health, attractiveness, and physical ability are of great significance, not only for self-perception, but also in regard to developing friendships and romantic partnerships (Fuhrer 2013).

Adolescents enter into their first intimate relationships in order to satisfy their basic psychosexual needs, such as acceptance, emotional security, and closeness. Many teenagers are nevertheless only rudimentarily informed and are not able to draw on real sociosexual experiences. Contrary to the assumption that teenagers are becoming sexually active increasingly earlier, only 27% of 16-year-olds and 47% of 17-year-olds have already had sex in Germany (cf. BRAVO 2016). Approximately half of 14- to 17-year-old boys have already had experience with petting. Although two thirds of all 14-year-olds feel themselves to be generally well informed, a third of them are uncertain on the subject of love and sexuality. A fifth of male 14- to 25-year-olds has experienced insufficient information on sexual violence. With female adolescents, it is more than a third, which attests to the urgency of the subject (Bode and Heßling 2015).

Above all, sexually inexperienced adolescents must receive sex education that gives information about sexual myths, pubertal development, sexual communication, and sexual functions in order to dismantle misconceptions regarding sexuality and romantic partnerships (Beier 2012). Many adolescents who violate sexual boundaries have not been able to acquire socio-sexual experiences with others their own age and do not exhibit sufficient sexual knowledge. This often leads to these mostly-male adolescents being very insecure in their identities (Machlitt 2004). Comprehensive sexual knowledge can also be effective against cognitive distortions (cf. Module 2) and maladaptive convictions.

Goals

- Developing age-appropriate sexual knowledge
- Developing prosocial attitudes toward sexual behavior
- Attaining knowledge about the definition of the term "sexual assault"
- Being able to differentiate between sexual contact with mutual consent and sexual contact without mutual consent
- Learning how to tell the difference between hands-on and hands-off acts
- Being made aware of one's own sexual preference structure
- Attaining a biopsychosocial understanding of one's own sexual preference development
- Internalizing: Your sexual preference is fate, not a choice!
- Reaching acceptance in order to reduce psychological strain

Interventions

Introducing Sexuality

Try to get an impression of whether your patient understands sexual acts as such. Take sufficient time to ascertain what kind of sexual knowledge your patient has. If necessary, use

Table 1 Typical developmental tasks of adolescence (cf. Fuhrer 2013)

Identity	Gaining clarity about what one wants and who one is
Body	Accepting changes in one's body
Gender role	Coming to terms with one's gender role
Relationship building	Building and maintaining close and mature relationships with peers of one's own and the opposite sex
Detachment	Achieving emotional detachment from one's parents
Career	Thinking about one's education/career
Values	Developing one's own world view
Finances	Learning how to handle money independently

the flipchart and create a mind-map together with the patient.

- **Discussion: What do you understand the term *sex* or *sexual acts* to mean?**
Have the patient come up with examples and supplement them if necessary:
  - Unnoticed observation of another person (voyeurism, colloquially "peeping")
  - Making sexual observations or comments
  - Exhibiting and posing (showing one's clothed body in suggestive poses or showing one's naked body demonstratively), with or without masturbation
  - Masturbating to one's own fantasies
  - Intimate touching, e.g., "feeling-up," frottage (colloquially, rubbing), kissing, stroking
  - Inserting one's penis, tongue, finger, or object into someone's vagina, rectum, or mouth
  - Looking at pornographic or erotic material (images, sounds, text), using them for masturbation, making them, or showing them to others
  - Causing someone else to do sexual acts
- **Psychoeducation: Working out the definition of sexual acts:** Sexual acts are first and foremost all acts that are sexually motivated and serve to increase arousal. At least one person is aware of the sexual act. Sexual acts can take place with or without physical contact. With ambiguous acts (e.g., a gynecological exam, or punching a woman in the breast), the deciding factor is whether the act was carried out with the goal of increasing arousal (Otto 2005).

Love, Sex, and Friendship

- **Discussion: Why do people have sex?**
- **Psychoeducation:** Sort the reasons the patient comes up with according to the **3 Dimensions of Sexuality:** *Desire, Attachment, Reproduction* (Beier and Loewit 2011) and clarify them (→ IS *Sexuality*). The learning outcome should be for your patient to understand that sexuality means far more than just the satisfaction of physical-sexual arousal.

- **Discussion: What is the difference between sex, love, and friendship?** If necessary, you may use illustrative examples, e.g.:
  - An 18-year-old goes to a club. He is out looking for a one-night-stand (sex).
  - A married couple is happily celebrating their 20th anniversary with a nice dinner. After the meal, they sleep together (love, sex).
  - A 19-year-old daughter is moving out of her parents' house. Mother and daughter are crying as they say goodbye, and they hug each other tightly (love).
  - Two girls greet each other with a kiss on the mouth (friendship, love, sex?)
- **Discussion: Whom would you like to have sex with? Who do you love? Who do you consider a friend?** The goal is for the patient to learn how to differentiate between the terms *love, sex, and friendship*, and to internalize the respective concepts.
  - *Love* is a very powerful feeling. It is the strongest form of affection toward other living creatures, things, or activities. You might love your parents, your partner, friends, pets, etc. Love is therefore "just" a strong feeling and not a behavior. Love can occur alongside sex or friendship or without them (e.g., parents).
  - *Sex* takes place because of physical attraction or arousal toward another living creature or thing. This can come from love, but it doesn't have to. One can also have sex with oneself (masturbation).
  - *Friendship* is a deep connection between two people where sexuality usually does not play a role. The basis of a friendship can be sympathy, trust, or common interests.
- **Psychoeducation:** Sometimes two people want different things. For example, one wants friendship and the other wants sex. That is why it is important to be able to recognize the difference and not to incorrectly interpret the desire for friendship as sexual attraction or take advantage of it for sex. Check whether it is clear to your patient where and when touching is sexual and where/when it is not sexual.

If you get the impression that the patient is not sufficiently sexually educated, refer to available sex-pedagogical materials and take the time for comprehensive sex education.

Dissexuality and Sexual Assault

- **Discussion/Psychoeducation:** Together with the patient, work through the concepts of *dissexuality* and *sexual assault*. Pay particular attention to cognitive distortions and missing concepts.
  - What does mutual consent mean?
  - What does mutual consent depend upon during sexual contact?
  - How can I tell that the person I'm with wants to be sexual with me?
  - How can I tell that the person I'm with DOES NOT want to be sexual with me?
  - What might dissexuality mean in this context?
- Use the → IS *Dissexuality* as well. The following examples may be helpful in addition:
  - A ten-year-old child who has had sex education lessons in school strips naked and tells you to touch him/her in his/her genital area.
  - A 24-year-old woman with a mental disability asks a neurotypical man to have sex with her.
  - A 15-year-old boy offers oral sex in exchange for money.
  - A 12-year-old girl initiates a plan to meet up with an adult man on the Internet and presents the prospect of spending the night together.
  - A 12-year-old boy is being filmed while masturbating.
  - A 7-year-old girl and a 10-year-old boy are being photographed while the boy puts his finger in her vagina.
- **Psychoeducation:** Explain the following concepts to the patient:
  - *Hands-on* (sexual contact that involves physical contact, such as "feeling up" a child; oral, vaginal, and anal sex).
  - *Hands-off* (telling a child to carry out sexual acts on themselves or on a third person, showing pornography to children; having

sexually suggestive conversations with children; observing children in intimate situations; exposing oneself to children and/or masturbating in front of them; consuming, distributing, possessing abuse images).
- **Psychoeducation:** Discuss with the patient what it means when we talk about child sexual abuse in a legal sense and what this involves (→ IS *Child Sexual Abuse*). Explain to the patient with the aid of → IS *Sex – When and With Whom?* when one is allowed to have sex with people of a different age and under what conditions. Explain the different stages of the COPINE-scale to the patient and explain what it means when we talk about indirect child sexual abuse in the legal sense, according to the current state of affairs (as of May 2017) (→ IS *Illegal Visual Material*). Have the patient sketch out a gradation for this, for example.
- **Discussion: Who commits sexual assault on children and adolescents?** Supplement as necessary:
  - People from all social classes and walks of life
  - People of all ages
  - Women and men
  - As a replacement act for the sexual contact people actually desire with an adult partner
  - People who are not aware of what they are doing (e.g., mental disability)
  - People who have a psychological disorder (e.g., personality disorder, schizophrenia, etc.)
  - People who have a sexual response to the child developmental body scheme

1.2 Module 1-2: Sexual Responsiveness to the Child Developmental Body Age

Theory

A person's sexual preference can be roughly described along three axes: 1) the gender of the desired partner; 2) the physical developmental age of the desired partner; and 3) the nature of the sexual interactions with the desired partner.

These characteristics can be understood on three levels: 1) on the level of sexual fantasies; 2) on the level of sexual behavior; and 3) on the level of one's individual self-concept, whereby self-concept and behavior are often oriented toward social values and can be impacted by social desirability.

Sexual behavior can be further divided into three forms: 1) genital interaction; 2) non-genital interaction; and 3) masturbation (cf. Beier et al. 2005).

Each person has their own individual manifestation form somewhere along the three axes in which they can reach their highest level of desire. If the stimulus pattern deviates from the individual arousal pattern, the same level of intensity of desire cannot be reached. It is assumed that the definitive expression of one's sexual preference occurs during adolescence and remains categorically stable over the course of one's life.

Along the axis of physical developmental age, one differentiates between the sexual preference for the adult, fully developed body scheme (teleiophilia, from the Greek *teleos* – complete, fully grown); the sexual responsiveness to the sexually immature or partially sexually-mature developmental age before the onset of puberty (pedophilia, from the Greek *pais* – child); and the sexual preference for the early pubescent developmental body age (hebephilia, from *Hebe*, the Greek goddess of youth).

Various combination forms frequently occur on the axis of developmental body age preference. Alongside a possible exclusive responsiveness for the child or early pubertal body schemes, arousing fantasies about other developmental body schemes may be present as well. An individual may be, for example, a pedohebeteileiophilic (with responsiveness to all three developmental body ages; Beier et al. 2013; cf. Fig. 1).

Goals
- Gaining knowledge about the general structure of human sexual preference
- Gaining knowledge about one's own sexual preference structure
- Understanding what responsiveness to the child developmental body scheme is and which forms it takes

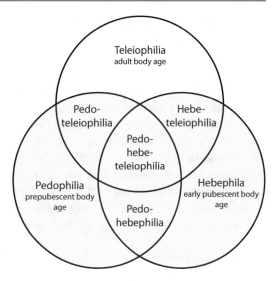

Fig. 1 Sexual Preference for Developmental Body Ages according to Beier et al. (2013)

Interventions
Human Sexual Preference

- **Discussion: What do you understand the term *sexual preference* to mean?**
- **Psychoeducation:** Explain in detail the axes, levels, and forms of the sexual preference structure to the patient using examples and have him fill out the categories with his individual content on the flipchart (→ IS *Sexual Responsiveness to the Child Developmental Body Age*). Use the illustrations of the three developmental body ages according to the Tanner scale for clarification.
- **Discussion: What do you understand "sexual responsiveness to the child developmental body age" to mean?**
  Use the → IS *Sexual Responsiveness to the Child Developmental Body Scheme* for this as well.
- **Homework:** Have the patient repeat the content of the session once more at home. Use the →WS *My Sexual Preference Structure.*
- **Homework discussion:** The patient should present his sexual preference structure during the next session. If any uncertainties having to do with axes, levels, or forms arise, help him out through targeted questioning.

1.3   Module 1-3: The Individual Disorder Model

Theory
There is as of yet no conclusive, generally applicable theory on the etiology of sexual preferences. Different theories include behavioral-theoretical, psychodynamic, or biomedical considerations on the development of paraphilias. In all likelihood, a multidimensional approach will be brought forward that includes biological as well as psychological and social influencing factors (Briken et al. 2013).

Because sexual preference remains stable in its general characteristics over the course of one's life, many people with a sexual responsiveness to the child developmental body scheme experience psychological distress and have already had to come to terms with the impossibility of change. Adolescents in particular often find themselves in the middle of a conflict between the conviction that their sexual interests are just part of a phase and will pass, and the recognition that it may not be as easy to influence their fantasies as they might initially have hoped. While the stability of this orientation is still in dispute, there is at this point no evidence of therapy having the ability to change preference – neither for sex, nor gender, nor for a developmental body age (Seto 2012). Even if we cannot be 100% certain that a preference will never change, the only way out of this psychological distress is acceptance of the current situation. The concept of radical acceptance goes a step further, and involves acceptance of the situation, conditions, needs, thoughts, feelings, and desires (Schwarze and Hahn 2016). Radical acceptance represents an inner attitude that requires a conscious decision. It is a decision in favor of a new path. It is important to recognize that acceptance is not the same thing as endorsement. Suffering comes about only when pain or uncomfortable emotions are not accepted. Thus, once every form of intentional change is avoided, the experience of suffering is unintentionally reduced (Armbrust and Ehrig 2016).

There are three different types of problems or emotional reactions to problems:

1. Solvable problems that provoke uncomfortable emotions
2. Unsolvable problems that provoke uncomfortable emotions that can be modulated
3. Unsolvable problems that provoke uncomfortable emotions that cannot be modulated

Solvable problems should be identified as such and then dealt with. The uncomfortable emotions will dissipate accordingly. Problems that cannot be solved demand a targeted modulation of the emotional reaction. Problems that cannot be solved and whose emotional reactions cannot be changed form a third category. Here, radical acceptance functions as the only way out of suffering ("My child has leukemia. I am horribly afraid. That is the way things are."). Radical acceptance is therefore the ability to be aware of oneself and one's environment, but not to expect that one's person or the environment should be different (Stiglmayr, Lammers, and Bohus 2006).

Goals
- Reaching a biopsychosocial understanding of one's own sexual preference development
- Learning that one's own sexual preference is fate, not a choice!
- Arriving at acceptance in order to be able to make changes

Interventions
The Individual Etiological Model

- **Discussion:** Discuss the following questions with the patient. Make sure to take sufficient time.
  - Since when have you sensed that you are attracted to children?
  - How were you able to tell?
  - Have you ever tried to change something in regard to this?
  - What explanation(s) do you have for your having a particular interest in and being sexually attracted to children?

The Biopsychosocial Model

- **Discussion/Psychoeducation:** Discuss the individual causal areas with the patient by helping them to fill in the three empty circles (biological, psychological, social) with personalized content, in order to be able to come up with hypotheses concerning the development of their own non-normative sexual preference. (Flipchart.)

Can Sexual Preference Be Changed?

- **Psychoeducation:** Explain to the patient that evidence from working with adults with pedophilia indicates that the individual sexual preference structure develops during adolescence and most likely remains an unchangeable part of one's personality. **BUT we do not know this with absolute certainty! We strongly suspect it to be the case!** First, it is important to accept the situation as it is NOW ($\rightarrow$ IS *Can a Sexual Preference for Children Change?*).
- **Discussion/Psychoeducation: What does acceptance mean?** Supplement if necessary:
  – Not fighting against reality.
  – Facing the facts.
  – Taking the situation as it is. Being okay with it.
- **Discussion:** Come up with a list of examples with the patient so that they can come to terms with the idea that there are some goals that are unreachable. Some everyday examples you might use are:
  – "I want to be able to run 100m in two seconds."
  – "I would like to be 2.2m tall."
  – "I would like to be ten years old again."
  – "I would like to get a good report card without having to go to school."
  – "I would like it to be hot and sunny outside, even though it's February and snowing."
- **Psychoeducation:** Explain the model for radical acceptance according to the $\rightarrow$ IS *Radical Acceptance*. **You can use the following wording guide, for example, for clarification**: In order for the suffering to stop, you have to accept the situation as it is. Allow yourself to come to terms with the way things are in this moment. Stop fighting against reality. Acceptance is the only road out of hell. Pain only leads to suffering when you refuse to accept the pain. Acceptance is a decision to endure the moment. Acceptance is recognizing what is. Accepting something doesn't mean that you think it's good. Accepting reality as it is requires a conscious decision. It is as if you have come to a fork in the road. It is then necessary to take the new road of acceptance and to leave behind the road of denying reality (cf. Armbrust and Ehrig 2016).

- **Psychoeducation**: There are three types of problems or emotional reactions to problems:
  1. Solvable problems that provoke uncomfortable emotions.
  2. Unsolvable problems that provoke uncomfortable emotions that can be modulated.
  3. Unsolvable problems that provoke uncomfortable emotions that cannot be modulated. With this kind of problem, radical acceptance functions as the only coping strategy.
- **Use the following examples to illustrate:**
  1. A boy has lied to his friend. He told him that he also wasn't invited to the birthday party of one of their classmates in order not to make his friend sad, but he feels bad about it. He has such a bad conscience that, the day before the party, he calls his friend and says sorry. His friend forgives him. They ask the classmate whether both of them can come. She agrees. The boy is happy and relieved.
  2. A young woman is dumped by her boyfriend. He breaks up with her because he has fallen in love with someone else. She is devastated, stays at home for days, and cries herself to sleep. She thought he was the love of her life. A few days later, she agrees to meet up with her friends and isn't quite as sad anymore. They agree to meet up again the very next day to play volleyball. She notices that the distraction helps. Her broken-heartedness quickly gets better enough that soon she can smile again.

3. A person is confined to a wheelchair after a car accident. She will never be able to walk again. She will have to rely on other people to help her for the rest of her life and will always be confronted with daily challenges. She is furious at the driver who did this to her. She is very sad and wishes she could play soccer again. That is the reality. And those are her thoughts and feelings. It is how it is.

2   Module 2 – Cognitions, Emotions, and Behavior

Cognitions, emotions, and behavior are unavoidably connected. Interpreting situations leads to emotions, and emotions lead to modes of behavior that people display (Dolan 2002). People can have no influence over whether they are in a particular situation or not – not even in therapy. In fact, people often find themselves constantly being in certain situations, e.g., when arriving someplace, when leaving someplace, when meeting people, etc. You also cannot influence whether stimuli reach your sense organs; you see, hear, feel, and taste something at all times. It is only with difficulty that you can influence what you are feeling when you have a particular thought. It is also very difficult for a person to influence how they behave when they feel a certain way. If you are sad, you cry. If you are furious, you scream or rage. If you are happy, you smile. What one can change, however, is how one evaluates a situation and thereby which emotion is triggered within oneself. Working cognitively means having a premise and a goal of being able to evaluate the same situations differently and thereby being able to experience different feelings and modes of behavior (Hofmann 2012).

In order to be able to process the environmental stimuli they receive via the sensory channels, humans must perform an act of interpretation. This is influenced by an individual's attitudes, experiences, personality, but also by sexual preference structure. A person constructs their own subjective reality for themselves (Dember 1990; Margraf and Schneider 2008). Human perception is therefore not objective. Because our perceptions and interpretations are affected by our sexual preference structures (among other things), a person with a sexual attraction to children must be particularly careful not to interpret situations incorrectly. People who feel sexually attracted to children have a tendency to perceive children's neutral interactive behaviors as signs of affection or expressions of (sexual) interest. The very same mechanisms are activated as when a teileiophilic-oriented person is interacting with an adult person they find sexually attractive. This therefore does not (yet) have to do with cognitive distortions, but rather with preference-typical perception errors that primarily occur in people in the state of being in love. Such perception errors should be identified and reflected upon with the patient. The patient must learn to recognize that he perceives these situations in this way because of his own sexual preference and particular need, and that it is not and will never be the case that a child is sending out any kind of communicative request for sexual physical contact. Children never intentionally seek out sexual stimulation, arousal, or desire with adults. These impulses originate solely from the person who is sexually attracted to children, who is often not even aware that this is happening. Being able to understand, correctly perceive, and process this and being able to control one's behavior accordingly is a central cognitive therapy goal.

Therapists know these dysfunctional interpretations as "cognitive distortions," dysfunctional and often automatically occurring thought processes that frequently bring with them unhelpful thoughts and negative emotional states (cf. Ellis 1977). Cognitive distortions (or thinking errors) are systematic distortions in our thinking (Haselton, Nettle, and Andrews 2005). They can help reduce an inner imbalance or inner tension. These can arise, for example, when people are confronted with things that are uncomfortable or that they know are not right. This distorted cognitive reevaluation of perceived reality allows one to endure the state of discomfort, to unburden oneself, and to restore one's internal balance. However, cognitive distortions can also lead to self-deception. According to Wilken (2008), dysfunctional cognitions are different from functional cognitions primarily in that functional cognitions are reasonable, in touch with reality, helpful, and productive. Opposite to these are dysfunctional cognitions or thinking errors. These are unreasonable, not in touch with reality, possibly self-harmful, and neither helpful nor productive.

Cognitive distortions are often present in cases of sexual assault. Specific cognitive distortions serve to stave off responsibility for one's own criminal behavior, as well as the feelings of shame associated with it. In addition, attitudes that enable sexual abuse have a high predictive value for a future-related relapse, and also count among the relevant dynamic risk factors for juvenile offenders (Becker 1990; Kahn and Chambers 1991; Worling and Langton 2012; Bosley and Hiscox 2014).

The process of examining and changing a patient's preference-related cognitions is a facultative element of therapy. It should be brought into play when indications of individual cognitive distortions are deduced during the diagnostic investigation. The overarching goal is to identify cognitions that are (potentially) relevant to the offense and to subsequently dismantle them. These may be:

1. Sexual myths in connection with dissexual behavior
2. Trivializations/minimizations
3. Denial
4. Justification/excuses
5. Attributing blame to the victim

Attributing blame to the victim, above all, is a cognitive distortion that can frequently be observed in juvenile sex offenders (Kahn and Chambers 1991). Motivate your patient to work with you in challenging the cognitions associated with child sexual abuse. The goal is to transform dysfunctional cognitions (e.g., ones that cause harm to oneself or others) into functional cognitions through restructuring interventions. It is also pertinent to tease out the processes that have led to these distorted cognitions. According to Hanson and Bussiere (1998), denial tendencies represent a specific form of cognitive distortions and indicate that the offender is indeed highly aware of his wrongdoing. If the offender were unaware of the problem, he would have nothing to deny. From this perspective, a denial of the offense can also be understood as a resource – in the sense of being an indicator of an awareness of guilt – that can be drawn upon during the therapeutic process.

Cognitive distortions in people with a sexual responsiveness to children can also have a self-esteem-maintaining function, however: "If the child was flirting with me, that means it wanted it that way – I'm not some kind of monster who makes passes at children." If patients did not have this or similar kinds of cognitive distortion, they would be confronted with various negative emotions that they would have to process. If emotions are regulated in a maladaptive way, mental disorders (such as depression or anxiety) may develop as a result. The purpose of psychotherapy is, among other things, to face up to negative emotions and to learn how to process them. The mere act of consciously perceiving or verbalizing one's own emotional state is already very difficult for many people, however. As long as one is unable to correctly assess one's emotional state, one is also unable to choose appropriate coping strategies and put them into practice. It is important to strengthen patients' ability to choose and utilize coping strategies, as Letourneau et al. (2004) have shown that juvenile persons who offend sexually exhibit deficits of (emotional) impulse control. In addition, some juvenile persons who offend sexually have reported that emotional states that are experienced as uncomfortable (boredom, annoyance, rejection, frustration, etc.) function as situational triggers for dissexual behavior (Gray and Pithers 1993).

If people find it difficult to recognize or place their emotions, identifying their physiological reactions may provide a point of access. This is however always merely an indicator that offers additional information, but does not represent a sole source of information for the identification of emotions, as different emotions can be accompanied by the same physiological responses. One's heart rate increases along with fear, for example, but also with happiness or surprise. The goal of psychotherapy is also for patients to become experts on themselves and their problems and to be able to deal with problem situations in the future as independently as possible. For this, it is helpful to know oneself and one's body as well as possible, including one's own physiological responses during sexual arousal.

The overarching **goals** of the **Cognitions, Emotions, and Behavior** module are:

- Elucidating the causal relationships between thoughts, feelings, and behavior for the patient
- Making the reciprocal effect between thoughts and emotions in connection with behavior "come alive"
- Translating this into the context of sexual assault and the use of child abuse images

As the following sub-modules are closely related in terms of content (that has already been illustrated at a higher level), the decision was made to leave out a single representation of the theoretical background.

2.1   Module 2-1: The Behavioral Model

Goals
- Learning to understand that emotions are not caused by situations but, rather, are the result of individual thoughts (i.e., cognitions)
- Building up knowledge about the basic principles of processing information
- Learning and becoming aware of the differences between sensory impressions, interpretations, emotions, and behavior
- Differentiating between self-perception and that of others
- Gaining proficiencies in external perception, increasing the ability to take on the perspectives of others

Interventions
Understanding the Behavioral Model

- **Psychoeducation:** Work through the behavioral model with the patient. Situations lead

to sensory impressions, and these sensory impressions are processed in the brain, from which arise thoughts. These thoughts lead to emotions and physiological reactions/physical sensations that accompany the feelings that arise. Because one is thinking about something and from that a particular emotion arises, one displays a behavior that other people perceive (→ IS *The Behavioral Model*).

- **Discussion:** Remind the patient of your initial session: the first time that both of you walked into the therapy space. That is a situation. In the therapy space, your patient would have seen chairs, perhaps a table. Ask him what else they saw in the therapy space or what they noticed about you as a therapist. These sensory impressions were sent to the brain. What thoughts arose from that? Many patients may have thought, "In a moment, I'll have to tell the whole truth." Others may have thought, "I'll for sure be rejected because of who I am." Others still might have thought, "I need to finally get some help." These thoughts can bring about nervousness or fear in some people. The heart rate increases, one starts to sweat (= physiological reaction/physical sensation). In terms of behavior, someone on the outside might see that the person is fidgeting with his fingers or shifting back and forth in their chair.

- **Psychoeducation:** For the discussion of the individual components of the behavioral model, the definitions introduced in Table 2 may be used.

Consequence of the Behavioral Model

- **Psychoeducation:** Simply being in a certain situation does not lead – as many people assume – to a particular feeling. If you are giving a presentation and everyone laughs, you do not immediately feel nervous or happy – only once you have started thinking and have made an evaluation does a feeling set in. If you are giving a presentation and everyone laughs because you said something wrong, then you evaluate that as being laughed at and feel unsure or anxious because of it. But if you

Table 2 Example definitions for the individual components of the behavioral model

Sensory impression	A sensory impression is the intake and processing of information or environmental stimuli via the sensory organs. The different sensory organs and their functions are:
	Nose → Smelling
	Eye → Seeing
	Ear → Hearing
	Skin → Feeling
	Tongue → Tasting
Thoughts	A thought is the thing that is thought about, or the act of thinking about something, an opinion, a point of view, or a notion/idea.
Physical sensations	All bodily reactions are considered to be physical sensations.
Emotions	Emotions can be described as comfortable or uncomfortable feelings that are only partially consciously experienced. Some examples of emotions would be fear, happiness, or surprise.
Behavior	All actions that can be immediately perceived by others are considered to be behavior, that is, everything that other people can see.

are giving a presentation and everyone laughs because you say something funny, then you evaluate that as reinforcement and feel secure or happy. It should be made clear to the patient that human behavior is a reaction to our feelings. The feelings are in turn the result of (evaluating) thoughts. For the most part, we do not notice these thoughts, because our brain produces them very quickly without our reflecting consciously on them or having to focus our attention on them. The process and consequences of the behavioral model can be worked through in a very vivid way using the example of "receiving a birthday present." This example is a good one for demonstrating that the situation ("receiving a birthday present") does not change. The experienced emotion (e.g., disappointment vs. happiness) is however dependent on the evaluation of the gift ("What's this? A homemade scarf? Again?" vs. "Awesome! I've been wanting this smartphone for ages!"). This means that

the same person can experience different feelings in the same situation – depending on how he evaluates the situation.

- **Discussion:** Once you have worked through the **Consequence of the Behavioral Model** with your patient, go through the model again using a personal example that has to do with sexual fantasies or already-exhibited behavior in connection with sexual contact with children.
- **Homework:** On the worksheet (→ WS *Self-Observation Report on the Behavioral Model*), your patient should describe four situations using the behavioral model that have led to thoughts, emotions, and behavior. The homework should not repeat situations that were used in the session.

2.2 Module 2-2: Perception

Goals
- Acquiring knowledge concerning the principles of perception and processing information
- Gaining skills in perception-control
- Working through the concept of perception
- Learning how to differentiate between perception and evaluation
- Identifying influencing variables on perception

Interventions
Review and Psychoeducation

- **Psychoeducation/Discussion:** Have your patient review the definition of the term **"sensory impression"** and the different sensory organs. Afterwards, work through the difference between a pure sensory impression and the evaluation of this sensory impression together using an example
- **One possible example of how to work through this can be seen in** Table 3.
- **Psychoeducation:** Together with the patient, come up with a list of adjectives for the other sensory impressions that describe the interpre-

Table 3 Example work-through of the difference between a pure sensory impression and its evaluation

Therapist:	"Can you please review for me again which sensory organs we have as humans?"
Patient:	"We have eyes, ears, skin, a tongue, and a nose."
Therapist:	"Very good. Thank you. The nose is a good example; it is a sensory organ. But what do we do with our nose?"
Patient:	"You smell with your nose."
Therapist:	"Absolutely! We smell with our nose. That is a sensory impression. Some smells we find pleasing, others not so much. Can you come up with any examples?"
Patient:	"Some flowers smell good. Or my deodorant. Not so good… burnt plastic. Or vinegar."
Therapist:	"How would you describe the smell of your deodorant? Is it fragrant? Fresh?"
Patient:	"I wouldn't exactly say fragrant. But fresh is about right. Yeah, it's fresh."
Therapist:	"And what does vinegar smell like to you?"
Patient:	"Vinegar smells sharp. Or burning."
Therapist:	"Ah, okay. So you had the smell in your nose, it gets sent to your brain, and there, you evaluated that smell: You interpret your deodorant as fresh and vinegar as sharp or burning. Is that right?"
Patient:	"Yes, exactly."

Table 4 Example evaluations for sensory impressions

Sensory organ	Sensory impression	Evaluation
Nose	Smell	Fragrant, fresh, sharp, burning, rotten, etc.
Eye	Seeing	Light, dark, blinding, glistening, etc.
Ear	Hearing	Loud, quiet, shrill, muffled, etc.
Skin	Feeling	Hot, cold, scratchy, soft, pointy, dull, etc.
Tongue	Taste	Spicy, sweet, salty, sour, umami

tations of these impressions qualitatively. A couple of examples for the interpretation of different sensory impressions can be found in Table 4.

- **Psychoeducation:** Your patient should understand that the evaluation of sensory impressions is a part of human perception. Perception is itself a process by which we interpret the world and the things around us. It is a complex process of gaining information through processing environmental stimuli according to subjective criteria. Perception is never objective, due to individual experiences and previous learning processes. Every perception is automatically associated with an evaluation (= thought, in the behavioral model). Work through the idea with the patient that there are additional factors that influence our perception, e.g., health, mood, traits, immediate needs like hunger or thirst. The information sheet → IS *Perception* may be used.

- **Discussion:** One can also differentiate between undirected and directed perception.
  - **Undirected Perception:** Typical situations would be the first day at a new school, or arriving at a birthday party where you only know the person whose birthday it is and none of the other guests. What would you perceive? The gender of the other guests, how many of them there are, what they're wearing, whether they're heavy-metal fans, hipsters, nerds, athletes?
  - **Directed Perception:** A typical example is when you are out walking and you desperately have to go to the bathroom: You are on the look out for a bathroom and are trying to decide which shop, take-out place, restaurant might have one – you might easily fail to notice how many women in a red skirt have walked by, or how many people were talking in a foreign language.

Sexual Preference and Perception

- **Psychoeducation:** Your patient now knows that perception is the subjective evaluation of sensory impressions. These evaluations vary from person to person – although sometimes many people will arrive at a similar evaluation. Have your patient discuss whether a person's sexual preference also influences his perception.
- **Discussion:** Your patient will, with some guidance, come to the conclusion that sexual preference does indeed have a significant influence on perception. A man attracted to the opposite

sex might pay attention to a woman's breasts, while a man attracted to the same sex might ignore them. Many people pay more attention to people with dark hair because they find this to be "hot," "sexy," or "good-looking." In turn, these people might not notice the children playing on the playground, or see them differently from your patient. The influence of sexual preference is also an example of directed perception. This can extend to someone interpreting situations differently depending on their sexual orientation. It is sometimes the case that people who are sexually attracted to children incorrectly interpret the behavior of children as sexual interest. Non-sexual situations are then interpreted by adolescents or adults as sexualized. A classic example is the statement: "If the seven-year-old didn't want me to get an erection, why did she sit on my lap?" – Have your patient come up with an answer. What possibilities could there be? Was she scared and came and sat on your lap because she needed protection? Did she want to play?

- **Homework:** Using the worksheet (→ WS *Self-Observation Report on Perception*), have your patient analyze his behavior in at least two situations in which they noticed their sexual arousal in response to children.

2.3   Module 2-3: Thoughts and Thought Biases

Goals
- Changing dysfunctional perception, thought, and attitude patterns
- Getting better at taking responsibility for one's own behavior and learning to establish this in everyday life
- Understanding that psychological stress, emotional strain, or problems arise through subjective interpretation and evaluation processes
- Identifying and modifying attitudes that facilitate sexual assault

Interventions
Working on the Concept of Cognitive Distortions (Mistaken Thoughts)

- **Psychoeducation**: As learned in the behavioral model, human behavior is influenced by thoughts and/or assessments of situations. The way you think about something also influences how you feel about it. These processes happen very quickly so that one can make an assessment of situations in a very short time. Therefore, sometimes automatic thoughts or evaluations can occur that are not helpful (i.e., dysfunctional) (→ IS *Mistaken Thoughts*). A mistaken thought is a distorted thought or belief that has little to do with truth or reality. It is a mistake, a wrong conclusion, or a misjudgment. Errors in thinking often lead one to do things that only give pleasure, are irresponsible, and may possibly hurt oneself and others. Mistaken thoughts assist one in avoiding responsibility, persuading oneself to do something, or justifying selfish actions (according to Stuyvesant et al. 2014).

- **Psychoeducation**: Automatic thoughts and cognitive distortions arise from basic assumptions that every person develops in the course of his or her life ("How do I explain the world and other people to myself?"). Usually these dysfunctional thoughts are not the result of reasoning or logical thinking and therefore will not be examined for their truthfulness and validity. Often these thoughts are not conscious. However, these thoughts are followed by feelings that one is very well aware of and that one will remember. Therefore, it is often wrongly assumed that a situation leads to a feeling, when in fact a situation leads to a thought, and this thought leads to a feeling.

Working on the ABC Scheme

- **Psychoeducation**: According to Wilken (2008), the process of cognitive restructuring consists of five steps:
  1. Communicating the cognitive model
  2. Revealing the dysfunctional cognitions
  3. Interrogating the dysfunctional cognitions
  4. Developing appropriate functional cognitions
  5. Training of the functional cognitions as part of a coping strategy

- **Discussion**: A suitable way to deal with cognitive distortions is the ABC scheme (→ WS *The ABC Scheme*). Work with the patient to develop alternative thoughts and alternative feelings for an example situation that involved cognitive distortion. In practice, it has been shown that for patients, it is easiest to work in this order "situation (A), feeling (C), evaluating thought (B)." The following examples can be helpful for your patient and provide psychoeducational information about typical distortions:

  1. **A student is given the problem sheet for the math test by the teacher. He looks at the first problem and thinks: "I am a failure."** (Arbitrary conclusion: self-deprecation occurs without checking whether the task or other subsequent tasks are at all solvable. The conclusion is made arbitrarily, without any evidence.)

  2. **A student interprets the fact that her classmates do not ask her if she would like to have lunch with them as "my classmates do not like me." She overlooks the fact that everyone greets her regularly.** (Selective generalization: Individual facts are taken out of the whole context and overemphasized. Other facts that contradict them are ignored.)

  3. **One teenager is the only person who doesn't dare jump from the 3-meter diving tower in the swimming pool and thinks to himself: "The others think I'm a loser**." (Mind reading: You assume you know what other people think about you without sufficient evidence.)

  4. **A trainee is criticized by his boss for a mistake and thinks to himself: "The boss doesn't like me. It must be because of me."** (Personalizing: External events are taken extremely personally without any evidence.)

  5. **A young person is about to take an important exam and thinks to himself: "If I don't pass this exam with an "A," I will never get an internship."** (Catastrophizing: People always think of the worst that could happen. Extremely

negative predictions are made without considering other possibilities).

- **Psychoeducation**: The patient should be made aware that feelings and behavior do not arise from situations, but from the assessments of these situations. After working through general everyday examples, you should now discuss concrete, (in)direct abusive behavior with your patient. Make the patient understand that sexual assault is preceded by motivation and planning. This often includes cognitive error chains (a series of flawed evaluations that preceded the sexual assault). The patient should learn that recognizing and changing dysfunctional cognitions is the basis for identifying future risk factors.

- **Homework**: Give the patient the → WS *The ABC Scheme* and ask them to document two situations for the next session, in which they observe their own thoughts and then tries to find an alternative, possibly more-helpful way of thinking about the same situations. Only then should the patient work through the → WS *Mistaken Thoughts in Child Sexual Abuse*. Only after this should the patient should work on the → WS *Mistaken Thoughts in Child Sexual Abuse*.

Handling the Denial of Sexual Assault

A special case presents itself when patients deny having committed sexual assault. O'Donohue (2014) proposes the following scheme for classifying the degree and nature of the denial:

- Complete denial of assault
- Denial regarding the extent of the assault
- Admitting the assault, but denying responsibility for the assault
- Denial of intent (for example, the touch was unintentional)
- Denial of the negative degree of the assault
- Denial of having planned the assault
- Denial of the possibility of relapse
- Denial of any problem related to the assault (e.g., alcoholism, problematic cognitions)
- Denial of the need for therapy

If the patient denies his offense out of shame, you as a therapist can use the following strategies:

- Differentiating the perpetration from the rest of the person: The act is only one aspect of you!
- Proceed by taking small steps using only a slightly-confrontational approach without pressing for details.
- Positive reinforcement of any efforts on the part of the patient.
- Examining the feared consequences of disclosing the crime.
- Assure the patient you will not reject him.

2.4   Module 2-4: The Emotions (Part I: Constitutive)

Goals
- Recognition of one's own feelings
- Working through basic feelings and the meaning and function of feelings
- Learning and/or strengthening of intervention skills

Interventions
Repetition and Psychoeducation

- **Discussion**: Have the patient repeat the definition of the term "feeling." Work together with your patient to demonstrate that a person''s ability to feel is innate (even people born blind smile when they are happy).
- **Psychoeducation**: However, many people find it difficult to admit, feel, or name their feelings. A division into "good" and "bad" feelings is too unspecific and provides too little information. Many people would say that fear and anger are "bad feelings," but only when one recognizes these two feelings in others can one know how to behave. If one only recognizes a "bad feeling," one does not yet know how one can behave.
- **Discussion**: Gather feelings from your patient that they know well about themselves. If the patient finds it difficult to name feelings on

their own initiative, they should use the → IS *List of Feelings* to help. How does your patient recognize these feelings? What physical sensations are associated with them? Work with them on the chart represented on → WS *Perception of Feelings* regarding a feeling he or she knows best. What are their physical sensations? What is their posture? What do they notice in their voice? What expressions do they make? What thoughts do they have, and how do they behave?

- **Discussion**: Afterward, read the individual examples to your patient on the → WS *Identifying Feelings*, and they should name the feelings of the underlined persons. The aim here is to identify the primary feelings. According to Ekman (1982), seven primary feelings are assumed, which people all over the world, regardless of culture or language, feel: anger, disgust, joy, sadness, contempt, surprise, and fear.

The Importance of Feelings

- **Discussion**: Ask your patient to repeat how feelings arise. Discuss with them what feelings are useful for. Why do people feel fear? What if you were not afraid? The meaning of feelings can best be worked out using the example of a Stone Age man meeting a saber-toothed tiger. What does the Stone Age man see and hear (sensory impression)? What does he perhaps think ("The animal can tear me to pieces," "I am going to die")? What feeling does this thought (fear) lead to? What physical symptoms does this feeling trigger? And what behavior is demonstrated? Feelings have a function: they show that something is important. If you are afraid of a predator, then something important is at stake: life. If you are afraid of an exam, then it is also about something important: your grade. If you love someone, then that person is important. If you mourn for someone or something, it is because the person or thing was/is important (→ IS *Importance of Feelings*).
- **Psychoeducation**: Your patient should understand that feelings...

– Motivate us to do or not do something
– Activate or suppress our behavior
– Help us with our orientation and, if necessary warn us
– Help us to communicate and interact with other people
– Confirm our perception

Attitude Toward Dealing with Feelings

• **Discussion**: Ask the patient to read the → WS *Attitudes Toward Dealing with Feelings* and check off any statements they agree with. If necessary, ask the patient to add further attitudes of their own. The → WS *Attitudes Towards Dealing with Feelings* can also be given as homework. Then afterward, discuss with your patient what consequences follow from the respective attitudes on the worksheet when one finds them convincing. This step can also be diagnostically valuable: If your patient affirms one of these statements, it is recommended that you work on these attitudes using cognitive techniques. Through guided discovery, your patient will realize that these statements represent dysfunctional ways of dealing with feelings.
• **Homework**: The patient should complete the → WS *Perception of Feelings* using three other basic feelings, and also work on the WS *Feelings in Conflict Situations with Children*.

2.5   Module 2-4: Regulation of Emotions (Part II: facultative)

Goals
• Learning to functionally manage strong emotions
• Learning exercises for emotion control and establishing these in everyday life
  In this section, the patient is taught skills to deal with strong emotions in a functional way. This is only therapeutically indicated if, to your knowledge, the patient has deficits in the regulation of emotions.

Interventions
Psychoeducation

• **Discussion**: Discuss with your patient how they react in emotionally difficult situations. Which strategies (inner dialogues, time-out, thought stop, distraction, relaxation strategies) does your patient use to stay calm and controlled? Do they use any at all?
• **Psychoeducation**: Explain to your patient that there are different strategies they can use to not lose control or "freak out," and that they should choose one or two options that they find appealing and wants to learn.
  – Calm oneself
  – Leave the situation (change of scene)
  – Consciously stop the thoughts that, for example, are making one angry
  – Do relaxation exercises (e.g., progressive muscle relaxation)
  – Create a counter-stimulus.
  – Exchange the negative feeling.
  – The safety-vault drill.
  – The examination of strong feelings.
  – Wait, i.e., do not follow the first impulse.
  – – Creating distance: reality check, observation and description, imagination (black-and white-technique, magnifying glass technique, etc.).
  – Encouragement through a positive self-instruction: "I am not the feeling, but I have a feeling that I can influence."
  – Change via imagination (making good memories), shifting attention, acting in the opposite direction.
Some of the exercises mentioned are explained in detail below.

Example Exercise (1) for Emotion Control: Setting Up a Counter-stimulus

• Give the patient a bag of pop rocks or something similar. Explain that now an exercise will follow in which the patient's own perception of feelings can be changed by means of a counter-stimulus.
• Inducing relaxation: Sit upright but comfortably. Try to have contact with the floor with

your feet. Can you feel the floor? Now close your eyes. Take a deep breath and allow yourself plenty of time to exhale. Concentrate on your breath. Breathe in and out calmly.

- The patient should now remember a situation with a strong feeling: Now try to remember an event that is associated with a strong feeling for you. Which situation do you remember? Do you have a picture in mind? Take a good look. Where are you? What do you see, feel, and smell? Now concentrate on your feelings. If you feel several, choose one. Stay with the feeling. It can be a pleasant or an unpleasant feeling. Which bodily sensation do you associate with it? If you have the situation clearly in front of you and the feeling is clearly perceptible for you, then take the effervescent tablet (or alternative) in your mouth. What do you taste now? How does it feel in your mouth? Concentrate completely on your experience in your mouth; when sucking, swallowing. What are you thinking? What would you like to do most now? Which feeling do you have now? How intense is the feeling from the memory journey now? Come slowly back into the room. Pay attention to the noises around you. You can open your eyes now.
- Evaluate the exercise with your patient. The following questions may be helpful:
  - What was your initial feeling?
  - How well were you able to experience this feeling?
  - What happened when the counter-stimulus (effervescent tablet) came?
  - What happened to the initial feeling?
  - Were there any difficulties?
  - What was helpful?
  - What could be additionally helpful?

Example Exercise (2) for Emotion Control: Exchanging the Feeling

- **Discussion**: Ask the patient to remember a situation in which they felt a very strong feeling and then together carry out an emotional analysis using the following criteria:
  - What was the feeling?

- How strong was the feeling (on a scale of 0–100%)?
- How did you know that it was exactly this feeling?
- Why did you get exactly this feeling in this situation? What effects did this feeling have on you?
- Which thoughts did you have?
- Did these thoughts amplify the feeling? Were these thoughts helpful?
- What kind of behavior did you exhibit?
- What were the negative consequences of the feeling/behavior?
- What were the positive consequences of the emotion/behavior?

- **Discussion**: Now ask the patient to consider whether they could have felt differently in the same situation, and ask the same questions again. Make it clear to the patient that one and the same situation can trigger different feelings, which is related to a different evaluation of the situation and consequently leads to different behavior and, therefore, different consequences.

Other Methods/Exercises for Dealing with Strong Feelings

- If necessary, you can now teach the patient further ways to control his or her strong feelings independently or to deal with them functionally. These include:
  - Safety-Vault exercise (→IS *The Safety-Vault Exercise*)
  - Progressive muscle relaxation(→IS *Progressive Muscle Relaxation*)
  - Checking strong emotions (→IS *Checking Strong Emotions*)
  - Wait, i.e., do not follow the first impulse
  - Creating Distance via: reality check or observation and description
  - Imagination exercises
- **Homework**: The patient should repeat the recently learned exercise using a different situation. Please also use the next sessions to keep asking about the newly learned exercise and its effectiveness. The aim is to enable your patient to regulate his emotions.

2.6   Module 2-5: The Body Experience

Goals
- Become an expert on your own body and its reactions
- Learn to understand that feelings are always involuntarily accompanied by physical symptoms
- Learn to recognize that there are no specific physiological reactions to emotions

Interventions
Development of Physiological Reactions Through Repetition

- **Psychoeducation/Discussion**: Repeat the behavioral model with your patient. This time the starting situation is the repetition of a familiar example: a Stone Age man who suddenly finds himself in front of a saber-toothed tiger. Have the patient repeat what sensory impressions the Stone Age man probably has, what he probably is thinking, and to what feeling this thought could lead. What physical symptoms are associated with this feeling and what behavior results from it? Expected physical symptoms of fear are: rapid breathing, sweating, pupil dilation, dizziness, dry mouth. Not only do feelings have a function, but the physical symptoms associated with feelings also have a meaning: the Stone Age man had to make a choice: Do I fight the predator or run away? Fight or Flight? For both behavioral options, you need your body and your muscles (similar to sports), and these physical symptoms are the preparations, the warming-up of the body, so to speak.

Working on Physiological Reactions to Sexual Desire

- **Psychoeducation/Discussion**: With the → WS *Bodily Experience with Sexual Desire* the physical sensations of the patient during sexual desire should be worked through. Where does your patient feel sexual desire? How do they notice their sexual desire? A typical response in males is: "Because I have an erection." Discuss with your patient in a psycoeducative way that an erection is the dilation of the blood vessels in the erectile tissue, thus increasing blood flow into the penis. Ask him if he is familiar with situations where he experiences sexual arousal or pleasure but has not had a full erection (e.g. because attention has shifted and a new sensation has occurred). Sexual desire can lead to an individual combination of physiological reactions in every person. Your patient should understand which symptoms accompany his sexual desire. This can also be linked to the homework assignment for the next session of observing what happens to his body during masturbation when desire increases and orgasm occurs or shortly after orgasm (increased heartbeat, sweating, faster breathing, etc.)

2.7   Module 3-1: Sexual Fantasies and Behavior

Theory
Studies on adults have shown that sexual particularities are a risk factor for committing or relapsing into sexual assault. Therefore, the non-normative sexual-particularity characteristics occurring in adolescents should be given as much attention. However, several factors determine whether fantasy turns into behavior, such as socio-affective deficits, abusive attitudes, and problems of emotional regulation (Kuhle, Schlinzig and Beier 2015). In premodern societies, the cognitive preconditions for the understanding of law as it prevails today were missing. It was considered perfectly normal to punish people for their fantasies and attitudes without any action having been taken. However, fantasies are not dangerous if one has learned to recognize them early on, to assess them, and to control one's behavior accordingly (Holmes 2006). In addition, according to studies from the *Hellfeld*, about 60% of sexual assaults on children are committed by people who have no sexual response to the child developmental body age and who sexually abuse the child as a "substitute"

for adult partners who are actually the ones desired (Seto 2008).

Goals

- Become an expert regarding your own sexual fantasies
- Learning that sexual fantasies can and must remain on the fantasy level if they include potentially harmful content to others
- Learning to recognize when sexual fantasies potentially harmful to others are forcing their way onto the behavioral level and how to interrupt this
- Working out the role of various external and internal influences (triggers) that lead to sexual fantasies that are dangerous to oneself or to others pushing onto the behavioral level and how they can be a preparatory element for the offense
- Identifying resources for sexual impulse control

Interventions

Sexual Fantasies – Intensity

5 Psychoeducation/Discussion: By means of the thermometer or traffic light method explained above, the therapy process is continuously provided with a visualized measure of the action relevance and intensity of the patient's fantasies (Sect. 4 in chapter "BEDIT-A Manual for Adolescents"). Together with the patient, repeatedly establish an overview of the progression of the curve. Work out factors that lead to an increase or decrease in the intensity/action relevance of the fantasies.

What Increases the Urge to Act on Sexual Fantasies?

- **Discussion**: Why could it be useful, to know one's own sexual fantasies well? Work out the following points for the patient to memorize. You can also use → IS *Sexual Fantasies*.
  1. Becoming an "expert" on your own sexual fantasies protects you from surprises. This reduces fear.
  2. Knowledge means gaining competence and entails an increase in self-awareness.
  3. In this manner, you can monitor if fantasies change or stay the same.

4. The more you know about your sexual desires and needs, the sooner you'll also recognize when a wish arises to want to realize fantasies. Because if fantasies just remain fantasies, nobody gets hurt. But only you can make sure of this.
5. With masturbation to the most exciting fantasy you have the greatest gain in pleasure.

- **Discussion**: The following questions should be worked through in detail with the patient. Particular attention should be paid to cognitive distortions and/or abuse-enabling attitudes.
  - **To what extent have you already succeeded in controlling your desire for sexual contact with children and managed not to live out your child-related sexual fantasies in your behavior?** (So is there already an awareness of the distinction between fantasy and behavior?)
  - Have you ever had the impression that the urge to live out your child-related sexual fantasies becomes stronger when you are in an unpleasant emotional state? In other words, is there a higher risk of actually living out your child-related sexual fantasies (i.e., committing a sexual assault) when you are angry, lonely, or sad?
  - **Have you ever had the impression that the urge to live out your child-related sexual fantasies becomes stronger when you get into certain situations**, e.g., when you are alone at home or passing by a playground?
  - **Psychoeducation**: It is important for your patient to learn about the inner and outer "triggers" that can lead him to live out his sexual fantasies at the behavioral level. These triggers can represent his own personal risk factors.
  - **Internal Triggers**: Triggers within a person that no one else can perceive (for example, feelings such as anger, fear, hopelessness, loneliness, etc.)
  - **External Triggers**: Triggers outside of a person that other people can also perceive (for example, the presence of a child).
  - Now work out with the patient his individual internal and/or external triggers for fan-

tasies involving sexual contact with a child that amplify the urge to act on them (→ WS *My Triggers*). Identify which factors weaken or increase the urge to act in these fantasies (situations, emotional states, actions, thoughts, etc.) To do this, the patient should evaluate each trigger again according to its risk potential.

- **Homework**: For the next session, ask the patient to write down a sexual fantasy with children that is well known to him. For this task, hand out the → WS *My Sexual Fantasies with Children* and discuss the homework instructions.

Sexual Fantasies – Analysis

- **Homework Review**: Ask the patient to read aloud his sexual fantasy. Make sure that the 5-W questions and the 5 levels have been taken into consideration. If necessary, ask more detailed questions to get an even more vivid picture of the described sexual fantasy. If the patient states that he has no sexual fantasies or cannot remember them, you can ask, for instance:
  - Report on the sexual fantasies that arose during your last masturbation.
  - What do you think about when you see a child you find sexually attractive? What do you like about the child? What would you like to do with the child?
  - What sexual thoughts or fantasies did you have when you were younger?
- **Discussion/Psychoeducation**: Now use the patient'\'s written description to analyze, for example, the following aspects of the sexual fantasy by asking the patient for more details. (Urbaniok and Endrass 2006):
  1. **Action Threshold:** How **recognizable** is it for the patient (and the therapist)? How constant does the threshold remain depending on internal and external influences? If an action threshold is low or permeable, the risk is higher that the fantasy gains action relevance in the short or long term.
  2. **Degree of Concretization**: Does the sexual fantasy refer to a real existing child

who may be well known to the patient? Or are children that are known to the patient from media (photos, videos, magazines) incorporated here? Does the perpetrator in the fantasy overcome real potential obstacles, thus including in the fantasy a preparatory run-up to the crime? Are the fantasies becoming more and more differentiated? A high degree of concretization indicates that the patient is already imagining what it would be like to live out this fantasy in behavior.

There are other characteristics of sexual fantasies (Urbaniok and Endrass 2006) that can be checked in order to assess whether and when the patient's child-related sexual fantasy becomes action-relevant:

3. **Quantity**: the time spent on certain fantasies and the duration of a fantasy, restriction of fantasy activity to certain situations, e.g., only when the patient is at home, or increased impairment of certain activities, etc.
4. **Quality**: the degree to which the fantasy is developed – from simple isolated thoughts to highly differentiated scenarios
5. **Intensity**: affective impact produced by a sexual fantasy
6. (previous) **Predictive Quality**: if assessable, the influence that the sexual fantasy or the estimated urge to act had on criminal behavior that has already taken place
7. **Controllability**: the degree to which a patient is able to control impulses to act that relate to offense-relevant fantasies
8. **Control Motivation**: the extent to which the patient is willing to control his impulses to act

2.8 Module 3-2: Consequences of Behavior

Theory

Decision-making processes take place continuously and lead to desired and/or unwanted, short-term and long-term, positive and/or negative behavioral consequences. With operant conditioning, one achieves a change in the probability of occurrence of certain behavior through its consequences. More precisely, positive consequences, or the elimination of negative consequences, increase the probability of occurrence of certain behavior. While negative consequences, or the disappearance of positive consequences, lead to the suppression of behavior (Rinck and Becker 2011). Thus, in order to suppress a certain behavior (direct sexual assault or the use of abuse images), it is first necessary to make visible and analyze short-term and long-term consequences. Child sexual abuse always has emotional, psychological, and social consequences for perpetrators, victims, and the respective environments (Kuhle, Schlinzig and Beier 2015).

Although operant conditioning has been studied primarily in animals, it is also omnipresent in humans. In order to survive, every organism must learn to identify connections between its own behavior and its consequences and then to optimize its behavior in such a way that agreeable consequences are maximized and negative are consequences minimized. One factor that should not be neglected is that short-term consequences influence us more than long-term consequences, which is why smokers, for example, repeatedly reach for a "relaxing" cigarette, even though this increases their risk of lung cancer in the long term. Over time, however, our ability to cognitively process these connections, to expect them, and to make them accessible through observation increases (Rinck and Becker 2011).

Goals

- Every behavior/decision has consequences
- Increasing sensitivity to the consequences of one's own actions
- Being able to distinguish between short- and long-term positive and negative consequences
- Recognizing that positive short-term consequences are often the trigger for action, but that negative consequences predominate in the long term
- The long-term negative consequences of direct/indirect sexual assault are more significant than the short-term positive consequences

Interventions
Introduction to Consequence Analysis

- **Discussion/Psychoeducation**: What do you understand by the term "consequence"? Every decision has consequences. Decisions can always have positive and/or negative consequences. These could be the reactions of other people or other kinds of results. Short-term consequences can be very different from long-term ones. Example: "I studied a lot (behavior), which is why I did not have time to play (negative short-term consequences). For this I got an "A" on the math test (positive long-term consequence)."
- **Discussion**: **What effect do a lack of self-control or impulsive decisions ("from the gut") have on daily life?** If necessary, include: harming yourself and others (e.g., starting a fight), coming into contact with the legal system (e.g., stealing), delays in achieving long-term goals (e.g., snacking although you want to lose weight). Explain the consequence analysis scheme to the patient using → IS *Consequences of Behavior*.
- **Discussion**: Use concrete examples to work out together what short-term and long-term advantages and disadvantages or positive and negative consequences behavior can have (flipchart). Use the 4-field schemata for this purpose (→ IS *Consequences of Behavior*). Start with general examples:
  - Eating a whole box of cookies
  - Truancy
  - Giving someone a gift
  - Studying for an exam
  - Getting drunk
  - Smoking
  - Stealing something
- **Continued Discussion**: In the next step, continue the discussion with terms relating to responsiveness to the child body age:
  - Playing with little girls/boys
  - Masturbation
  - "Hands-off" assault
  - "Hands-on" assault
- **Useful Examples of Short-term Advantages and Disadvantages Are:**

- **Advantages**: sexual gratification, power, feelings of relaxation and relief; avoidance of loneliness, emptiness, and boredom; pleasure in life, bonding and closeness, tenderness, security, love, curiosity, creativity
- **Disadvantages**: guilt, bad conscience, shame, fear of being discovered, disgust, defeat, loneliness, no time for other hobbies, sleeplessness, damage to victims, punishment
- **Useful Examples of Long-term Advantages and Disadvantages are:**
  - **Advantages**: pleasure in life, bonding and closeness, tenderness, security, curiosity, creativity
  - **Disadvantages**: Depression, guilt, damage to victims, panic attacks, criminal charges, imprisonment, fines, disappointed community, social ostracization or exclusion, loneliness, placement in a home
- **Discussion**: This can also be externalized using the two-chair method: as the therapist, you sit on the "pro" chair, and the patient sits on the "con" chair. The advantages and disadvantages can now be discussed together. Then the roles are reversed. Alternatively, your patient can sit once on the "pro" chair and once on the "con" chair, and you remain in a neutral, interviewing position in each case.
- **Psychoeducation**: The result should be the realization that the short-term advantages usually trigger action, but often do not last very long. In the long term, the disadvantages often outweigh the impulsive actions. Therefore, it is important not to immediately give in to one's immediate need for sexual contact with a child (directly or indirectly), but to first consider what immediate and subsequent consequences this may have for oneself and for others.
- **Homework**: Give the patient the → WS *Consequences of Sexual Contact with Children* and ask him to delve deeper into the topic of the lesson by thinking further about short- and long-term advantages and disadvantages and writing them down.

- **Discussion**: Is there anything about your own current behavior, associated with a sexual preference for children, that could be problematic? For example, babysitting, going to the swimming pool, acting as youth-coach for children, etc. Again, you can use the 4-field scheme if necessary.
- **Homework Review**: Go through the consequences found by the patient once again and add to them if necessary.

2.9   Module 3-3: Self-Observation – The Therapy Journal

Theory

Problem behavior does not occur without prior and subsequent conditions. To be able to change a behavior and its enabling factors, both aspects must first be analyzed in detail. Regular self-observation as a form of cognitive processing is particularly suitable for this purpose, as it allows for a differentiated breakdown of the underlying conditions over time. A favorable side effect is that just the increased engagement with the behavior and its circumstances often leads to an increased perception of the problem structure and an incipient change in behavior through self-regulation, which increases personal responsibility (Lauth and Mackowiak 2009). Cognitive therapy methods for adults (simplified) can also be applied to adolescents.

In order to accurately capture the functional condition model, it is necessary to include the different components: The external or internal situation as a temporally preceding condition, the internal processing as mediating condition (thoughts, feelings, bodily sensations, etc.), the exhibited behavior in its different modalities as a dependent variable, and the external and internal short- and long-term consequences as subsequent conditions. Self-observation is helpful in the diagnostic as well as in the therapeutic context, since recently acquired evaluations or behaviors can also be practiced (Bartling et al. 2008). In order to maintain motivation and personal responsibility, the patients' self-observation homework must be reinforced on a continual basis through follow-up discussions and evaluations. If the patient's commitment is not appreciated, he will very likely lose interest in conducting the self-observation.

Goals

- Applying/practicing the acquired knowledge of behavioral and consequence analysis means:
  - Becoming an expert on your own visible and hidden experience and behavior
  - Anticipation of behavioral consequences and thus
  - Increasing the control over one's actions
- Perception-training for preceding, accompanying, and subsequent conditions that provoke sexual impulses toward children (in fantasy and behavior)
- Early detection when sexual fantasies regarding children threaten to emerge at the behavioral level

Interventions

Introduction to Self-Observation

- **Discussion/Psychoeducation:** Read aloud to the patient the following situation: "A neighbor – a single mother – calls your parents and asks if you can babysit her 6-year-old daughter on Friday night. She would like to attend the office party." *Should your patient have a sexual interest in boys or the early pubescent body age, modify the example to fit this situation.* Then discuss the following questions with the patient:
  1. What thoughts would you have in this situation?
  2. What would you feel?
  3. How do you imagine you would behave?
  4. What consequences of this behavior (positive/negative, short-/long-term) would be likely?
- **Psychoeducation**: Repeat the interrelationships within the behavioral model. Above all, repeat that a different evaluation of a situation (thoughts) can lead to different actions (behavior).

- **Discussion**: Extend the situation to include alternative feelings and thoughts; clarify the results on the flipchart:
  1. What thoughts could you have in this situation?
  2. What would you feel *then*?
  3. How do you imagine you would behave *then*?
  4. What consequences of this behavior (positive/negative, short-/long-term) would be likely?
- **Discussion**: **Why might it be important for you to be able to effectively observe yourself and your sexual daydreams, fantasies, and sexual behavior?** Use the → IS *Therapy Journal* and, if necessary, add the following: By observing your sexual fantasies and sexual behavior you can practice...
  1. Paying attention to the connections between feelings, thoughts, and behavior
  2. Getting to know yourself better
  3. Identifying problems in their early stages
  4. Controlling your own actions more effectively
  5. Recognizing the difference between behavior and subsequent reactions (consequences)
  6. Finding good solutions
  7. Perceiving when your sexual fantasies increase the urge to act
  8. **All this forms the basis for your future prevention plan!**
- **Homework**: Now inform the patient that he/she will keep a therapy journal in the future and explain the standardized self-observation log (→ WS *My Therapy Journal*). From now on, provide the patient with sufficient self-observation logs each time. Explain to the patient how to work through the therapy journal (→ IS *Therapy Journal*). The patient must take time every day to consider whether (or which) moments were relevant. If possible, at least one situation per day should be documented, but at the minimum, more than one situation per week. If this is difficult for the patient, you can help him in the following session by asking questions: e.g., "Were there everyday situations in the last week in which

you met children (bus/tram, on the street, school, playgrounds, parks, etc.)? Or: "Have you seen children on the Internet or television in the last week? What was going through your mind?"

The patient should concentrate on the following aspects:

– Real contact situations with children
– Child-related sexual fantasies during masturbation
– Child-related (sexual) daydreams
– Situations in which he encountered children in the media

3   Module 4 – Controlling Behavior

In the controlling behavior module, the reconstruction of criminal offences and the formulation of preventive strategies are dealt with. The focus here is on the ability to assume a different perspective, the development of solution-oriented coping strategies, and a detailed examination of the crimes committed. With the exception of working through offences, this module can be applied to both sex offenders and non-criminals. Please note that working through offences is only indicated for young people who have already engaged in sexually assault.

The overall **objectives** of the module **Controlling Behavior** are:

• Prevention of (repeated) sexual offenses
• Improving the ability to adopt the perspectives of imagined and actual victims of child sexual abuse and victims of abuse images,
• Development of solution-oriented coping strategies

3.1   Module 4-1: Empathy

Theory
Empathy is the ability to perceive, understand, and feel the thoughts and feelings of others. Empathy helps us to assess the quality of a relationship and to show understanding and compas-

sion, and is thus an important part of social interaction (Schuler et al. 2016).

It is assumed that the inability or unwillingness to assume the victim's perspective is conducive to (sexual) assault (Finkelhor and Lewis 1988; Blake and Gannon 2008) and can increase the risk of renewed (sexual) assault (O'Donohue 2014). Studies on pedophilic men, for example, have shown a reduced ability on the part of perpetrators to adopt a different perspective when compared to non-perpetrators (Schuler et al. 2019). In addition, a lack of empathy for one's own victims (= victim empathy) could be demonstrated among adult (sexual) offenders (Fernandez et al. 1999; Marshall et al. 1998; Tierney and McCabe 2001)). Reports on juvenile sex offenders (Halse et al. 2012) also show that they are often not able to describe the effects of their sexually assaultive behavior on their victims. A higher level of empathy is associated with increased impulse and behavioral control (Ward and Hudson 2000). Accordingly, training to improve one's capacity for empathy is considered a core element in the treatment of sex offenders (McGrath et al. 2010).

Goals
• Fostering the ability to put oneself in other people's shoes
• Applying this ability to imaginary or actual sexual contacts with children and victims of abuse images
• Understanding the emotional, social, and psychological consequences of one's own actions for the victim
• Identifying and correcting misinterpretations of victim behavior

Interventions
What is Empathy?

• **Discussion**: Describe on an everyday situation in which someone typically reacts with empathy, such as a child falling off a bicycle and hurting himself. Take time to describe this scenario in detail: "It is a sunny and mild Sunday afternoon. You are sitting with someone you like on the balcony; kids are playing.

Suddenly you see a 6-year-old child fall off a bicycle in front of the house, scraping his hands and knees bloody, and then he starts to cry etc." Discuss with the patient afterwards: **What would you do and why?** Typically, it is reported that the observer approaches the child, helps him up, and comforts him. Make it clear that these reactions are based on empathy.

- **Psychoeducation – Characteristics of empathy:** Empathy is the ability to perceive the feelings of others, to understand these feelings, to imagine how it feels to experience these feelings, and finally the ability to show concern and respect for the individual. Empathy can be weakened by errors in thought, negative emotions, and sexual arousal. Compile **characteristics of empathy** with the patient on the flipchart:
  - Being able to see things from a different perspective
  - Being able to put oneself in someone else's place
  - Being able to understand how others think and feel
  - Being able to understand how one's own behavior can affect other people

Importance of Empathy for the Therapy?

- **Discussion**: Let the patient work out the importance of empathy for therapy. **Why is it important to talk about empathy in this therapy?**
- **Psychoeducation** (→ IS *Empathy*): Empathy is an important precondition for
  - Having positive relationships.
  - Understanding how a child feels and thinks. Then I can better make sure I don't do anything to a child that he or she does not like.
- **Discussion**: Ask the patient to assume the "victim's perspective" in the context of simple examples (being fired, celebrating a birthday and nobody comes, having a quarrel with one's best friend, etc.) and describe his experience. If the patient finds it difficult to empathize with others, as a therapist you can provide a model of an empathetic reaction.

Letter to a Victim

- **Psychoeducation/Discussion**: Work initially with letters from victims of child sexual abuse and abuse images (→ IS *Letters from Victims*). For example, have the patient read the letter and ask the patient to share the feelings and thoughts that arise. **How will the victim feel shortly after the abuse? What are the short-term consequences? How will the victim feel after a longer period of time (weeks, months, years) after the abuse? What are the long-term consequences? Are there differences between short-term and long-term consequences?** Ask the patient to fill out the → WS *Report on Letters from Victims*.
- **Homework**: Ask the patient to write a letter to a child with whom he has already had sexual contact. The letter will not be sent. Patients without previous sexual contact with children are asked to write a letter to a child who appears in their sexual fantasies. They should imagine how the child would feel if they were to live out their sexual fantasies with the child in behavior. Use the → WS *Letter to my Victim(s)*.
- **Discussion: What criteria should the letter to the child fulfill?** Work out the following aspects together with the patient, and record the results on the flipchart:
  1. Apology
  2. Taking responsibility for one's own actions
  3. Recognizing one's own behavior as inappropriate
  4. Acknowledging the victim's pain, suffering, and harm
  5. No use of justifications
  6. No self-pity
- **Homework Review – Discussion of the letter**: Ask the patient to read out aloud his letter to the victim. Then ask the patient to tell you how he feels and what he thinks. Then give your patient feedback on the letter. Take into consideration how the aspects of responsibility and empathy are dealt with. Does the letter claim full responsibility for the patient's own behavior, or does it attempt to justify the situation? Is the child held responsible in any

way? Does the patient apologize for his behavior? Does the letter show the patient's ability to imagine how the victim may have felt and thought (before and after the imaginary or real sexual contact)?

Letter From a Victim

- **Discussion**: Ask the patient to write a letter addressed to himself. The letter should be written from the perspective of a victim with whom the patient has had sexual contact in fantasy or in reality. In the letter, the victim should convey what he/she wants to tell the patient.
- **Discussion: What characteristics should a letter written by a victim to you have? What will the victim convey?** (→ IS *Characteristics of a Letter from a Victim*) Work with the patient through the following aspects and record the results on the flipchart. The victim could:
  1. Express anger
  2. Use a hateful tone of voice
  3. Describe a good life before the abuse
  4. Convey feelings from during the abuse
  5. Describe the short-term and long-term consequences of the abuse
  6. Name the details perceived to be the worst
- **Homework**: As homework the patient will be asked to work on the → WS *Letter to me from my Victims*.
- **Homework Review**: Ask the patient to read aloud to his letter from the victim. Then the patient should tell you how he's feeling and what he's thinking at the moment. Pay attention as to whether the letter reflects an understanding of the consequences for the victim. Can the patient imagine the feelings of the victim? Is the letter realistic?

3.2   Module 4-2: Problem Solving and Coping Strategies

Theory

When dealing with both external stressors (e.g., homework, arguments) and internal stressors (e.g., sexual fantasies, negative feelings), people employ different coping strategies (Lazarus and Folkman 1984). There are 3 basic types of coping strategies:

- Problem-oriented coping
- Emotion-oriented coping
- Avoidance

In problem-oriented coping, action strategies are adopted in order to solve a problem or reduce the consequences of a problem. Emotion-oriented coping primarily involves improving one's own emotional state. Thus, for example, others are blamed or one imagines things to happen or to disappear. With avoidance, strategies are used to avoid the problem, e.g., by engaging in other activities (distraction) or by seeking out other people (social alternatives).

The initially mentioned coping mechanism should be seen as a positive adaptation to the stress situation, while the other two coping mechanisms tend to be ineffective. Even though an immediate improvement in well-being may occur, the latter coping strategies usually do not lead to a solution to the problem and may even amplify the problem (Weber 1994). Furthermore, these coping strategies are associated with depression, anxiety, or delinquent behavior (Seiffge-Krenke 2007; Metzke and Steinhausen 2002).

Scientific studies indicate that adult sex offenders tend to use maladaptive coping strategies in conflict situations and try to regulate negative emotional states such as boredom or loneliness through sexual activity (Marshall et al. 1999; Feelgood et al. 2005). There is also evidence that maladaptive coping strategies contribute to the risk of relapse. In order to regulate stress situations, adolescent sex offenders also seem to use emotionally focused coping strategies significantly more often than non-perpetrators (Pagé et al. 2010). Therefore, an improvement in the ability to use problem-focused coping strategies in order to achieve a lasting reduction in aversive states of being is a significant goal in reducing the risk of abuse (Cortoni and Marshall 2001).

Goals
- Identification of dysfunctional problem-solving strategies in social interactions
- Development of problem-focused coping strategies

Interventions
Dealing with Stressful Situations

- **Discussion**: Collect examples with the patient of experienced problematic or stressful situations. Discuss with him: **How did you react in such stressful situations? What did you do to make the stressful or problematic situation more bearable?** Consider with the patient the short- and long-term consequences of the strategies used. Explain that short-term relief can be helpful to restore well-being in stressful situations, but that problems still require a long-term solution.
- **Discussion**: Hand out the → WS *Problem Solving – New Behavior*. Use this worksheet to work together to develop examples of alternative behavior for the stressful situations noted by the patient. Determine the resources that the patient has that are supportive in the context of the problem. **Which of your characteristics could help you to behave differently in similar situations? What else could help you to deal with such situations? What if you were to no longer have this problem in your friendship/partnership anymore?**

Coping Strategies

- **Discussion: What do you understand by the term "coping strategies"?** Work out a concept of coping with your patient.
- **Psychoeducation**: Coping strategies are thoughts and behaviors used to manage unpleasant, stressful, or overburdening stressors. Stressors can be internal or external:
  - Internal stressors: negative feelings, deviant sexual fantasies, sexual impulses
  - External stressors: workload/school-stress, arguments with friends/family
- **Discussion: What causes stress in you? What role do sexual fantasies with children**

play in this? Are these internal stressors for you? Explain to the patient that each person has very different strategies for handling stress and/or problems. There are strategies that are more appropriate, i.e., positive, and there are strategies that are not appropriate and can even amplify a problem.
- **Discussion**: Can you describe or define positive coping strategies?
- **Psychoeducation**: A positive coping strategy addresses a problem in such a way that one benefits from it both in the present and in the future. Positive coping strategies are also called problem-focused coping strategies.
- **Discussion**: Do you know of any examples of positive or problem-focused coping strategies? Compile examples on the flipchart together with the patient. Possible starting points are:
  1. Talking about the problem with another person
  2. Positive self-instructions (inner conversations with oneself)
  3. Accepting a situation
  4. Recognizing and expressing one's own needs and wishes
  5. Recognizing and preventing faulty perception
  6. ...
- **Discussion/Psychoeducation: Can you describe or define negative coping strategies?** Negative coping strategies lead to feeling better in the short term, but they do harm in the middle and long term. These are strategies that do not effectively address the problem or may even amplify it. A distinction is made between emotionally oriented coping strategies and avoidance. Emotional coping involves an emotional response to the problem, such as becoming angry or brooding. With avoidance, the problem is not addressed but avoided.
- **Discussion: Do you know of examples of negative coping strategies for avoidance or emotionally coping?** Work out examples together with the patient and record them on the flipchart. Examples include:
  1. Avoidance
  2. Postponing something

3. Physically hurting someone
4. Substance abuse
5. Insulting someone
6. Brooding
7. Pretending that everything is fine
8. Distraction
9. ...

- **Discussion**: Hand out the → IS *Coping Strategies* and explain the 3 strategies again. Think of a problem or conflict situation, and have the patient describe what the consequences of using the different strategies might be.
- **Homework**: To delve more deeply into the principle of effective coping strategies, the patient should complete the → WS *My Coping Strategies*.
- **Homework Review**: Discuss with the patient the → WS *My Coping Strategies*. Pay particular attention to what coping strategies were described, i.e., whether they were negative or positive strategies. Ask the patient to imagine how the problem would have developed if the other two strategies had been used.

3.3   Module 4-3: Sex Offender Treatment

Theory

This module is exclusively intended for patients who have already engaged in sexually assault. This applies both to the use of abuse images and to direct sexual assault on children. In order to enact a long-term change in behavior, it is important to examine criminal offences that have already been committed. Here, the course of events around an act of assault is analyzed in detail, and accompanying thoughts, feelings, perceptions, bodily sensitivities, and sequences of action are put together in context. By working through the offence, any cognitive distortions that may still exist should be uncovered, cognitive and emotional restructuring processes should be further enhanced, and the assumption of responsibility is to be heightened. At the same time, the precise reconstruction of the offense allows the development of preventive strategies (Worling and Langton 2012).

The patient should be made aware that a sexual assault represents targeted behavior and follows a certain amount of planning. The patient does not necessarily have to be aware of the planning. Some assume that a sexual offense "just happens." In the reconstruction of the offense, it is important to work out with the patient how certain decisions between different behavior options led to the offense. The patient should be able to visualize the individual decision options and be aware of the associated negative consequences. During the next step, the patient should imagine the positive consequences which could result from the abandonment of this behavior.

Goals

- Insight into individual dynamics of the offense including fantasy activity and planning
- Taking responsibility for the act
- Early recognition of risk developments
- Understanding the negative consequences of delinquent behavior
- Working out positive consequences of a change in behavior
- Acquiring strategies for how to break the offense cycle

Interventions

The Reconstruction of the Offense

- **Psychoeducation**: Explain to the patient why the reconstruction of the offense is important: The analysis of (direct and/or indirect) sexual assaults on children that have already taken place is important because it allows you to ...
  - Become an expert on your own criminal behavior
  - Discover possibilities for how you can control your behavior in the future
  - Identify offense-related mistaken thoughts
  - Understand the negative consequences of your assaultive behavior
  - Understand the positive consequences that a change in behavior would bring
  - Acquire strategies for how to recognize and the offense cycle early on in the future
- If the patient has already committed several sexual assaults, you will choose one of these

sexual assaults together with him. This does not have to be the first, last, or most-serious offense; it is only important that it is an offense that the patient can remember well and about which he is also willing to talk.

The Three Phases of Sexual Contact

- **Discussion**: How does sexual contact with another human being usually occur? Does it happen suddenly or does something else happen before or after? How does it happen that people consume pornographic material? Does it happen suddenly or does something else happen before or after?
  Work out the 3 phases of sexual contact with the patient and record the results on the flipchart:
  1. Preparation phase
  2. Sexual contact
  3. Post-phase
- **Psychoeducation**: Sexual behavior (direct or indirect) does not just happen. There is always a preparation phase: I make a date with a woman/man who is sexually attractive to me in a hotel room and buy condoms beforehand, or I check to see if I am alone, then I start the computer and open a porn site on the Internet. The same applies to sexual assaults or the use of abuse images – these do not just happen either. They are often pre-fantasized or pre-pared for concretely. Early recognition of this preliminary phase increases the time window in which you can stop your actions.

The Offense Cycle

- **Psychoeducation**: The offense cycle is particularly suitable for reconstructing the course of the crime in detail (after Bessler 2008). Here it doesn't matter whether it concerns direct or indirect sexual assault on children. Working out an offense cycle is time-consuming and will probably take several therapy sessions (→ WS *My Offense Cycle*). The offense behavior in each phase of the offense cycle – analogous to the behavioral model – is represented with 5 levels:

1. Sensory perception
2. Cognition
3. Emotion
4. Physical experience
5. Behavior
- **Discussion**: Together with the patient, go through the offense cycle phase by phase, taking into account both the phase-specific suggestions, as well as the 5 levels (sensory perception, cognition, emotion, body experience, behavior). Record the results of the offence cycle on the flipchart, and ask the patient to document the findings from the analysis on the → WS *My Offense Cycle*. If the patient is cognitively overwhelmed by the offense cycle model, you can also use the offense staircase model. Here, each step represents a step toward sexual assault (→ WS *My Offense Staircase*). Make sure that you do not trigger any resistance from the patient. You are not in the position of an investigating authority, and you do not have to "prove" guilt to the patient or critically question every detail as to its veracity. Ask open questions at the beginning and avoid your own interpretations. Promote the memory of details (e.g., weather, mood, color of certain objects). In this way you support the patient in condensing the experience (Urbaniok 2003).
- **Discussion**: The following questions are suitable for analyzing a sexual assault (according to O'Reilly 2014):

Direct Sexual Abuse

- **Preliminary phase – trigger, lead-up, planning**
  - When did you start thinking or fantasizing about an act of sexual abuse?
  - How did you choose your victim for the act of sexual abuse?
  - Where were you right before the act of sexual abuse?
  - What were you doing right before the act of sexual abuse?
  - What were your thoughts immediately before the act of sexual abuse?
  - How did you approach the victim?

- What steps did you take in advance to prevent the exposure of your act of sexual abuse?
- **Crime phase – committing the crime, implementation**
  - Where did the sexual abuse take place?
  - What exactly happened during the sexual abuse?
  - How did you feel during the sexual abuse?
- **Post-phase – behavior after the offense**
  - What did you do immediately after the sexual abuse?
  - How did you feel immediately after the sexual abuse?
  - What thoughts did you have immediately after the sexual abuse?
  - Did you say anything else to your victim?
  - How did your sexual abuse come out into the open?
  - How did you feel when everything came out?
  - How do you feel about it now?

The Use of Child Sexual Abuse Images

- **Preliminary phase – trigger, lead-up, planning**
  - When did you start thinking or fantasizing about consuming child abuse images?
  - How did you choose the abuse images of children? How did you find them?
  - Where were you right before you consumed the child abuse images?
  - What were you doing just before you consumed the child abuse images?
  - What were you thinking just before you consumed the child abuse images?
  - What steps did you take in advance to conceal your consumption of child abuse images?
- **Crime phase – committing the crime, implementation**
  - Where did you consume the abuse images of children?
  - What exactly happened during this? Did you masturbate?
  - How did you feel during this?

- **Post-phase – behavior after the offense**
  - What did you do right after the consumption of abuse images of children?
  - How did you feel immediately after consuming the child abuse images?
  - What did you think about immediately after consuming the abuse images of children?
  - How did it come out into the open that you consumed child abuse images?
  - How did you feel when it all came out?
  - How do you feel about it now?

Contact Cycle in Repeated Sexual Contact

- **Discussion/Psychoeducation**: If your patient has already engaged repeatedly in sexually assault, a cyclical process can be observed. The post-phase can again lead into the preliminary phase and thus trigger the offence cycle. First, explain the cycle using a fictitious example on the flipchart. Once the patient has understood the model, the scheme should be applied to his offenses.

---

4 Module 5 – Social Competencies and Intimacy

Due to limited social competencies, patients may display a lack of intimate relationships. A low level of intimate relationships may in turn be connected with increased emotional loneliness and limited satisfaction with life (Whitaker et. al 2008). The following module accordingly aims to strengthen interactional skills and intensify trusting relationships in order to achieve a higher degree of psychological stability and quality of life.

The primary **goals** of the module **Social Competencies and Intimacy** are:

- Improvement of social competencies and overcoming social isolation
- Understanding of the connection between a lack of intimacy and emotional loneliness, and their effect on quality of life

4.1 Module 5-1: Social Competencies

Theory

Demographic studies suggest that juveniles with sexual particularities and behavior tend to live in social isolation and are not as developed as their peers in their social competencies (Awad and Saunders 1989; Hunter et al. 2003). They tend therefore to show increased emotional loneliness and experience a marked insufficiency in the formation of social contact (Letourneau et al. 2004; Thornton et al. 2008). The inability to build and maintain relationships with others of the same age, along with social isolation, have proven to be relevant predictors for repeat sexual assault committed by juvenile offenders (Worling and Langström 2006).

This module thus aims to improve social competencies. The patient should learn skills helpful to the establishment of pro-social and satisfying relationships to same-age peers. It should be assessed which social-communicative skills are in need of improvement. These might be, for instance, working with critique, giving feedback, saying "no," leading conversation, or conflict management.

Goals

- Improvement of interactional skills
- Identification of important partners in social interaction and their emotional relationship quality
- Increase of self-efficacy in contact with emotionally-important partners in interaction
- Establishment of a social network with stable relationships
- Comprehension of rules for feedback

Interventions

My Social Competencies

- **Discussion:** Ask the patients to evaluate themselves using →WS *My Social Competencies.* **In what areas have you recognized problems for yourself? Have you recognized your strengths? Is there anything in particular you would like to work on?**

- **Competency training:** Following the profile from →WS *My Social Competencies,* pick out an area of social competency that needs support. Role play can assist in this task. You may additionally look to other current manuals to help work on identified weaknesses.

Social Relationships

- **Discussion:** Hand out the →WS *My Social Competencies* and with the patients, get an overview of their current social relationships. **How would you assess your current social network? Are you happy with it? Do you feel alone? If yes, what can you do about it? Do you want to make new contacts? If yes, how can you achieve that?**
- **Discussion:** Hand out →WS *The Quality of My Relationships.* **Are there people in your life from whom you have thus far experienced acknowledgment, acceptance, and security? Are there people from whom you have experienced rejection and refusal? How is it currently?** Consider with the patients if there are patterns in their relationships to same-age peers that might place a burden on the quality of these relationships.
- **Discussion (Patients Without a Partner):** What situations come up again and again in your relationships to friends of the same age that place strain on you and your friendships?
- **Discussion (Patients with a Partner):** What situations come up again and again in your relationship to your same-age partner that place strain on you and your partnership?
- **Discussion:** Using the following questions, work out the functionality of patients' current behavior on a flipchart:
  - What unpleasant consequences do you avoid through this behavior?
  - What agreeable situations do you reach through this behavior?
  - What sort of quality do the long-term consequences have?
  - Do you see a connection between the degree to which you experience your relationships as pleasant or unpleasant

and the difficulties you encounter in your relationships?

Rules for Feedback

- **Discussion:** Hand out the →WS *Rules for Feedback,* and ask the patients to read the rules for responses out loud. **What could be appropriate times for feedback? When could feedback be "too much" for other people? What can be understood as "concrete" behavior? What does the word "immediate" mean?**
- **Discussion:** Ask the patient to imagine that he has studied for a math test and inexplicably got a "C," even though he deserved an "A." Now the math teacher would like to talk about this grade. The following points should be paid attention to during the feedback (compile the results on a flipchart):
  1. What concrete behavior is my feedback related to?
  2. What did I perceive?
  3. What did I assume?
  4. What did I feel?
  5. What goal does my feedback serve?
     Ask the patient to formulate their feedback in I-statements.
- **Homework:** Hand out the →WS *Positive Feedback in Relationships.* In the coming weeks the patient should give one positive response to a person in their surroundings.
- **Homework Discussion – Discussion of the →WS *Positive Feedback in Relationships*:**

Ask the patient to clarify in which situations and to whom a positive response is given. Was it difficult for them? What reaction did their response receive?

4.2   Module 5-2: Intimacy and Sexual Preference

Theory

From the beginning of life humans have a fundamental need for acceptance, security, and safety. These needs can be met in interpersonal relationships – particularly intimate relationships. Intimacy in relationships can lead in turn to greater personal satisfaction with one's life and a higher degree of emotional well-being (Beier and Loewit 2011). Intimacy means feeling trust and closeness with someone. Intimacy is in principle independent from the existence of a sexual relationship and, therefore, cannot be equated with one. Sexuality may, however, be an important factor in communicating and deepening intimacy within an interpersonal relationship.

Sexual responsiveness to the child body age limits or makes it impossible for a juvenile to use and experience sexuality as a means of intimacy in a partner relationship. However, sexuality plays no role in the great majority of trusting relationships (e.g., in friendships) and is therefore not a precondition for experiencing intimate relationships. Adult pedophilic men often lack intimate relationships to other adults and thus commonly display a high degree of emotional loneliness (Marshall 1989). There is no evidence to suggest that it is any different for juveniles who experience sexual attraction to children. An insufficient feeling of belonging to same-age peers' experiential world and a high degree of loneliness may lead the affected juvenile to seek contact with the world of children more intensively in order to satisfy their needs for intimacy, closeness, and sexuality.

The initiation or deepening of trusting – and thus intimate – relationships to persons of similar age can reduce feelings of loneliness and lead in turn to higher quality of life, improved psychological stability, and finally, to higher impulse control regarding the sexual molestation of children.

Goals
- Communication of the connection between insufficient intimacy and loneliness, and its effect on quality of life
- Development of the meaning of intimacy and emotional closeness as they relate to the (prior) sexual molestation of children
- Improvement of skills for the appropriate regulation of closeness and distance in interpersonal contact

- Strengthening of competencies in appropriate communication of feelings
- Communication of knowledge about the impact of one's own sexual preference on relationship formation.

Interventions

What Does Intimacy Mean?

- **Discussion:** Together, work out the characteristics of intimacy. Questions such as the following might be used: **What does the word "intimacy" mean to you? Can you name some characteristics of an intimate relationship?**
- **Psychoeducation:** "Intimacy" is a condition of deep trust. The concept of "intimacy" is frequently equated with sexual relationships, but this is incorrect. With the patient, compile the following aspects, and write them out on the flipchart (→WS *Intimacy*). Intimacy means:
  - A feeling of security, trust, and emotional closeness.
  - Shared experiences (e.g., shared free-time activities).
  - Caring for the other person.
  - Confirmation/recognition of one person by the other.
  - Mutual support in crisis situations.
  - The feeling of a familial bond.
  - Functional verbal and nonverbal communication.
  - Opening oneself.
  - Conflicts can be solved.
  - Sometimes, also consensual sexuality.

Intimate Relationships with Same-Age Persons

- **Discussion:** Hand out →WS *Intimacy in My Relationships*. Be critical if your patient names intimate relationships to children. The relationships identified in the previous module on →WS *My Social Relationships* can be used here as a basis. **Are there people in your life with whom you feel intimate?**
- **Psychoeducation/Discussion:** Elicit the patient's attitude toward relationships and discuss advantages (e.g., the feeling of leading a

fulfilling life, better self-esteem, better resistance to stress, better psychic and physical health) and disadvantages (e.g., risk of being hurt, disappointed, or jealous; the necessity of one's own initiative and efforts; compromises must be met; the necessity of opening oneself) of intimate relationships with same-age persons. You can make a pros-and-cons list on a flipchart.

- **Discussion:** What do you think about relationships? Do you want a relationship? Have you had experiences in relationships? What role do fundamental needs like acceptance, trust, and security play in relationships? What are the advantages and disadvantages of intimate relationships with same-aged persons?

Intimate Relationships with Children

- **Discussion:** Think of problems that could arise in a relationship between juveniles or adults and children.
- **Psychoeducation:** Work out the following aspects on a flipchart:
  - A relationship between a child and a juvenile or adult is always asymmetrical. That means it is never equal.
  - Children do not yet understand the worlds of juveniles or adults. Children live in a world of their own.
  - Sexuality is never a way to experience intimacy in relationships with children because it implicitly means committing sexual molestation.
  - An intimate relationship with a child is never possible – even when it is desired.

Sexual Responsiveness to Child Bodies and Sexually Intimate Relationships

- **Psychoeducation:** It is at this point recommended to begin with a refresher on the dimensions of sexuality (Module 1). With the patient, work out the influence their sexual preference has/could have on current and future sexual relationships. Take note of whether your patient experiences and exclusive or non-exclusive sexual responsiveness to the child body-age scheme. To aid in this, hand out →IS *Sexual Responsiveness to the Child Body Age and Partnership.*

- **Discussion:** Into which of these two groups would you currently place yourself? Does a sexual relationship with a same-aged person represent an actual or just a desired a possibility for you? Do you have sexual fantasies about adults?
- **Discussion:** Now think about the influence of a sexual responsiveness to the child body on the formation of relationships between same-aged persons. **What impact can a sexual responsiveness to the child body age have on the formation of relationships between same-aged persons?**
- **Psychoeducation:** Together with the patient, consider the following on a flipchart:
  - A person has a "secret" that they cannot share with their partner.
  - A person can develop feelings of guilt toward their partner because they have, for instance, looked at abuse images online, are sexually interested in children in their surroundings, or had (sexual) contact with children.
  - It may be necessary for a person to fantasize about a prepubescent child during sexual contact with their partner in order for them to become sufficiently aroused.
  - Sexual dysfunction (e.g., erectile or orgasm dysfunction) can occur when a person does find their partner sexually attractive. This can lead to a person becoming distant from their partner.

5   Module 6 – Relapse Prevention

In this module, prevention measures, as well as future planning for the purposes of relapse prevention, will be addressed. With the aid of a prevention plan, the patient will be given a feeling of control and influence over the development of risk situations for child sexual abuse. In addition, as a reinforcement to these resources, a future plan will be put together based on the patient's

own strengths, future perspectives, and fulfilling activities.

The overarching **goals** of the **Relapse Prevention** module are:

- Putting together a prevention plan to inhibit (renewed) sexual assaults on children and the use of abuse images
- Working out life goals

6   Module 6 – Relapse Prevention

In this module, prevention measures, as well as future planning for the purposes of relapse prevention, will be addressed. With the aid of a prevention plan, the patient will be given a feeling of control and influence over the development of risk situations for child sexual abuse. In addition, as a reinforcement to these resources, a future plan will be put together based on the patient's own strengths, future perspectives, and fulfilling activities.

The overarching **goals** of the **Relapse Prevention** module are:

- Putting together a prevention plan to inhibit (renewed) sexual assaults on children and the use of abuse images
- Working out life goals

6.1   Module 6-1: – Prevention Plan

Theory
The concept of relapse prevention in addiction treatment (Marlatt and Gordon 1985) represents the theoretical framework for this module. It shall be made clear to the patient in the following content that sexual assaults on children and the use of abuse images are consequences of events, thoughts, feelings, and behaviors that can be recognized and controlled early on. As such, an ostensibly unimportant decision can lead to an increase in readiness for and probability of a relapse, such as, for example, in the case of an adolescent who has molested a child in the past

and is about to take on a job as a babysitter (Steen and Bromberg 2014). The goal is for the patient to learn to be aware of his individual risk factors for sexual contact with children and the use of abuse images, and to develop strategies for functional coping (i.e., not harming oneself or others) with risk factors. Risk factors are conditions that increase the probability of one's committing an act of child sexual abuse. Risk factors may include a visit to a public swimming pool, for instance, or to a playground, or feelings such as worthlessness or dejection. With patients who have not molested a child, situations may be analyzed in which they see/saw themselves as being in danger of sexually molesting a child or of using abuse images of children.

Psychotherapeutic methods that are suitable to this module are stimulus control (e.g., specific risk situations, such as avoiding contact with children, are actively controlled by the patient); thought-stopping (recognizing one's own thought processes and modes of behavior that could lead to an act of abuse in a certain situation; stopping those thoughts by imagining negative consequences); and self-management (e.g., the patient is made aware that he is capable of controlling his behavior). Situational and behavioral analyses as well as self-observation are also suitable.

Goals

- Creating awareness of ostensibly unimportant decisions that can increase the risk of sexual abuse towards children
- Identifying and managing individual risk factors
- Developing coping strategies in order to break potential offense patterns
- Coming up with a prevention plan

Interventions

The Risk Ladder – Steps on the Way to Sexual Abuse

- **Psychoeducation/Discussion:** Explain to the patient that an act of sexual abuse does not happen in an uncontrolled and impulsive way, but rather usually builds up over a longer period of time (hours, days, or even up to several years). On the way to an act of abuse, several steps have to be climbed or taken that bring one closer to the next act of sexual abuse. External situations, thoughts, or feelings can take one further in the direction of sexual abuse. Work together with the patient to come up with a possible scenario for an act of sexual abuse. Hand out the → IS *The Risk Ladder – Steps On the Way to Sexual Abuse* and explain the individual steps that lead toward an act of sexual abuse.
- **Discussion:** Have the patient fill out the → WS *My Risk Ladder,* based on an act of sexual abuse they committed. If your patient has not committed an act of sexual abuse, use a situation in which the patient saw/sees himself as being in danger of committing an act of sexual abuse. Work out from the fictive as well as the patient's own example that the ability to make decisions becomes increasingly limited as the patient's sexual arousal increases.
- **Psychoeducation**
  - The Risk Ladder begins on the lowest rung with a lower degree of sexual arousal. The further up the ladder they are, the stronger the patient's sexual arousal will be. This makes it increasingly difficult to interrupt the risk development process.
  - It makes a difference whether one has to take "just" one step down the ladder (interrupting the risk development process at an early stage) or whether one has to "jump down" multiple rungs at once (interrupting the risk development process at a late stage).

Risk Factors on the Way to Abuse

- **Psychoeducation:** Go over the concept of risk factors on the way to direct or indirect sexual abuse in detail (→ IS *Risk Factors*).
- Risk factors are conditions that increase the probability of one committing an act of sexual abuse. These can be internal (i.e., within you and not visible to others) or external (i.e., outside of you and visible to others):
  - **Internal risk factors:** thoughts and feelings such as dejection, worthlessness,

hopelessness, anger; increase in fantasies about child sexual abuse
- **External risk factors:** increased porn consumption, visiting swimming pools or playgrounds, end of a relationship, a conflict
• Explain that the earlier a patient identifies his risk factor and the earlier he does something to prevent it, the greater the window (of time) will be that he will have to decide how to act; and the greater his chance of success will be of preventing an act of sexual abuse from taking place. Work out his individual risk factors. Refer to the concept of internal and external triggers that was just introduced.
• **Discussion:** What do you think – could the risk of you committing a (repeated) act of sexual abuse toward a child increase? How can you tell (feelings, thoughts, behavior) that you are already headed in the direction of committing an act of sexual abuse on a child? Which negative states of feeling are associated with an increased risk of committing child sexual abuse (again) for you? What do the first steps leading up to sexually abusing a child look like for you?
• **Homework:** Ask the patient to write in the risk factors that are applicable to him on the → WS *My Risk Factors*.

Dealing with Risk Factors

• **Psychoeducation:** Explain to the patient that there are three types of possibilities for managing risk factors, thereby hindering (repeated) sexual assaults:
- **Avoidance:** staying away from or stopping yourself from doing something
- **Escape:** removing yourself from a dangerous situation at a certain point
- **Coping:** actively doing something to prevent yourself from molesting a child in risk situations, such as by putting alternative thoughts into practice
• **Discussion: Can you come up with any advantages or disadvantages to these strategies?**
• **Psychoeducation:** Hand out the →IS *Examples for Dealing with Risk Factors* and

discuss what dealing with risk factors might look like. Examples for sensible coping strategies might be:
- Leaving the situation
- Alternative behavioral strategies, e.g., talking with someone, listening to music
- Strenuous physical activity
- Weighing things up in your mind by analyzing the consequences (see Module 3)
- Talking encouragingly to yourself (positive self-instruction)
- Putting stress regulation skills into practice

Confidants

• **Discussion:** Inform yourself about possible people that you could confide in. The following questions may be helpful:
- Do you have friends, acquaintances, or family members who are informed about your sexual interest in children?
- How did you inform them of this?
- What were your experiences with this?
- Did you experience rejection or understanding?
- Do your confidants help prevent you/are they able to help prevent you from having sexual contact with children?
- If you haven't yet had anybody, whom you could confide in, whom would you consider?
• **Discussion:** Ask the patient to fill out the →WS *My Confidants*. If he is unable to name anyone, this is where he can list people whom he would consider for that role. If the patient has not yet confided in anyone, use a role-play, and act out a situation in which the patient reveals his sexual attraction to the child developmental body age to someone close to him.

My Prevention Plan

• **Discussion:** Work together to come up with the content and structure of a prevention plan for avoiding sexual molestation of children and the use of abuse images. **What does your prevention plan have to look like so that it can help you avoid sexual contact with chil-**

dren in the future? What does the plan have to contain in order for you not to consume abuse images?

- **Psychoeducation:** Explain the core elements of a prevention plan to the patient using the flipchart:
  - Knowledge about one's own risk factors (e.g., a visit to the public pool, disappointment)
  - Strategies for managing risk factors
  - Identifying individual dangerous and non-dangerous contact situations with children,
  - Informing confidants (e.g., for support, possibility of sharing your concerns with someone)
- **Discussion:** Hand out the → IS *Coming Up with a Personal Prevention Plan* and go through it together with the patient. Work with the patient to come up with an example of a prevention strategy for at least one risk factor from his own list (with at least a moderate level of danger, if possible). For this, use the →WS *Strategies for Dealing with Risk Factors.*
- **Homework:** Ask the patient to write out strategies for each of the risk factors on his list, using the →WS *Strategies for Dealing with Risk Factors* for help. Make sure to give the patient sufficient worksheets.
- **Homework Discussion – Presenting the Strategies for Dealing with Risk Factors:** Have the patient delineate his strategies for dealing with risk factors. Take sufficient time for each risk factor. Give feedback as to whether the strategies are sufficiently detailed and concretely formulated.
- **Homework:** Ask the patient to fill out the → WS *My Prevention Plan*. The result should include a list of all the risk factors and their respective coping strategies.
- **Homework Discussion – Prevention Plan Presentation:** Have the patient present his prevention plan. Give feedback on each of the strategies, considering the following points:
  - Practicability/feasibility
  - Goal orientation
  - Presence of intermediate goals
  - Problem-focused coping strategies

The goal is for the patient to leave therapy with a list of functional behaviors in order to be able to reduce or avoid risk-heavy interactions and relationships. The individual prevention plan should be kept with the patient at all times after this. Alternatively, a pocket-sized emergency card may be written out.

6.2   Module 6-2: Plan for the Future

Theory

Positive psychology or resource-oriented approaches set the focus on promoting human well-being and supporting human needs. Risk and avoidance-oriented approaches are considered necessary here, but insufficient for a comprehensive therapy program. With that in mind, while putting together a future plan, attention should be paid as to whether the targeted strategies are practicable in regard to the resources at hand. In order to be able to effect long-term changes, the respective strategies should be problem-focused. While developing goals, one must keep in mind that approach-oriented goals (e.g., eating an apple) are easier to achieve than avoidance-oriented goals (e.g., not eating any more chocolate). It can also be helpful when the avoidance-oriented goal of "not committing child sexual abuse" is reformulated into an approach-oriented goal, for example: "I would like to live a happy, fulfilling life, without causing harm to others." Working out small, intermediate goals can make the path towards the actual goal easier; in reaching an intermediate goal, a partial goal is always already achieved, which can have a motivating effect on the overall goal.

Goals

- Identifying and strengthening resources
- Increasing self-efficacy
- Developing life goals, while considering goal orientation, cost-benefit analysis, and intermediate goals

Interventions

Resources and Strengths

- **Discussion:** Work together with the patient on the definition of resources. **What does the term "resources" mean to you? What use are resources?**
- **Psychoeducation:** Resources are a set of accomplishments or strengths that help a person to reach his or her goals and to make it through hard times (Flipchart).
- **Discussion:** Work together on identifying your patient's resources and ask him to fill out the →WS *My Resources*. Discuss with the patient how these resources could help him to reach the therapy goal of abstaining from these problem behaviors.

My Personal Goals

- **Discussion:** Take down your patient's life goals on the flipchart. **What might be important in your life in the future? What goals do you have for the future?**

Approach and Avoidance Goals

- **Discussion:** Ask the patient to consider how the goal of "freeing yourself from loneliness and spending more time with other people" can be achieved. Stimulate the process by naming two conceivable goals as an example, such as:
  1. "I never want to say no to meeting up with someone again."
  2. "I want to join a sports club."
- **Discussion: How do you feel about the first goal? How about the second? What would you estimate the likelihood is of being able to achieve each of these goals? Which goal do you like better, and why?**
- **Psychoeducation:** Hand out the → IS *Approach and Avoidance Goals* and explain the respective concepts. Emphasize that approach goals are often easier to achieve than avoidance goals. Accordingly, the goal of *not committing any more acts of sexual abuse* is more difficult to achieve than goals that lead to a happier and more fulfilling life and, in this way, help reduce the need to bring about sexual contact with children. Help the patient as

he goes through his stated goals to reformulate them as approach goals on the flipchart, as needed. Refer to his set of resources that he identified while doing this.

Intermediate Goals

- **Discussion/Psychoeducation:** Work through the pros (easier to achieve than the ultimate goal, as you already have some sense of achievement on the way to your goal) and cons (it can take more time) of intermediate goals. Use the image of a goal staircase, in which every step represents a sense of achievement. Use a simple example (e.g., getting a good grade in math, losing 5 kilos), and divide the ultimate goal up into intermediate goals.

Costs and Benefits of Goals

- **Psychoeducation:** Review the concept of consequence analysis. Emphasize that every goal and the efforts that go with it come with benefits but also with costs that can play out very differently in the short and long term. Use searching for abuse images on the Internet as an example.
- **Discussion: Name the short- and long-term consequences of searching for abuse images on the Internet. Try to name positive and negative consequences.**
- **Psychoeducation:** Work together with the patient on short- and long-term positive and negative consequences. Use the flipchart as a visual aid:
  - **Short-term consequences:**
    Positive: sexual arousal, sexual satisfaction
    Negative: costs time and money
  - **Long-term consequences:**
    Positive: ???
    Negative: feeling of not being satisfied, loneliness, fear of/actually being charged with possession and/or distribution of abuse images
- **Psychoeducation:** Explain that the short-term gains can "block out" long-term consequences, even if the latter would be much

more significant. In addition, changes in behavior can be made more difficult when the costs are initially high and there is a delay before the benefits kick in, such as with learning to play an instrument, for example, or a new sport.

- **Discussion: Why do people who have understood this problem still not change their behavior?** Explain that instant gratifications can be more difficult to resist in emotionally demanding situations or conditions.
- **Discussion: Which short- and long-term costs and benefits do the personal goals written down on the flipchart have?**
- **Homework:** Hand out the → WS *My Plan for the Future* and ask the patient to complete a drawing with his goals for the future.
- **Homework Discussion:** Ask the patient to present his drawing and explain his goals. Go through the following questions with him:
  - Is the goal you're aiming for realistic?
  - How likely is it that you will achieve the goal?
  - Will the goal make you happy?
  - Is this an approach or an avoidance goal?
  - How can avoidance-oriented goals be reformulated into approach goals?
  - Can this goal reduce the risk of an act of sexual abuse taking place, or could it even increase it?
  - Are there intermediate goals?

6.3 Module 6-3: Review and Send-Off

Theory
A successful send-off is of great importance for a successful treatment. For this, it is important to make the patient aware of the upcoming end of therapy and to make enough time and space for thoughts and feelings about the therapy coming to an end.

Goals
- Writing down negative and positive feedback

- Visualizing achieved goals (review) and the future (outlook) goals

Interventions
- Communicate to the patient that he must continue to put what he has learned in therapy to use in order to live up to his goal of long-term abstinence from abusive behaviors.
- Write down positive and negative feedback.
- Give the patient the opportunity for a review (what have I achieved?) and an outlook (what is my next goal?).

7 Module 7 – Working with Caregivers

Theory
According to current empirical literature on the subject, a multi-systemic approach is the most promising in the treatment of juvenile offenders for the purposes of relapse prevention (Borduin and Schaeffer 2002). The integration of family into the therapy process increases the chances of a successful treatment outcome for juvenile sex offenders (Heiman 2002; Zankman and Bonomo 2004; Halse et al. 2012; Jones 2015).

Nevertheless, the decision as to the degree to which the primary caregivers should be informed and, above all, what they should be informed about, ultimately lies with the juvenile himself. As has been addressed above, while working with adolescents, their significant need for autonomy must be respected and reinforced. Should an adolescent show no readiness whatsoever to integrate his caregivers into the treatment process at the start of the psychotherapeutic connection process, this should be initially accepted by the therapist. It is necessary to work with the teenager on what benefits there might be to opening up to one's parents and to what degree the system can be integrated into his prevention and relapse plan. In principle, the authors of this manual recommend that the parents or other primary caregivers be brought in – but not against the will of the patient. Exceptions to this are when there is an acute danger to oneself and to others (see Sect. 8.5 in chapter "The Berlin Prevention Project Dunkelfeld").

In addition, sexual assaults perpetrated by juveniles frequently take place within the family systems in which the juveniles live. This makes it more than necessary to bring the families into the treatment process, also, for example, as a means of figuring out the extent to which parental dysfunction plays a role in additionally increasing the risk of relapse. Analogously, families must also be brought in in cases where the adolescent has not yet committed a sexual abuse offense, in order to analyze the degree to which intrafamilial mechanisms might be present that should receive primary preventative therapeutic treatment.

It should be kept in mind that juvenile sex offenders, compared to other juvenile offenders, experience a higher degree of general familial dysfunction as well as intrafamilial violence. The following intrafamilial deficits have been reported, among others: few psychosocial resources, poor problem-solving skills, parental rejection of the adolescent, limited sexual boundaries, a high degree of conflict, low intrafamilial cohesion, as well as a high mutual dependency and a tendency towards social isolation (Bischof et al. 1992; Blaske et al. 1989; Thornton et al. 2008). Above all, family systems in which the sexual molestation takes the form of sibling abuse are under a particularly high degree of stress (Worling 1995). Subsequently, these juveniles experience less emotional support within the family and are less adept at building positive connections (Righthand and Welch 2004).

We must also consider the fact that a great number of juveniles do not remain in the family after committing sexual assaults, but rather end up residing in youth care institutions, which, due to the lack of specific facilities, are often inadequately equipped to deal with this topic. Supervisors there must also be brought into the treatment process, not least in order to support adequate interactions with the juvenile within the facility. Caregivers, therefore, as a term refers henceforth to parents as well supervisors, including all of the important people in the patient's social environment.

If the juvenile has already sexually molested children, the primary caregivers will need support in dealing with a sexual offense that has been committed by their child. The realization that one's own child is a sex offender comes with an immense degree of emotional stress. The goal is to help them learn to accept what has occurred, to cope, and to support their child in the therapeutic goal of continued abstinence from abuse behavior. The apportioning of responsibility and blame to the juvenile that often arises must be openly addressed. Understanding and accepting the fact that one's own child displays a sexual particularities that includes a desire for sexual contact with children demands professional support. At the same time, it is necessary, as a therapist, to keep in the back of one's mind that the sexual preference structure is not considered an excuse for any mode of behavior, but rather that it is necessary to strengthen a sense of responsibility in the patient for his own past and future behavior.

Through their behavior, family members can contribute, consciously and unconsciously, to the reestablishment of entrenched patterns of behavior, from which (new) acts of sexual abuse may follow. Parents of sexually molesting adolescents often rationalize the offenses of their children, for example, in that they display the same cognitive distortions with respect to the victim, or, alternatively, characterize their children on the basis of their sexual offense as "evil" (Steen and Bromberg 2014).

The task of the therapist is to critically interrogate the familial factors in relation to possible or already-occurring sexual molestation of children, to check whether they continue to be present, and to determine what influence they might have on the therapy outcome. At the same time, stress factors affecting the parents or primary caregivers should also be met with a neutral, validating therapeutic approach. It is critical to take them seriously in regard to their worries and fears and to win them over to the treatment of the adolescent so that he is able to see his social system as a resource, rather than a risk factor.

Uncovering and changing familial mechanisms that stabilize the inadequate behavioral patterns of sexual offenders is vital to the

Table 5 Mal-/adaptive parental reactions

Adaptive parental reactions	Maladaptive parental reactions
Acceptance of the child's sexual problem	Cognitive distortions, e.g., trivialization, denial, etc.
Demanding that the child assume responsibility	
Reduction of the probability of relapse through appropriate monitoring of the child and appropriate setting of boundaries	A chastising, aggressive attitude towards the child
	Rejecting the child
Assuming a supportive attitude toward the child	Poor control of their own emotions
Appreciation of the child's resources	
Positive reinforcement of the child's resources	
Maintaining a positive child-parent relationship	

therapeutic process. The therapist's task within the context of the interventions is to strengthen the adaptive strategies of the parents or to help them to develop them. At the same time, mal-adaptive strategies should be teased out and openly talked about, as well as appropriate strategies developed for dismantling them.

Table 5, drawing on Bennett and Marshall (2005) as well as Heiman (2002), offers an overview of the parental reactions to be either supported or dismantled that should be paid attention to.

The frequency of appointments made with caregivers should depend on the necessity of each individual case. Generally, in the field of child and adolescent psychotherapy, one may take the prevailing ratio of 4:1 as a guide; this should be catered to each individual patient, however, and adjusted to the particular requirements that come up while working with caregivers over the course of therapy.

Goals

- Supporting the juvenile in the transfer of the content learned into everyday life
- Changing negative familial influences (e.g., behavioral patterns, attitudes, relationships, assignation of roles, etc.)
- Improving familial functionality
- Increasing parental skills
- Learning to understand the developments of the juvenile's delinquency

- Processing and, if necessary, reconditioning of accompanying emotions in the caregivers
- Identifying and modifying potential familial cognitive distortions
- Becoming aware of the model function of the one's own partner- and sexual-relationship structures
- Inclusion in the patient's safety plan: monitoring, recognizing, and interrupting the development of risks

Rationale

It is necessary to take a primary resource-oriented approach while working with parents (Blasingame 2014):

- As a therapist, induce hope, and communicate to the parents that people are capable of changing and surpassing themselves.
- Positive developmental steps on behalf of the patient should also be highlighted and emphasized to the parents.
- Encourage the parents to appreciate their child's strengths (again)!
- Avoid having a purely deficit-oriented focus and make this a topic of conversation!

The following points should also be considered while establishing a therapeutic relationship with the parents of the patient (after Borg-Laufs 2009):

- Reliable availability of the therapist – also for crisis situations between therapy sessions
- Preparation of parents by the therapist for the possibility that confrontation and critiques may come up over the course of conversations with parents – e.g., regarding existing family rules, or parenting deficits – as a means of reducing resistance. Example: "I have the hypothesis that your child…, because you, as parents…."
- Communication of basic knowledge about the foundational principles of a positive upbringing and strategies for changing behavior
- Communication of etiological knowledge about the background and motives behind sexual assaults already perpetrated by your child
- Communication of a comprehensive knowledge about disorders, in respect to the sexual particularities of your child

Interventions

The order as well as the selection of the interventions introduced below is to be determined by the therapist according to the individual need, as not every set of parents requires support in all subject areas. It is recommended however to make use of the → IS *Integrating Parents into the Prevention Plan* in any case.

Parental Emotions

A common necessity in working with parents of juvenile sex offenders or patients with sexual particularities is picking up on, recognizing, reflecting on, and normalizing the emotional reactions triggered in the parents. Typical emotions upon confronting the fact that one's own child feels a sexual attraction to children or even has already sexually molested children are: disbelief, anger, guilt, shame, and fear.

One of the first goals of the therapeutic work should therefore be to motivate the parents to speak openly with the therapist about their own emotional experiences. Helpful questions may be:

- What kinds of feelings does the thought that your child has committed child sexual abuse and/or feels a sexual attraction to children trigger in you?
- How does the thought that sexual assaults have taken place within your family make you feel?
- How does the thought that other people might find out about your child's make you feel?
- Which of these feelings (that you mentioned) do you express openly?
- Which feelings are still present?

The therapist should explore exactly which emotions dominate in each individual case, and not allow him- or herself be put off by superficial answers. It is often difficult for parents to verbalize negative emotions about their child. Answers that create the impression of a still-intact "happy family" environment should also be critically interrogated. The emotions being worked out should be authentically validated in the interests of building this supplementary relationship, although the specific dominant emotion in each case should be subsequently worked on together with the therapist.

Disbelief

Many parents refuse to believe that their child has committed sexual abuse (Pierce 2011). A similar reaction can occur if the therapist attempts to communicate to the parents that their child is sexually oriented towards children. In most cases, it is necessary to explore specific cognitive distortions on the part of the parents, such as denial mechanisms. The accompanying feeling is usually that of being overwhelmed. It is necessary to communicate to the parents that it is normal to question behavior displayed by one's own child that violates sexual boundaries. No parent expects his or her child to become a sex offender and/or display a sexual interest in children. Reacting with disbelief when learning that your own child that you have raised desires sexual contact with prepubescent children is to be validated as a completely understandable reaction. Many patients initially do not tell their parents all of the details or deny their sexual desires and/or the details of their acts of sexual abuse for various reasons, including as a way to avoid negative consequences or even out of a profound sense of shame. In this way, parents are denied the opportunity to get an overview of the extent of the acts of sexual abuse or the core issues with their child's sexual preference structure.

Therapists should communicate the following aspects to parents (after Schmid 2014):

- The parents' reactions are understandable and relatable.
- The parents should not put pressure on their child, but rather communicate to him that they love him as their child above all else and value him.
- The parents should carefully, but also authentically and openly appeal to their child's sense of responsibility and honesty so that he can gradually open up to them and gain trust in his parents as a resource.

Additional potentially helpful strategies for reducing parental disbelief are (after Heiman 2002):

- To grasp what the parents understand about what has happened and which explanatory model they have

Examples of possible questions:

- What exactly do you understand to have happened?
- What do you understand your child's desires to be, in regards to sex?
- To fill gaps in knowledge by communicating information:

Examples of possible questions:

- What do you need in order to be able to give up your disbelief?
- What can you understand, and what is more difficult for you to understand?
- To clarify what the function of their resistance is

Examples of possible questions:

- What would happen if you were to accept that your child feels a sexual attraction to children?
- What would such a sexual particularities mean for you as parents or for the family?
- What kinds of consequences do you think this kind of sexual particularities might have?
- To see the situation in a new light

Examples of possible questions:

- What would be the advantage of acknowledging that which has been said/has happened in its entirety?
- What would the negative consequences be of acknowledging what has been said/what has happened?

Anger

Anger or resentment most often arises in parents when their child has already been sexually abusive, something that usually occurs within the family system. It should be signaled to parents at the outset that resentment and anger are common emotions for parents in their position. One should work psychoeducationally with parents to communicate to them that positive changes in their child – those they experience themselves, as well as those they are actively told about by the therapist – will lead to a reduction of feelings of resent-

ment and anger in the long run. It is important to communicate to parents, however, that they should not let their anger out on the patient directly, as this reduces the chances of his feeling secure enough to confide in his parents comprehensively. Parents' impulses to punish must be spoken about openly and deemed unhelpful. The therapist should validate anger and resentment as such; however, he or she must focus on the functional handling of these emotions by the parents and work on them if necessary with the inclusion of the patient as appropriate. The overarching objective should be for them to be able to allow themselves to love their child again (Schmid 2014).

Guilt

Many parents of sexually molesting adolescents see themselves as having failed (Pierce 2011). In the case of patients with a sexual particularities for the child developmental body age who have thus far abstained from abuse, as well, many parents ask themselves to what degree they are responsible for their child's sexual impulses. Classic verbalized questions on the part of parents are: *What did I do wrong? Could I have prevented this?*

These attitudes should be interrogated in an active and targeted way during therapy.

Examples of possible questions:

- What could you have done better, in your opinion?
- Would you really have been able to foresee the sexual assault?
- How have you actively contributed to what happened, in your eyes?

As part of the psychoeducational sessions, the therapist should talk about the following points with parents, if necessary, as part of communicating a model for this disorder:

- Developing a realistic view of their part in what happened.
- It is never possible to be 100% in control.
- Sexual preference cannot be built up or broken down by parenting measures.
- The patient – the parents' child! – bears the responsibility of his sexual preferences and his (sexual) behavior.

Shame

Some parents internalize what has happened and experience a great sense of shame (Pierce 2011). In particular, there is a distinct fear that people within the larger family system and/or the social environment of the parents will find out about the sexual history or preferences of the patient and that the family will face social stigmatization. The therapist should explore the reasons behind parents' feelings of shame in detail. One must work together with the parents on the question of who needs to know about their child's sexual assaults and to what extent, and on what points the family should and can be protected. The child's sexual particularities should be dealt with according to the same procedure as for sexual assaults. One needs to determine who really needs to know about it and what positive or negative consequences could accompany this.

Fear

Parents' fears primarily have to do with the potential harm to others that this sexual particularity poses, and with the probability of relapse for sexual assaults. Parental fears should be normalized using an objective approach – empirical knowledge about the frequency of sexual assaults or recidivism rates, for example, can be useful here. Care should always be taken, however, on the part of the therapist not to trivialize or minimize, but rather to work toward a realistic image regarding possible future acts of sexual abuse!

Psychoeducation

It is necessary to work not only with the patient himself, but also with the parents on an individual model for this disorder. This means making their child's sexual particularities understandable for the parents, in order to make it possible for them to deal with it. First, the parents' existing level of knowledge should be recorded in detail. Parents often ask questions about the reason or the abuse and desperately search for answers. In the beginning, one should orient oneself in terms of the content using the following questions:

- What do the parents know about their child's sexuality?
- What do the parents imagine a sexual particularities to mean?

- What do the parents imagine *their* child's sexual particularities to mean?
- What kinds of hypotheses do the parents have about its origins?
- What kind of an attitude do the parents have in regard to its changeability and exclusivity, but also regarding its causal relations to dissexual behavior?

Depending on the parents' individual needs and previous knowledge, it may be necessary to go through a psychoeducation on the following topics with them:

- Psychosexual development in adolescence
- Sexual preference structure
- Dissexuality
- Risk factors
- How offenses occur
- Relapse prevention

Above all, it is recommended to emphasize the communication of the following aspects and to explicitly point them out as part of psychoeducation:

1. Differentiating between the planes of fantasy and behavior: Communicating the difference between a sexual responsiveness to the child developmental body age (expression of sexual preference) and child sexual abuse (expression of dissexual behavior).
2. Individual sexual preference has to do with fate, not choice. An affected person is not responsible for his sexual preference, but he is responsible for his sexual behavior.
3. Due to the lack of empirical knowledge about the stability of sexual preference in adolescence, it is impossible to make a final statement about it; however, a cure in the sense of extinguishing the sexual impulses should not be promised. The relevant literature contains retrospective knowledge drawn from working with adult pedophilic men above all, so that, according to the current state of knowledge, it should be assumed that a sexual responsiveness to the child developmental body age becomes manifest in adoles-

cence and remains categorically stable. However, a definitive statement cannot be made.

Offense-Supportive Factors on the Part of Parents

It is important to work together with the parents to make clear whether and in what form mechanisms exist within the family system that contribute to the juvenile patient being hindered in his effective management of risk situations or even whether abusive behaviors are in fact being supported. The first task of the therapist is to understand the intrafamilial structures and their functionality in order to subsequently modify them, if necessary.

In terms of content, one should be concerned above all with the following foundational questions:

- What can the parents change themselves?
- Which parenting style do they exhibit?
- How do the parents communicate with their child?
- How would you evaluate the general parenting competency?
- Are age-appropriate boundaries being set for the child?
- Are there age-appropriate rules in place?
- How would you evaluate the overall familial atmosphere?
- How are conflicts and problems dealt with?
- Would the intensity of attachment within the family be considered age-appropriate?
- Do the parents display any cognitive distortions in respect to the juvenile's (potential) sexual assaults?
- Are the parents actually making the juvenile accountable for his sexually abusive behavior? Do what degree?

The current state of the familial situation should be recorded in detail in light of these aspects, and, building on this, one should work together with the parents to find possibilities for change or potential needs. The following subject areas should be discussed with parents as needed and varied in their therapeutic intensity according to need.

1. **Working on Parents' Parenting Style**

Generally speaking, one can differentiate between four parenting styles (after Maccoby and Martin 1983):

1. **Authoritarian:** A strong exercising of power on the part of the parents is central, often combined with parental rejection. This is expressed in the frequent use of commands, as well as the expectation of obedience from the child. Rules must be strictly adhered to by the child. Misbehavior is often sanctioned with drastic punitive measures. The needs of the child are of little interest to the parents.

2. **Neglectful:** Neglectful parents often treat their child with rejection and offer only little guidance. Only the bare minimum of time is dedicated to the child, who receives very little to no emotional affection. The child is given no direction, nor judged – positively or negatively – on his behavior.

3. **Permissive**: Permissive parents behave toward their children with a great deal of acceptance and few demands. The child is barely controlled, he or she is allowed to develop without restrictions, and misbehavior remains unsanctioned.

4. **Authoritative**: An authoritative parenting style is characterized by the child being met with acceptance and clear structure. The child's spontaneous activities are condoned, and he or she is encouraged to develop self-reliance. Positive behavior is reinforced (praise), help is offered in difficult situations, misbehavior receives appropriate sanction. A "healthy degree" of control is exercised along with warm and open communication.

The goal is authoritative parental behavior, as this increases the probability of a supportive parent-child relationship. Compared with children whose parents exercise one of the other three parenting styles, children of authoritative parents are on the whole more socially competent, more emotionally adjusted, higher-achieving, display higher impulse control, and have fewer behavioral problems (Baumrind 1991; Görlitz 2010). First, the therapist should ascertain which parenting style is exhibited by the patient's parents. Standardized surveys may be used as a support, e.g., "The Parenting-Style Inventory (ESI)" [„*Das Erziehungsstil-Inventar (ESI)*"] by Krohne and Pulsack (1995) or the "D-ZKE Zurich Short Survey on Parenting Styles" [„*D-ZKE. Zürcher Kurzfragebogen zum Erziehungsverhalten*"] by Reitzle (2015).

Should there be any indications of an unsupportive parenting style, the following interventions are appropriate:

- Psychoeducation on the styles of parenting: definitions, working out pros and cons
- Standardized parental self-observation, e.g., through daily documentation of one positive and one negative interaction with one's child, using a journal
- Behavioral analyses of critical parenting situations (e.g., using a SORKC-model)

2. **Working on Intrafamilial Communication**

In many families, problems are not talked about openly; instead a climate of avoidance dominates. It is of crucial importance that the parents and the patient learn how to speak openly with each other about the subject of sexuality as well as (if applicable) the patient's sex offenses. Therapeutically, use should be made above all of the many available materials and manuals on communication training. Among other things, the primary features of communication should be taught, such as active listening and constructive feedback. In addition, we recommend analyzing the difficult conversational situations with the parents – ideally with the parents and the patient together – in role-plays and with video feedback and practicing alternative communication structures.

At the same time, parents should be prepped for upcoming conversations on the topics of sexual particularities and/or sexual assault. It can be helpful to go over the following questions with them in advance (after Heiman 2002):

- What does your child need for him to be able to open up to you in conversation? How can you guarantee connection, support, security, etc.?
- What exactly do you want to communicate to your child?

- What concrete things can you do to prepare for this conversation? What exactly do you want to find out?
- How do you think your child will react when you actively address this topic?
- What attempts have you made thus far to engage in conversation with your child?
- How does your child usually react to confrontation with problems?
- What are your (worst) fears regarding what might happen if you address the topic directly (running away, becoming suicidal, aggression, etc.)?
- Are you worried that you won't be able to do a good job of controlling yourself?
- How would you react if your child denies certain aspects or everything? Why might your child do that? What function might this have?

It is necessary to show the parents that they should not just sporadically signal to their child that they are ready to have this conversation, but rather that they should actively approach their child about it. Subjects must be addressed directly. Parents should also not avoid uncomfortable topics, as they are the role models that serve as a guide to their child. Parents must in some cases learn to actually listen to the adolescent and not to judge him. In this way, the patient is able to experience not having to feel uncomfortable about talking with his parents about sexuality. This is a crucial aspect, as it is only when the patient can place trust in his parents that there is a realistic chance of being able to incorporate the parents into the prevention plan.

3. **Working on the Parent-Child Relationship**

Should deficits in the parent-child relationship already reveal themselves at the outset or over the course of therapy, e.g. if the parents noticeably distance themselves from the patient, or if they aggressively reject him, strategies should be developed for how the parents to become close with their child again. The following measures are effective for this (after Jones 2015; Thornton et al. 2008):

- Strengthening perception of desired behavior
- Establishing positive reinforcement of desired behavior

- Spending time together
- (Re)discovering the patient's resources
- Positive reinforcement of the patient's resources
- Conveying moral support
- Inducing hope and communicating to the child that his parents believe in him
- Guaranteeing emotional availability
- Perceiving the child independently of his acts of sexual abuse, so that the child is not reduced to his delinquency and/or his sexual preference.

4. **Working on and with Boundaries**

   Should it become evident that no age-appropriate boundaries have been set within the family system, the focus should be put on establishing them. This involves, among other things, granting privacy to each family member, agreeing upon consequences for the violation of boundaries, establishing clearer general rules for behavior, forbidding verbal or physical violence etc. If it becomes necessary to establish new family rules, it is a good idea to make this official with a behavior contract. Depending on the state of the patient's cognitive development, it may be useful to introduce a reward system according to behavioral therapeutic principals for keeping to the rules. It is essential for all family members to be involved in the establishment of family rules and for (appropriate) compromises to be made on all sides.

5. **Working on the Intrafamilial Conflict Culture**

   If the family has marked difficulties with addressing their problems openly and/or solving them constructively, the completion of a problem-solving training may be a good idea. An example for the approach based on Görlitz (2010) can be found in the → IS *Solving Problems Together*.

   An example of a useful measure for getting families to regularly work together on problems is the establishment of a family council. For this, families come together on a regular basis to approach problems together in a structured context and solve them constructively. An overview of the formal framework and content structure of a family council and more can be found in Görlitz (2010).

Parents' Relationship and Sexual Satisfaction

An important aspect of working with parents or primary caregivers is their function as a model for the patient. By observing and imitating parental behavior, children learn new and complex behaviors. Depending on the positive or negative reinforcement of their behavior by the parents, the probability of occurrence of already-learned behaviors may change. In addition, by observing their parents, children and adolescents acquire the ability to recognize discriminative stimuli, in the sense of being able to better discern which situational cues demand which behavior (Alby and Schmidt-Bucher 2007).

The concept of model learning or social learning established after Bandura (as cited in Hautzinger et al. 2006) thereby represents one of the central concepts of knowledge and skill acquisition in the social context of young people. In the treatment of mentally ill children and adolescents, too, model learning is indicated as a therapeutic method for a number of disorders. The mechanism of model learning is also effective for the development and modification of attitudes regarding the formation of partner and sexual relationships. Here, the so-called *modeling effect* plays a role, according to which the new behavior is learned via pure observation of this behavior in the model (Alby and Schmidt-Bucher 2007).

Parents should be encouraged to engage in self-critical reflection with the support of the therapist as to what kind of model they offer their child in regards to the formation of partner and sexual relationships, as well as what suggestions and expectations they are conveying when it comes to roles. If an adolescent learns, for example, that he can effectively impose his will on a partner by means of aggressive behavior, he may possibly use this parental model behavior in his own relationships. Parents should be motivated to take on the perspective of their child and to ask themselves the following questions (for example):

- Which relationship values and norms am I passing on to my child?
- Is my child adopting potentially-dysfunctional behaviors that we as parents are setting as an example?
- How does our child experience our partner relationship?
- Which role models are we performing, and do we talk about gender roles?
- Is our child frequently confronted with parental conflicts?
- How do we deal with relationship conflicts as opposed to familial conflicts and which conflict-solving strategies are we conveying to our child?
- What kind of a concept of sexuality do I set as an example for my child?
- Is it possible that I am suggesting to my child that sexuality is taboo?

Should it become clear in the course of this that the parents are experiencing dissatisfaction with their own partner relationship and/or their sexuality together, the subject should be addressed openly and, if necessary, a recommendation that they seek out their own therapy should be voiced. It is important to elucidate to parents the responsibility that they have as a model for their child as far as his acquisition of social skills is concerned, and that attitudes as well as how they deal with subjects having to do with partner and sexual relationships are a part of that. If the parents are in need of therapy themselves, and they consent to this, the case should ideally be taken on by a therapist trained in sexual medicine. It is not recommended to serve as therapist to both the adolescent and the parents at the same time, as this may lead to role conflict. A particular concern is that the adolescent may begin to doubt the loyalty of the therapist and start to withdraw from the therapeutic process.

Inclusion in the Prevention Plan

As already explained at the beginning of the module on working with parents, the inclusion of the parents in the prevention plan should be obligatory with each patient. The parents should be motivated to support their child in the goal of future abstinence from abuse behaviors. The therapist should therefore – above all while the child is still living under his parent's roof – actively incorporate the parents into the individual prevention plan. Monitoring the patient usually comes with a great deal of stress for the parents which must be openly discussed and authentically validated.

The following questions may be helpful when getting started on this subject:

- What can parents do themselves in order to reduce the risk of sexual assaults being committed by their child?
- What degree of parental supervision is currently necessary in order to reduce the risk of (additional) acts of sexual assault being committed by the juvenile?
- Are there currently control mechanisms put in place by the parents? Which function do these serve?
- Which prohibitions exist? Which function do these serve?
- How often is the juvenile left unsupervised? How often does the juvenile have unsupervised contact with prepubescent children?
- From the parents' perspective: what are potential risk factors for the juvenile's sexually molesting behavior?
- What kinds of risk situations are there, e.g., babysitting, surfing the Internet unsupervised, etc.?
- What kinds of consequences, such as helplessness, social isolation, hostilities, etc., does the necessary degree of monitoring have for the juvenile, as well as for the family system as a whole?
- Are the parents even in a position to be able to provide the necessary degree of supervision and control?
- Which measures need to be put in place consistently?
- How can the parents' burden be lessened? Who can potentially be included as well?
- Must additional authorities be activated, such as child protective services?
- What should parents do if they suspect that their child is on the verge of committing an act of direct or indirect sexual abuse?

Concrete strategies should be worked out with the parents that they can put into use to support their child's abuse behavior. A useful basis is the → IS *Relapse Prevention Tips for Parents*. Parents can document their strategies with the help of the therapist using the → WS *Our Prevention Measures*.

8   Module 8 – Treatment of Comorbid Disorders

According to empirical results, juvenile sex offenders often display psychopathology that extend beyond boundary-crossing sexual behavior and sometimes take the form of clinically relevant symptoms requiring treatment. According to Seto and Pullman et al. (2014), a clinically relevant psychopathology represents a risk factor in juvenile sex offenders for repeat sexual assaults, most of all when anxiety, depression, and personality problems are present.

In a meta-analysis, Seto and Lalumière (2010) compared, among other things, the psychopathology of juvenile sex offenders with juvenile offenders who had not committed sexual offenses. The former showed significant and frequent psychopathological symptoms, in particular relating to anxiety disorders (principally social anxieties), as well as low self-esteem – but no higher levels of depression or neuroticism.

In a meta-analysis by Boonmann and colleagues (2015) that studied the prevalence of mental disorders in juvenile sex offenders compared to juvenile offenders who had not committed sexual offenses, it was shown that 69% of the juvenile sex offenders met the diagnostic criteria for at least one mental illness. 44% displayed additional comorbid disorders. The most frequent diagnoses were social behavior disorders, substance abuse, anxiety disorders, ADHD (Attention Deficit/Hyperactivity Disorder), and affective disorders. To summarize, juvenile sex offenders were diagnosed significantly less often with externalizing disorders than juvenile offenders who had not committed sexual offenses. Regarding internalizing disorders, there were no significant differences (Boonmann et al. 2015).

A study included in the meta-analysis of 't Hart-Kerkhoffs and colleagues (2015) similarly studied the occurrence of mental disorders in juvenile sex offenders, classified by age of the victims. The results showed that 75% of the total sample group displayed at least one mental disorder, with a comorbidity rate of 54%. In an exclusive consideration of the juveniles who sexually abused children, in 84% at least one, and in 74% one present comorbid mental disorder could be ascertained ('t Hart-Kerkhoffs et al. 2015).

The studies consulted as examples show that there is a high frequency of mental disorders in juveniles who have committed sexual offenses. Of principal interest is the heterogeneous distribution of the disorders ascertained, which has a direct effect on treatment.

The authors of this manual are not currently aware of any studies that deal explicitly with the occurrence of psychopathology in juveniles with sexual particularities for the child body age. On the contrary, our own analyses (Kreutzmann 2017) show that about half of the patients who have presented themselves to the project "Primary Prevention of Child Sexual Abuse by Juveniles" (PPJ) with some sort of sexual preference also display an additional mental disorder. In both self-evaluation and the evaluation of others, this group also shows externalizing and – in particular – internalizing psychopathology at a higher rate than a norm sample. A very heterogeneous spectrum of disorders present could also be ascertained (Kreutzmann 2017). The observable subclinical phenomena of mental disorders do not fulfill the diagnostic criteria, but nevertheless have an effect on the therapeutic process and the therapeutic relationship.

Accordingly, no concrete goals or interventions can be formulated for the treatment of comorbid mental disorders. Of greater importance in the context of a comprehensive child and adolescent-psychiatric diagnostic would be to initially ascertain possible psychopathological symptoms. A resulting assessment of the necessity of treatment should then be incorporated into the therapy plan. In order to reduce individual risk factors, the aim should be the improvement of the juvenile's general level of function. As the studies cited show, psychopathological symptoms appear to coincide with an increased risk of committing sexually-violent behavior.

It should furthermore be assumed that in the case of juveniles with externalizing mental disorders, which coincide by definition with reduced impulse control, other precautionary measures must be taken than with juveniles with internalizing disorders. No blanket measures can be formulated to this end. Rather, taking the system into account, an individual therapy – ideally with child and adolescent-psychotherapeutic expertise – must be developed. Should a supplementary medication be necessary to suppress impulses in the case of externalizing disorders, for instance, or for the medicinal improvement of affect in depressive disorders, this can only happen with child and adolescent-psychiatric oversight, in accordance with the guidelines.

Also to be integrated into the treatment plan is the onset of an acute comorbid mental disorder. Both the presence of a mental disorder before one is aware of one's own non-normative sexual preference, and the development of such a disorder as a reaction to process of integrating a deviant preference are conceivable, but imply different treatment goals.

Finally, the aspect of mental impairment must be considered. The modules contained in BEDIT-A were designed for juveniles of average intelligence. For juveniles with a markedly below-average intelligence or a present mental impairment, it must be considered on a case-by-case basis to what extent the manual is appropriate. In any case, a slower pace of work should be chosen and repetitions should be considered.

To summarize, value must be placed in the diagnostic framework on a comprehensive assessment of the juvenile patient, so that psychopathologies and present mental disorders can be ascertained as necessary. Only then can an adequate therapy plan be developed. Disorders acutely in need of treatment (e.g. from the schizophrenic spectrum of disorders or severe addiction disorders), especially when they coincide with real endangerment of the self or others, must be prioritized on principle.

9   Module 9 – Medicinal Treatment Options

Cave: Reading this chapter does not replace the consultation or collaboration with a specialist in child and adolescent psychiatry, or a doctor with supplementary training in child and adolescent endocrinology. Legally effective medicinal consultations may only be carried out by specially-trained medical colleagues.

Theory
In the treatment of sexual behavior disorders and non-normative sexual preference, the use of psychotropic drugs can be a sensible building block, but always adjuvant to a psychotherapeutic-sexual-medicinal intervention. Medications can minimize sexual impulses experienced as urgent and cumbersome, but do not, however, alter the content of fantasies. In other words: the quantity, not the quality, of sexual fantasies and impulses can be influenced via supplementary pharmacotherapy.

A precondition for an accompanying medicinal therapy is the ego-syntonic processing of currently-occurring sexual fantasies, i.e. the acceptance of current sexual fantasies involving children as a part of the self. If this is present and the occurring sexual impulses are simultaneously experienced as adversely urgent and strong, impulse-dampening medication can be considered.

Three classes of medication, each functioning through different mechanism, come into question:

- Selective serotonin reuptake inhibitors (SSRIs)
- Antiandrogen medications (cyproterone acetate and GnRH-analogues)
- Opioid antagonists.

SSRIs are primarily known for their therapeutic indications for affective disorders. The adverse medicinal effect of SSRIs that is well known from this indication, the reduction of sexual appetite, is a contributing factor to the efficacy of this class. There are clinical experiences and studies that show reductions in sexual impulses through the use of SSRIs (Bradford and Greenberg 1996; Greenberg and Bradford 1997). SSRIs are administered regularly to adult patients for the purpose of dampening sexual impulses (Thibaut et al. 1993), as – among other reasons – the effect of SSRIs on the sexual experience and behavior of adults is well studied (Guay 2009).

Cyproterone acetate (CPA, sold under the brand name Androcur®) is an antiandrogen that blocks androgen receptors as a competitive antagonist. Through this, androgens (i.e. testosterone) are unable to bind to receptors, halting its reaction on target cells. A result of this suppressed androgen effect is a marked reduction in sexual fantasies and sexual behavior (Bradford and Pawlak 1993).

Gonadotropin releasing hormone analogues (GnRH-analogues, sold under the brand name Salvacyl®) similarly lead to a sharp reduction in sexual fantasies and sexual behaviors. Unlike CPA, GnRH-analogues target the hormone-regulating centers of the brain and reduce the endogenous production of testosterone in the testicles.

Opioid antagonists: Naltrexone is a competitive antagonist that affects the opioid receptors in the brain. In case studies a naltrexone treatment showed an increase in control over sexual desire (Raymond et al. 2002, 2010; Ryback 2004). It is hypothesized that naltrexone indirectly influences the dopaminergic reward system. Up to this point naltrexone has only been usable for the reduction of sexual desire in the context of expanded access, but has – compared to the other

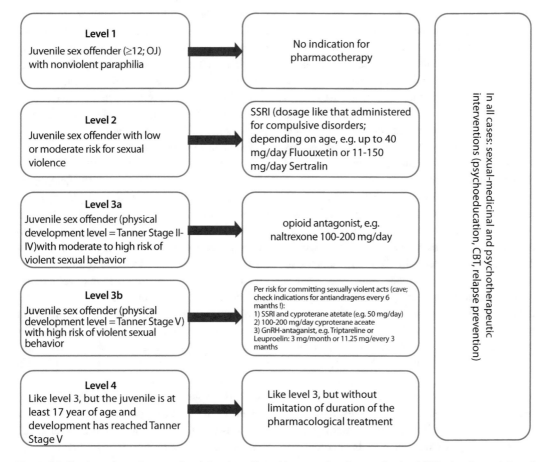

Fig. 2 Medication schema for sexually-violent juveniles with a sexual preference for the child body scheme (adapted from Thibaut et al. 2016)

pharmacological therapy options described here – a better side-effect profile.

The World Federation of Societies of Biological Psychiatry (WFSBP) has published guidelines for the treatment of adolescent sex offenders with paraphilias that can serve as a further source of information for professionals administering treatment (Thibaut et al. 2016). These guidelines contain a schematic of the medications, reproduced here and expanded to include opioid antagonists as a supplementary pharmacological option (Fig. 2).

Goals
- Acquisition of knowledge on the possibilities and limitations of medicinal therapy in the case of non-normative sexual preference.

Interventions
Shared Decision and Informed Consent

Discuss with your patient and their parents the option of supplementary administration of medication. Not all patients with a sexual particularities for children require (*indication*) or want (*participation/compliance*) medicinal treatment. An indication is present if your patient displays a high risk of committing assault, and compliance can be present if your patient experiences his sexual fantasies about children as urgent, and has the impulse to act on these fantasies.

Make it clear to the patient that medication can lessen the intensity of sexual fantasies, but that they will not fully cease. There is no "magic pill" that can make sexual preference disappear. Based on the current state of research, a "cure" in the sense of eliminating sexual preference cannot be brought about. Remind them of the goal of the therapy: to not commit dissexual behavior – and that medication can help with this. The patient should also understand that all medications have unwanted effects, known colloquially as "side effects," and will also come into question. Discuss the desired and undesired effects of medication with your patient (→IS *Medicinal Treatment Options*).

In connection with this, the patient should discuss with you what, from their perspective, could be an argument against medication (pros-and-cons list). This can be undertaken as a homework assignment, so the patient can think it over in peace and develop an opinion of his own.

Preparation for Medical Examinations

Should your patient decide in favor of supplementary medicinal treatment, it is important to prepare them for the recommended preliminary medical examinations. This should be done in cooperation with specialist colleagues. Should there be no one qualified working in the same facility, adequate consent from the patient and their guardian, in the form of a signed release from the obligation to confidentiality, will be necessary.

Explain to the patient that, from the medical perspective, a series of physical examinations must be undertaken in order to best rule out the possibility of complications. Among other tests, an EKG will be done, their blood pressure will be measured, blood will be taken to do bloodwork, and their Tanner stage ascertained, as the effective use of an antiandrogen medication only comes into question around or at the end of physical development. You may refer them here to →IS *Medicinal Treatment Options*.

Excursus: Tanner Stages

The term *Tanner stage* refers to James M. Tanner and describes the classification of physical development/the degree of physical maturity. The criteria for the classification in 5 different degrees of physical maturity are (a) breast development in those assigned female at birth, (b) testicle size and testicle volume in those assigned male at birth, and (c) the development/quality of pubic hair in both sexes.

Where *Tanner I* describes a prepubescent body, i.e. no palpable breast tissue or a testicular volume of <1.5 ml, and no pubic hair or vellus hair, *Tanner V* describes the adult body age, with fully-developed breasts or a fully-grown penis and testicles with a testicular volume of >20 ml, as well as thick, curly pubic hair extending over the mons pubis, thighs, and to the linea alba (cf. Marshall and Tanner 1969, 1970).

Worksheets BEDIT

Working Group of the Prevention Project Dunkelfeld

Fig. 1 Agreement for group work (participant)

I hereby agree to the following points:

1. I will take care to participate in sessions in way that allows all participants to feel comfortable and work together in a safe environment.
2. I will treat others and myself in a respectful and supportive way.
3. I will not behave in a verbally or physically aggressive manner.
4. I will regularly take part in the weekly therapy sessions.
5. Should I plan not to take part in a session, I will excuse myself at least 24 hours in advance.
6. I will arrive on time to all sessions, so as not to interrupt others or miss anything myself.
7. I will complete the homework assignments and the accompanying journal entries on self-observation and practice.
8. I will try to take an active role in group sessions and to open up in discussions.
9. I understand that I can speak freely about my sexual fantasies, past sexual contact with children/minors, my past offenses, as well as private information and therapy content, as the therapists are bound by legal confidentiality agreements.
10. I will keep all information shared in trust by other participants to myself. I will not share the content of the therapy, personal information, or names of participants.
11. I understand that explicitly-announced sexual contact with children/minors, other explicitly-stated offenses, or explicitly-stated suicidal intentions could result in therapists being forced to act in the interests of my safety or for the protection of other persons (e.g. through the administration of medication, temporary inpatient treatment, notification of social services).
12. I understand that any such steps will be discussed and agreed upon with me before their implementation.

Violations of this agreement endanger my own interests regarding success in therapy as well as the interests of others. Repeated violations of this agreement may thus result in expulsion from the treatment program.

By signing with my PIN I agree to the above conditions:

_____   _____
Date   Signature(PIN)

Working Group of the Prevention Project Dunkelfeld
Charité – Universitätsmedizin Berlin, Corporate Member of Freie Universität Berlin, Humboldt-Universität zu Berlin, and Berlin Institute of Health, Center for Human and Health Sciences, Institute of Sexology and Sexual Medicine, Berlin, Germany
e-mail: klaus.beier@charite.de

Fig. 2 Agreement for group work (therapist)

I hereby agree to the followingpoints:

1. I will accept the personality of the patient, with no spoken or unspoken judgment.
2. I will show the patient the same respect that I myself would want as a patient.
3. I will try to design the working conditions in such a way that it is possible for all patients to reach their therapy goals in a safe environment.
4. I will take care to administer a professional and effective therapy.
5. I will be available for the weekly therapy sessions and, should I be unable to be present for any reason, will excuse myself at least 24 hours in advance.
6. I will be punctual, concentrated, and prepared for the agreed-upon appointments.
7. I will treat patients' written assignments with respect and responsibility, and protect their rights.
8. I will regularly make use of supervision and the support of my colleagues.
9. I will heed the legal agreement to confidentiality. Furthermore, I will not communicate information or names of group members exchanged during therapy sessions with any third party.
10. I will follow the ethical and professional guidelines.

By signing I agree to the above conditions:

_____   _____
Date   Signature

Fig. 3 Regulation of testosterone levels in men

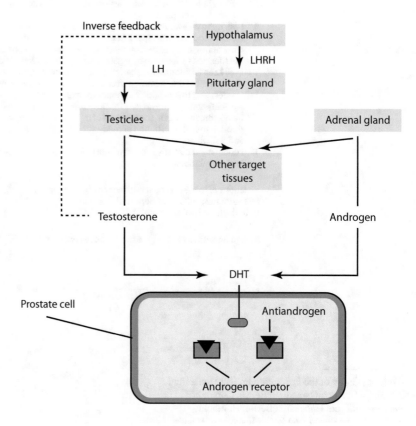

The concept of sexual abuse is used when no mutual consent to sexual behavior is present:

1. When the other person is incapable of giving consent, that is to say physically or mentally unable to make their own decision;
2. When a person is not fully informed about or has not understood the behavior's content, execution, and possible consequences;
3. When the other person has not agreed freely and without pressure.

Based on definitions of child sexual abuse, dissexual behavior toward children (with prepubescent or early-pubescent body schemes) encompasses the following sexual behavior (with no claim to being exhaustive):

1. Sexually-motivated observation in intimate situations (voyeuristic activities),
2. Sexually-motivated touching or stroking outside the genital area,
3. The use of abuse images of children for one's own sexual stimulation and/or preparation for or inducement of sexual stimulation,
4. Grooming, i.e. the initiation of sexual contact with children on the Internet (chatrooms, etc.), through other media, or in direct contact situations,
5. Revealing one's genitals with or without masturbating (exhibitionist acts),
6. A person inviting a child to sexually stimulate them,
7. Inviting a child to sexually stimulate him- or herself,
8. Taking part in the sexual manipulation or stimulation of a child,
9. Penetration with the penis, tongue, finger, or objects of the mouth, vagina, or anus of a child,
10. Creation of abuse images of children with one of the above-mentioned sexual acts with or in the presence of children,
11. Discussion of sexual themes for the purpose of sexual arousal in the presence of a child,
12. Display of pornographic depictions in the presence of a child for the purpose of sexual arousal.

Behaviors described in points 1. and 2. are viewed as dissexual/problem behavior. Behaviors described in points 3. to 12. correspond to judicially-relevant sexual behavior that can lead to criminal prosecution.

→ Masturbation to sexual fantasies about children is not regarded as dissexual behavior!

Sexual offenses and dissexual behavior against children occur because someone has made the decision to act.

Fig. 4 Dissexuality and child sexual abuse

	Category	Qualitative Description
1	Indicative	Non-sexual depictions of children in underwear/bathing suits doing normal activities or in normal situations (e.g. from advertisements, catalogues, photo albums)
2	Nudity	Depictions of nude or partially-nude children in normal situations (e.g. swimming pool, beach)
3	Posing	Depictions of (partially) clothed or nude children consciously taking on a pose or unusual posture
4	Erotic Posing	Sexualized or erotic depiction of (partially) clothed or nude children in stimulating or unnatural poses
5	Explicit Erotic Posing	Sexualized depiction of (partially) clothed or nude children with a focus on the genital area
6	Sexual Behavior Between Children	Depiction of sexual behavior between children without the participation of adults (e.g. touching, masturbation, oral sex, penetrative sex)
7	(Severe) Child Sexual Abuse	Depiction of sexual acts by one or more children with the participation or one or more adults (e.g. touching, masturbation, oral sex, penetrative sex)
8	Sadistic or Zoophilic Acts	Depictions of violent acts against children (e.g. with objects, bondage, whipping, experiences of pain) or l sexua acts by children toward animals

The consumption of <u>Categories 1 to 3</u> can be seen as dissexual/problem behavior. <u>Categories 4 to 8</u> represent legally-relevant abuse images, the dissemination, acquisition, and possession of which are punishable per § 184 German criminal code.

Fig. 5 Categories for the description of child sexual abuse images of children

	GnRH-Analogues (Synthetic Analogues of the Neurohormone Gonadotropin-Releasing Hormone, i.e. GnRH)	Cyproterone Acetate (Competitive Antagonist at the Androgen Receptor)	Selective Serotonin Reuptake Inhibitor (SSRI)
Group	Antiandrogen	Antiandrogen	Antidepressant
Brand Names	e.g. Salvycl®, Decapeptyl®, Enantone®, Trenantone®	Androcur®	e.g. Seroxat®, Tagonis®, Zoloft®, Cipramil®
Use	Used for the greatest possible suppression of the secretion of sex hormones. An important indication of this is in the inhibition of hormone-dependent tumor growth, e.g. in the case of prostate cancer. Further used in reproductive medicine to influence the organic regulation of egg cell maturation in women	Discovered through research on hormonal birth control. Administered to women in combination with sex hormones to treat symptoms of androgenization (e.g. increased body hair, acne), in the event that contraception is also desired	Originally developed for the treatment of depression. Most often-administered medications for the treatment of depression and other psychological illnesses (e.g. anxiety disorders, compulsive disorders)
Effect	The hypohpyse receives a signal through the medication that sufficient testosterone is present. The hypophyse then ceases production of messengers for the testicles and adrenal glands. The body thus stops producing testosterone	Cyproterone acetate blocks the body's testosterone receptors. It aims by these means for an effect similar to the reduction of testosterone levels	The concentration of serotonin, a neurotransmitter in the brain, is increased in the region of the synapses (nerve cells' contact points). This results in a change to the concentration of receptors and an antidepressant effect. This has no effect on people without depression. It is not fully known how SSRIs reduce sexual impulses and fantasies, as they have no effect on testosterone levels. It is believed that this effect might be explained by the resulting slower progression of emotional states
Effects on Sexuality	Nearly always: decreased sexual desire and fantasies, reduction of erectile and orgasmic function. Sexual impulses and fantasies are reduced, but are not qualitatively changed	Similar effect to GnRH-analogues, but generally less intensive. Nearly always: decreased sexual desires and fantasies, reduction of erectile and orgasmic function. Sexual impulses and fantasies are reduced, but are not qualitatively changed	Reduction of sexual impulses, sexual arousal, and orgasmic function (not in all patients). The effect is considerably less than that of GnRH-analogues or cyproterone acetate

Fig. 6 Medications for the reduction of sexual impulses

Medications for the Reduction of Sexual Impulses

	GnRH-Analogues (Synthetic Analogues of the Neurohormone Gonadotropin-Releasing Hormone, i.e. GnRH)	Cyproterone Acetate (Competitive Antagonist at the Androgen Receptor)	Selective Serotonin Reuptake Inhibitor (SSRI)
Unwanted Side Effects	Increased perspiration, hot flushes, bone pain, decreased bone density, weight gain, fatigue, joint and back pain, muscle weakness, reduced muscle mass, impaired sperm production, reduction of testicle size, depressive moods, asthenia, reduction of body hair. Rarely: testosterone levels do not reach their previous levels after cessation of the medication	Increased liver values, fatigue, weakened concentration, development of breasts (gynecomastia), weight gain, thromboses, impaired sperm production, depressive moods	In general SSRIs are safe and tolerable medications. Initial side effects such as restlessness, nausea, dizziness, and insomnia usually improve after 1-2 weeks
Distinctive Feature	At the beginning of treatment too much testosterone is produced. Androcur® (cyproterone acetate) must thus be taken supplementarily for 6 weeks		
Preliminary and Follow-up Examinations	Regular blood tests, bone density tests every 1-2 years (based on age and pre-existing conditions)	Regular blood tests (particularly for liver values), checks of bodyweight and blood sugar as necessary	Regular blood and liver value tests
Ingestion	Intramuscular injection every 3 months, e.g. in the upper thigh	Either via intramuscular injection every 2 weeks or as a daily tablet. The injection places less strain on the body than the tablets	As a tablet once or multiple times daily. Cannot be administered via injection
Assessment	Dependable reduction of sexual impulses and fantasies. Works better than Androcur® Generally good tolerability	Dependable reduction of sexual impulses and fantasies. Generally good tolerability	Generally good tolerability. Only unreliable and weak reduction of sexual fantasies and impulses

Fig. 6 (continued)

– "I didn't know I could think about things other than children […] I'm totally surprised by the other interesting activities I've discovered since taking medication."

– "I always felt like I was up to my neck in water and had to get up on my toes to even keep my head above the surface. Since taking medication I'm totally relaxed and can see what else is going on, since I'm not constantly busy just trying not to drown. My life has gotten totally relaxed. "

– "Before I started the drug therapy, I wasn't concerned with anything but kids. It was always about boys. I couldn't concentrate on anything else. I always looked for shows on TV with young boys and spent the whole night looking for photos of boys so I could save and archive them. I had to masturbate five or six times a day. I spent hours masturbating—until I couldn't anymore. Since starting medication I've got a clear head for the first time. I'm discovering other interests besides boys […] I think Amnesty International is great, and I can really get into their projects. I feel like a huge weight has been lifted. I only masturbate once or twice a day, and I can actually relax while doing it […] On the other hand it doesn't work so good with the medications. You hardly get an erection, your penis isn't as hard, it takes longer to reach orgasm, and over time there's less and less sperm. But you're not always in the mood to do it, and that's important to me."

– "I have the feeling that I'm more vulnerable since taking medication. I used to have armor on, lived in a shell, and tried to hide myself and my feelings. That need is gone now. And when I tell someone how I'm thinking and feeling, I'm more open and less afraid that someone could find me out, that someone could see who I really am. I'm also calmer and more relaxed around other adults, because I don't feel like I've got something to hide. It's still there, but it doesn't bother me as much. I even see chance encounters with boys with more distance […] At the same time you have to be careful not to try to leave everything to the medication and forget about your own responsibility […] It's about the limit, when you used to masturbate multiple times a day and then suddenly it's just once a week, and it's different than you're used to. But I'd keep taking the medication because you just get some peace and quiet. I threw away my whole collection of photos because I just feel dumb about it since taking medication. I couldn't understand why I'd saved 4000 images that don't mean anything to me anymore."

Fig. 7 Patient reports after medicinal treatment

Below you will find a few examples and key words that you can use to describe your current self

Self-Assessment

- What are my abilities?
- What are my strengths?
- In what areas am I an optimistic person?
- What attitudes and behavioral patterns do I have?
- What attitudes and behavioral patterns would I rather not have?
- What positive experiences do I have in interacting with others?
- What accomplishments can I share?
- What makes me laugh?

Appraisal By Others

- How would someone who knows and likes me describe me?
- What have I been praised for recently?
- What kind of acknowledgment and fondness do I receive from whom?

Preferences and Interests

- What is my life philosophy?
- What are my interests besides my job?
- Where do I want to travel?
- What do I have in common with my friends?
- How do I spend time with my friends?

Sexuality

- What is my sexual preference?
- What body scheme am I sexually responsive to?
- What sexual practices do I prefer?
- How much time per week do I spend on the Internet?
- How much time do I spend per week looking at pornographic material?
- How much time per week do I spend masturbating?
- How much time per week do I spend with children/minors?
- How do I feel about my sexual behavior and my sexual preference?

Fig. 8 My current self

Below you will find a few questions that you can use to summarize the contents up to this point.

1. What topics have been important to you up to this point?

2. What topics would you like to work on further?

3. What irritated you most during therapy?

4. Do you have any particular wishes regarding your further course of action?

5. What do you expect from the further progression of therapy?

6. What are your concrete goals?

8. What do you think your therapists are trying to achieve with the therapy?

9. How will the therapists know if you have reached your goals?

10. Which individual strengths and other factors (therapy, friends, medications, etc.) could help you reach your goals?

11. What will change once you've reached your goal?

12. What would you do if all your problems suddenly disappeared? How would your life change?

Fig. 9 My therapy goals and expectations

Situation	Thoughts and Assessments	Emotions and Physical Sensations	Behavioral Impulses	Actual Behavior	Consequences of Behavior (long-term and short-term)

Fig. 10 Behavioral analysis

I'd like to try an exercise with you that will require you to use your imagination. Anything that we humans can imagine becomes more vivid and realistic if we first release tension. So:

– Please sit up straight, but comfortably.
– Try to place both feet equally on the floor. Do you feel the floor under your feet?
– If you're comfortable doing so, close your eyes. If not, concentrate on one point on the floor in front of you.
– Breathe in deeply and then slowly breathe out. – And again…
– Concentrate fully on your breath. Breathe in and out again. Observe yourself precisely. How does it feel to sit on this chair?

Please imagine the following situation:

> It's a beautiful summer day. 26 degrees, a fantastic blue sky. You've got the day off. You sit on a meadow in the park, or on a bench, and read the paper. What does it look like there? Are there other people around? Are they laying in the sun? … How about you? Do you like to sit in the shade or in the sun? … How does it feel? Can you feel the warmth? … Can you smell the summer? Linden trees, maybe fresh-cut grass? Sunscreen? … Take a little time, observe until the situation becomes more real and you can feel where you are … Look around, everything … How do you feel? You see a 40-year old man you've never seen before. Picture him: he's tall, thin, and well-built. His hair is a little thin and gray, and he has a beard … Can you imagine him? Do you see him? What is he wearing? Where is he laying? Or is he sitting? The man looks over at you now and then. How do you feel?

Leave the situation and come back to this room. Stretch out and open your eyes. […] What did you experience?

– What did you think of this exercise? Was it easy to imagine this situation, or did you have trouble? Why?
– What did you think during the imagination exercise? What did you think when you realized the man was looking at you from time to time?
– How did you feel?

Fig. 11 Imagination exercise for self-observation (1)

I'd like to try an exercise with you that will require you to use your imagination. Anything that we humans can imagine becomes more vivid and realistic if we first release tension. So:

- Please sit up straight, but comfortably.
- Try to place both feet equally on the floor. Do you feel the floor under your feet?
- If you're comfortable doing so, close your eyes. If not, concentrate on one point on the floor in front of you.
- Breathe in deeply and then slowly breathe out. – And again…
- Concentrate fully on your breath. Breathe in and out again. Observe yourself precisely. How does it feel to sit on this chair?

Please imagine the following situation:

It's a beautiful summer day. 26 degrees. Gleaming blue sky. You're in the park again and have nothing to do. You have nothing but time. Can you see your surroundings? What's going on around you? Do you still see other people? How does it feel? Can you feel the warmth? What do you smell?t you now and again. How does that feel?

Take a little time, until the situation becomes more real and you can feel where you are. … Look around and observe everything. What do you feel now?

You notice a child that you like. Imagine the child: How old is it? A girl or a boy? What colour is the hair? How do the clothes look? Can you imagine the child? Can you see the child? What is the child doing? Lying down? Sitting? Playing?
Now you notice that the child is looking at you now and again. How does that feel?

Leave the situation and come back to this room. Stretch out and open your eyes. What did you experience?

- What did you think of this exercise? Was it easy to imagine this situation, or did you have trouble? Why?
- What did you think during the imagination exercise? What did you think when you realized the child was looking at you from time to time?
- How did you feel?

Fig. 12 Imagination exercise for self-observation (2)

Influencing Perception

In Order to help patients improve their self-observation capabilities and better handle their impulses, measures like the following can be useful. Be sure that the goal of this activity is to strengthen the patients´ feelings of self-efficacy.

1. Reciprocal Influence of Thoughts, Emotions and Behaviors

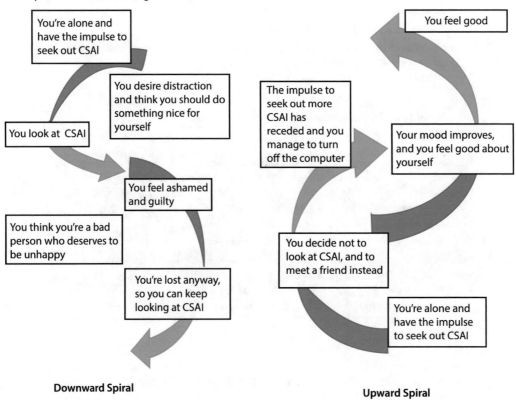

Downward Spiral   **Upward Spiral**

Fig. 13   Influencing perception

Influencing Perception

2. Dealing with Sexual Impulses – Go For It Or Let It Be

Assessment of Impulse's Intensity
1– 2– 3– 4– 5– 6– 7– 8– 9– 10

Go For it!	Let It Be!
Concentrate on your impulse […]	Give yourself 15 minutes […]
Imagine what you could do […]	Pick out a pleasant activity […]
Imagine how it would be […]	Think of something nice […]
Sense your sexual arousal […]	Go somewhere else […]
Block everything else out […]	Speak with someone […]

Assessment of Impulse's Intensity
1– 2– 3– 4– 5– 6– 7– 8– 9– 10

3. Using Sexual Arousal That Occurs During Group Work

When sexual fantasies or sexual behavior is spoken about in the group, it can happen that participants may feel sexually aroused. Therapists should not deny this arousal, but rather address it and use it for a live experiment in dealing with sexual impulses. The clients can be asked to assess the intensity of their sexual arousal. Different possibilities for dealing with it (ignoring it, talking more about it and considering it, taking a break for a few minutes, etc.) can then be discussed. The influence of these strategies on sexual arousal can be ascertained through assessing intensity again. Make sure the participants understand that they need to make a decision for or against one of the two options—going for the sexual impulse or letting it be—and thus having influence over their perception. If it seems sensible, therapists could explain the cycle of sexual arousal (excitement phase, plateau phase, orgasm phase, resolution phase) and emphasize that sexual arousal within the excitement phase comes and goes, dependent on behaviors and subjective psychological factors.

4. Importance of Situationally-Triggered Automatic Thoughts

It can be helpful to work out the importance of assessments and thoughts to the process of perception. The confrontation with sexually-arousing stimuli automatically triggers sexual thoughts and sexual arousal along with them. Whether patients confront their sexual impulses or decide against it is dependent on the situation. Therapists can illustrate these differences in behavior by comparing situations between a patient and a (nude) child that seem to be the same on first glance, but which are actually differentiated by the degree of external supervision. Say this interaction takes place in a sauna (external supervision: high), at a lake (external supervision: medium), or in front of the computer (external supervision: low). A comparative behavioral analysis shows that the same automatic thoughts are triggered in all three situations, e.g. "I like this child" and "I'm a pervert." As these automatic thoughts are first and foremost implicit, the participants will principally express explicit thoughts ("Hopefully no one notices") and require help in identifying the underlying assumptions and automatic thoughts.

Fig. 13 (continued)

Influencing Perception

Situation	Basic Assumptions/ Automatic Thoughts (implicit)	Thoughts (explicit)	Emotions	Impulses	Behavior
Sauna	"I like this child" "I'm a pervert"	"Hopefully no one notices anything" "Hopefully I don't get an erection"	Sexual arousal; fear; shame	To watch the child, to make contact To leave the situation	leaving the situation
Lake	"I like this child" "I'm a pervert"	"Hopefully no one notices anything" "What if I were alone?"	Sexual arousal; fear; shame	To watch the child, to make contact To leave the situation	leaving the situation
Computer	"I like this child" "I'm a pervert"	"No one can see me" "I should turn the computer off"	Sexual arousal; curiosity	To look at the pictures To leave the situation	looking at the pictures

This comparison of different situations can help both in recognizing the similarities between the situations and underlining the clear differences. Each participant is master of their own decisions. Therapists should make clear that participants are capable of deciding against impulses and have already made this decision many times in the past.

This exercise can be helpful in supporting acceptance of one's sexual preference, and can be repeated multiple times.

Fig. 13 (continued)

Fig. 14 Myths about the sexual abuse of children

1. I don't hurt anyone when I expose myself (in a sexual way), as long as I don't touch the child.
2. If a child doesn't show any resistance, they must want it too.
3. Some boys and girls are consciously seductive and want to come onto adults sexually.
4. Some children say they want to be touched in their genital area—so it must be good for them too.
5. Children want to experience their sexuality in the same way adults do.
6. If even the ancient Greeks had sex with children, it can't be so wrong.
7. Sex with a child produces a greater feeling of intimacy and closeness to adults in the child.
8. If a child doesn't tell anyone that they have been sexually abused, the experience can't have been so traumatic.
9. Some sexual relationships between adults and children are similar to sexual relationships to adults.
10. Sexual activities with children help them to learn about sexuality.
11. Children who have been sexually abused by more than one adult are clearly doing something to attract adults.
12. Sometimes adults suffer more from society's reaction to sexual contact between children and adults than the child does.
13. It's enough when a pedophilic man keeps his distance from children to avoid direct sexual contact.
14. Sexual abuse isn't usually planned; it just happens.
15. Children often invent stories of sexual abuse to get attention.
16. When someone decides never to abuse a child again, it's likely he will be successful in doing so.
17. When a child wants to see an adult's genitals, it means they want to have sex.
18. Some children initiate sexual acts on their own.
19. Some men feel sexually attracted to children because they've been rejected so often by adult partners.
20. Children can give an adult more acceptance and love than other adults can.

Further myths and false assumptions about the sexual abuse of children

| Myth | Sexual violence doesn't happen very often. |
| Fact | About 9% of all girls and 3% of all boys will become victims of sexual abuse. |

| Myth | When a child says NO, they actually mean YES. |
| Fact | All children have the right to be believed when they say YES or NO. When children say NO, they mean NO. |

| Myth | Children who are victims of sexual molestation provoked it. |
| Fact | No child desires sexual behavior with adults, or enjoys it. No style of clothing, no pose, and no behavior of a child gives an adult the right to enter into sexual behavior with a child. |

| Myth | Men commit sexual abuse because they lose control. |
| Fact | Studies of convicted sex offenders show that most sexual offenses were planned. Men can control their sexual impulses. It is their responsibility to do so. |

| Myth | Men who commit sexual abuse are emotionally and mentally unstable and imbalanced. |
| Fact | Studies show that most sex offenders are categorized as normal by friends, colleagues, and personality tests. |

| Myth | The victim doesn't know the offender. |
| Fact | In reality most victims know the offender. They could be friends, neighbors, acquaintances, or family members. |

| Myth violence | A child who has never been hit or injured cannot be the victim of sexual violence. |
| Fact | The absence of injuries does not mean that the child isn't a victim of sexual violence. The threat of violence or the use of weapons stuns a child and hinders resistance. In no way does that mean that the child consents to the interaction. If anything, that means that the child tried to protect him- or herself. Children (like adults) react differently to dire situations and thus to sexual violence. Some are obviously shocked and exhausted, while others will appear quiet and controlled. The quiet, controlled victim can be just as traumatized as the exhausted victim, but merely shows this in a different way. |

The belief in these myths indicates a shift in responsibility for the abuse from the perpetrator onto the victim. In cases of child sexual abuse, the adult is always the one responsible.

Fig. 15 Feelings in situations with children

Think of an everyday situation with a child: **Who** was the child? **Where** was it (a child known to you personally, in a normal contact situation, at the store, playing sports, in a bus or train, etc.)? **What** did you perceive? What did you experience? What were your thoughts in this situation? What was the impulse regarding your own behavior?

1. What thoughts/assessments contributed to your feelings during this meeting? Typical thoughts are

2. What feelings were triggered by contact with the child? Can you describe these more precisely? Try to name at least one of the seven fundamental feelings (fear, shame, anger, disgust, happiness, love, sadness).

3. Is this particular feeling influenced by the relationship with the child?

4. What differences are there between how you would like to behave and how you actually do behave? How would you explain these differences?

5. For each interaction with a child, try to form a statement that could help you in that situation (e.g. "I breathe deeply and can handle it when a child speaks to me," "I always try to help children," "No one can see my thoughts, I can act completely normally with a child").

Emotion:

1. ....

2. ....

Physical Sensation:

1. ....

2. ....

Posture:

1. ....

2. ....

Voice:

1. ....

2. ....

Verbal Expression:

1. ....

2. ....

Behavior, Behavioral Impulse:

1. ....

2. ....

Thoughts:

1. ....

2. ....

Fig. 16 Perception of emotions

Fig. 17 Regulation of emotions through strong physical sensation

Give each participant a sour candy, a hot chili pepper, a strong peppermint, or something similar that stimulates strong physical sensation.

Explain to participants that this exercise is about changing one's own perception by employing a strong counteracting stimulus.

Prepare the group with a short relaxation exercise:
– Please sit up straight, but comfortably.
– Try to place both feet equally on the floor. Do you feel the floor under your feet?
– If you're comfortable doing so, close your eyes. If not, concentrate on one point on the floor in front of you.
– Breathe in deeply and then slowly breathe out. – And again…
– Concentrate fully on your breath. Breathe in and out again. Observe yourself precisely. How does it feel to sit on this chair?

Now ask the patients to remember a situation with a child, during which they had an intense feeling.
– If you'd like to, close your eyes.
– Now try to remember a situation (with a child), during which you had an intense feeling.
– What situation are you remembering? Do you have images of it in your head?
– What do you feel in this situation? Where are you? What do you see? What do you smell? What do you sense?
– Now concentrate on your feelings, and pick out one feeling.
– Concentrate on this feeling, whether pleasant or unpleasant.
– What kind of physical feeling causes this emotion? … Take your time.
– When you can see and feel the situation, take the candy (or chili pepper, etc.) and place it in your mouth. If you'd like, close your eyes.
– How does it taste? How does it feel in your mouth?
– Concentrate on the feeling in your mouth. Swallow it. … Take your time.
– What are you thinking about right now?
– What would you like to do?
– How do you feel right now?
– How intense is the feeling?
– Come back to this room, turn your attention to the sounds around you. Open your eyes.
– Stretch your arms and legs.

Now assess the exercise with the group:
– What feelings did participants concentrate on?
– How well could participants engage with this feeling?
– What happened when the counteracting stimulus came into play? What happened with the initial feeling?
– Were there irritations? Were there feelings that were easier/harder to influence?
– What was helpful? What else might be helpful?

Tip: Participants need time for this exercise—both for the reconstruction of a feeling called up by a memory, as well as distracting the attention through the counteracting stimulus. Observe and guide the patients. Pay attention to their body language before moving on to the next step of the exercise!

Please describe what fantasies involving a child you experience as particularly arousing during masturbation. Narrate your imagined behavior, and describe your feelings and thoughts.

Should you have had actual sexual contact with a child, please describe this (e.g. the first or the most recent contact, or that which you can best remember). You may use the questions below as a guideline. Try to use complete sentences, and avoid bullet points to make your descriptions more clear to you and others. Correct grammar and spelling are unimportant here. This is about feelings and thoughts. We would ask you to please leave your report with us. You may of course also copy it for yourself.

Please keep the following points in mind in depicting your sexual fantasies:

1. Sex and age of the child.
2. Do you know the child personally (e.g. out of your circle of friends or neighborhood)? If not, do you imagine a child that you don't know, but have perhaps seen in a picture (magazine, TV, or Internet)?
3. Please describe the child. How do they look? How do they behave? Are they quiet or outgoing, trusting or distrustful?
4. Where does the encounter take place in your fantasy? In your apartment, outdoors, or elsewhere?
5. What do you say to the child, or what does the child say to you?
6. What do you do with the child? Where do you touch or caress them? Do you penetrate the child with your finger orally, anally, or vaginally?
7. How does the child react? Does he or she tolerate your touching or fight it off?
8. Where does the child touch or caress you?
9. What situation or fantasy situation is particularly sexually arousing to you?
10. What images do you have in your head just before you reach orgasm?
11. What are your feelings and thoughts before, during, and after the imagined sexual contact?

If you've already had sexual contact with a child, consider the following points:

12. Age and gender of the child at the time of first sexual contact.
13. What was your relationship to the child (e.g. father, neighbor, acquaintance of the family)?
14. How did it happen that you had sexual contact with this child?
15. What did you say and do, and what happened afterward?
16. What did you think, feel, perceive, and how did you behave: before (a week before, a day before, minutes before), during, and after the sexual contact?
17. Where did the contact (usually) happen?
18. Did you try to stop the child from telling someone about the contact? If yes, what did you say or do?
19. How often did you have sexual contact with this child and over what period of time?
20. Would you personally consider the contact in question to be sexual abuse?
21. How and why did you end the sexual contact? Did the police get involved? If yes, how did that happen?

Fig. 18 Guidelines for describing sexual experiences in fantasy and behavior

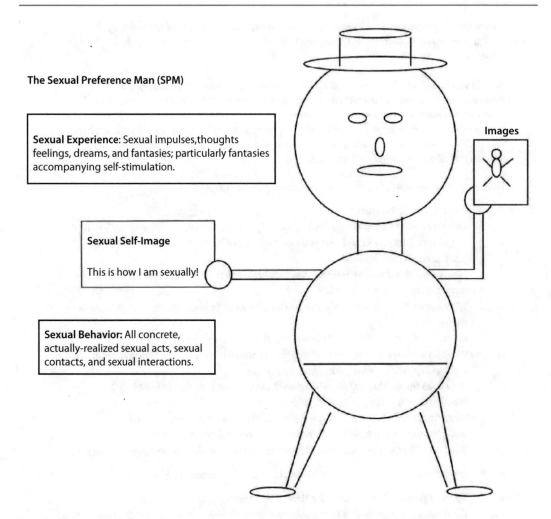

The Sexual Preference Man (SPM)

Sexual Experience: Sexual impulses, thoughts feelings, dreams, and fantasies; particularly fantasies accompanying self-stimulation.

Images

Sexual Self-Image

This is how I am sexually!

Sexual Behavior: All concrete, actually-realized sexual acts, sexual contacts, and sexual interactions.

Fig. 19 Sexual preference man

The Sexual Preference Man – Example for Processing the Questionnaire
(modified Sexual Preference Man, after Ahlers et al. 2008)

1.1 Children (before puberty)
a)   Girls: 0%, ages __to__

b)   Boys: 20%, ages 8 to 10

The person in this example experiences fantasies during masturbation that are overwhelmingly (50%) about early-pubescent boys between ages 11 and 13, followed by 25% of fantasies about adult women aged about 19 to 45. A further 20% of fantasies relate to prepubescent boys between the ages of 8 and 10. A smaller percentage (5%) of accompanying fantasies are about girls, aged 16-18, in late puberty.

1.2 Children (early puberty)
a)   Girls: 0%, ages __to__

b)   Boys: 50%, ages 11 to 13

Together the percentages make 100% and are represented in the circle below, labelled with the corresponding categories

1.3 Adolescents (late puberty)
a)   Girls: 5%, ages 16 to 18

b)   Boys: 0%, ages__to__

1.4   Adults (after puberty)
a)   Women: 25%, ages 19 to 45

b)   Men: 0%, ages __to__

This is an example of how to fill out the percentages according to the case above, generating a pie chart:

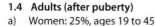

Fig. 19   (continued)

1. Fantasies Accompanying Masturbation

The following concerns the persons or partners who feature in your fantasies that accompany masturbation, and how these imagined partners can be organized into different stages of body development. By percentage, how do the persons in your masturbation fantasies vary in terms of body development phase, gender, and age span?

Please make sure that all the answers on this page total up to 100%!

1.1 Children (before puberty)

    a) Girls: ____%, ages ____ to ____
    b) Boys: ____%, ages ____ to ____

1.2 Children (at early puberty)

    a) Girls: ____%, ages ____ to ____
    b) Boys: ____%, ages ____ to ____

1.3 Adolescents (at late puberty)

    a) Girls: ____%, ages ____ to ____
    b) Boys: ____%, ages ____ to ____

1.4 Adults (after puberty)

    a) Women: ____%, ages ____ to ____
    b) Men: ____%, ages ____ to ____

Please fill out the circle below with your percentages. Label the corresponding segments to make a pie chart:

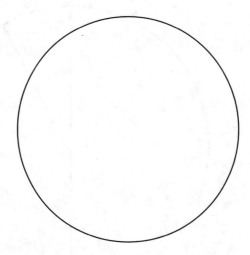

Fig. 19 (continued)

Sexual Acts and Modes of Behavior
The following concerns the sexual acts and modes of behavior that you have performed as an adult (e.g. petting, sexual intercourse, exhibitionist behaviors, etc.). By percentage, how do the objects of your sexual acts and modes of behavior vary by gender, and in which age span were your partners in previous real sexual contact?

Please make sure that all the answers on this page total up to 100%!

2.1 Children (before puberty)
a) Girls: _____%, ages _____ to _____, number of instances of contact: ca. _____

b) Boys: _____%, ages _____ to _____, number of instances of contact: ca. _____

2.2 Children (at early puberty)
a) Girls: _____%, ages _____ to _____, number of instances of contact: ca. _____

b) Boys: _____%, ages _____ to _____, number of instances of contact: ca. _____

2.3 Adolescents (at late puberty)
a) Girls: _____%, ages _____ to _____, number of instances of contact: ca. _____

b) Boys: _____%, ages _____ to _____, number of instances of contact: ca. _____

2.4 Adults (after puberty)
a) Women: _____%, ages _____ to _____, number of instances of contact: ca. _____

b) Men: _____%, ages _____ to _____, number of instances of contact: ca. _____

Please fill out the circle below with your percentages. Label the corresponding segments to make a pie chart:

Fig. 19 (continued)

3. Sexually-Arousing Visual Materials

The following concerns sexually-arousing visual materials (nude or erotic images, pornographic images or films, etc.) that you use, e.g. during masturbation. By percentage, how do the subjects depicted in these materials vary by gender and body development stage, and what age span is depicted?

Please make sure that all the answers on this page total up to 100%!

3.1 Children (before puberty)
a) Girls: ____%, ages ____ to ____

b) Boys: ____%, ages ____ to ____

3.2 Children (at early puberty)
a) Girls: ____%, ages ____ to ____

b) Boys: ____%, ages ____ to ____

3.3 Adolescents (at late puberty)
a) Girls: ____%, ages ____ to ____

b) Boys: ____%, ages ____ to ____

3.4 Adults (after puberty)
a) Women: ____%, ages ____ to ____

b) Men: ____%, ages ____ to ____

Please fill out the circle below with your percentages. Label the corresponding segments to make a pie chart:

Fig. 19 (continued)

4. Sexual Self-Portrait

How do you see yourself sexually? How are you, or how do you describe or define yourself with regard to sex or as a sexual being (e.g. "normal," "perverted," "macho," "softie," "fetishist," "lesbian," "gay," etc.)? Trying to find your own words and own description; formulate your sexual self-portrait below:

....

....

....

....

....

....

....

5. Other Sexual Fantasies and Activities

Should other content be present in your sexual experience (fantasies), sexual behavior, and in the visual materials you consume (e.g. pornography) that relates to your sexual interests, please write them down here: e.g. things/objects/materials, babies/toddlers (ca. 1-6 years of age), sick/injured persons, animals, specific practices, etc.

....

....

....

....

....

....

Fig. 19 (continued)

Letter from a victim

I'm a 19-year old girl and I'm a victim of child sexual abuse and child pornography. Even now I'm still in the process of discovering all the different ways the abuse and the exploitation has hurt me, sent my life down the wrong paths, and destroyed a normal childhood, my teenage years, and my time as a young adult that everyone deserves.

My uncle started abusing me when I was four years old. He used, I know now, the normal ways that offenders use to groom their victims for abuse and keep them quiet: he told me that I was special, that he loved me, and that we had our "special secrets." Since he lived near our home, my parents thought nothing of it when I went to spend time with him.

First he showed me pornographic films, then he began to do things with me. I remember that he put his finger in my vagina and it really hurt. I remember that he tried to have sex with me and that hurt even more. I remember telling him that it hurt. I remember that most of the time when I went to spend time with him I had no clothes on, and sometimes I had to dress up in lingerie. And I remember the pictures.

After the abuse he'd go with me to buy my favorite snack, potato chips. Still today when I eat potato chips, I have these feelings of panic, guilt, and humiliation. It's as though I'm never going to be rid of what happened. At the time I was confused and knew that it was wrong and that I didn't like it, but I also thought that it would be wrong to say something bad about my uncle, who said that he loved me and bought me things that I wanted. He even let me ride on his motorcycle with him. I'll never ride a motorcycle again. The memories are too awful.

There's a lot I don't remember but won't ever be able to forget because of the disgusting pictures of what he did to me that are still out there on the Internet. I've tried for so long to bury those awful memories in my mind. To think about them is still painful sometimes. Sometimes I just stare off in front me when I realize I'm thinking about it. And then I just can't pay attention to anything around me.

I spend every day of my life in constant fear that someone will see my photos and recognize me and I'll be humiliated all over again. It hurts me to know that someone's looking at them—looking at me—while I was still a little girl being abused for the camera. I didn't choose to be there, but there I am forever, in pictures that people use to do sick things. I want everything to be deleted. I want everything to stop. But I'm powerless now, just like I was powerless then to stop my uncle.

When they discovered what my uncle had done, I went to therapy and thought that I'd get over it all. I was totally wrong. The whole understanding of what had happened to me only came when I was older. My life and my feelings are even worse now because the crime never really ended and never really will.

It's hard to describe how it feels to know that at any moment, someone somewhere is looking at photos of me as a little girl being abused by my uncle, and getting sick enjoyment out of it. It's like I'm being abused over and over again.

Fig. 20 Letter from a victim

I'm unable to do simple things that other teenagers do easily. I don't have a driver's license. I always say I'm going to get it, but then don't. I can't plan things well. My thoughts just cut out when I think about how I'm going to move forward with my life. I've tried to find work, but I just avoid that too. The best I could do would be to forget that, even as a little girl, I was forced to lead a double life, and forget what happened to me. Before I know it I've missed a job interview or other things that would help me find one.

Sometimes I remember things about the abuse, and I don't realize it until it's too late. I failed anatomy in school, for instance. I just couldn't think about the body because of everything that happened to me. The same thing happened in college. Without knowing why I just stopped going to class. I failed out in my first year and moved back in with my parents.

It's easy for me to block out feelings and avoid things that make me uncomfortable. I don't know when I'll be ready to go back to school. I've got this huge problem where I just avoid everything that gives me unpleasant feelings or reminds me of my abuse. I'm always afraid that people can see it in me that I'm a victim of sexual abuse, that my abuse is public knowledge. I worry that my friends might stumble onto my pictures online, and it fills me with shame and self-consciousness.

Wherever I go I feel judged. Am I the kind of person that does that? Is something wrong with me? Is there something repulsive and disgusting about me? I'm too ashamed to tell people what happened to me. I'm afraid they'll judge me and think it's my fault. I live in a small city and feel that if one person knows, then everyone will know. I live in fear that someone will see one of these terrible pictures of me and then my secret will be out. It's like my life has been placed on hold waiting for this day, and I'm just stuck there.

I know those disgusting pictures of me will just be there for everyone to see forever. I had awful nightmares. I'd wake up bathed in sweat, crying, and I'd go to my parents so they could calm me. The memories still flare up sometimes. Memories of what my uncle did to me are still in my head. My heart starts racing, I break out in sweat, and then a clearer picture appears in my head and I just have to leave the situation. I've heard my uncle's voice in my mind: "Don't say anything, don't say anything, don't say anything." The thought that there are still pictures out there of all of it just makes everything worse.

It's like I can't escape the abuse, not now or ever. I've had so many nightmares that I can't sleep well in the dark. I like to leave the light on and think it protects me from the bad dreams. I hate horror films and sometimes have nightmares for days afterward. Sometimes I have this inexplicable fear that stops me from doing normal things that other young people do. My friend invited me once to go to an amusement park with her and her uncle. I couldn't get it out of my head that I would be abused. In the end I couldn't go. I asked myself if my friend's uncle had seen my photos. Did he know me? Did he know what I'd done? Is that why he invited me to the amusement park?

Trust isn't an easy thing for me, and I often feel uncomfortable around people. I had to quit my job as waitress after there was this guy there who I thought was always staring at me. I couldn't stop thinking that he recognized me. Had he seen my pictures somewhere? It was just too uncomfortable for me to keep working there. I have trouble saying no because I learned at a young age that I don't really have control over what happens to me. I'm trying to get better about it, because I know that not saying no just makes it easier for someone to hurt me again.

Fig. 20 (continued)

Since my uncle always bribed me to do sexual things in front of the camera, I have trouble accepting gifts from people. I always think they expect something in return if they give me something. That makes my relationships with friends difficult. I want to have kids someday, but I get this huge fear when I think about how I'd have to protect them. Who could I even trust? Their teacher? Their coach? I don't know if I could even trust someone else with my kids. And what happens if my kids and their friends ever found pictures of me on the Internet? How could I even begin to explain what happened to me?

I feel really confused about what love is. My uncle said he loved me, I wanted that love. But I know that what he did to me wasn't love. But how do I know in the future if it's actually love, or just another person trying to use me? The truth is I'm exploited and used every day by someone somewhere in the world. How can I ever get away from it when the crime that was done to me never ends? How can I get away from the humiliating abuse that I experienced when it's out there, being used by sick people for their entertainment? Are my pictures being shown to children, like my uncle showed me, to tell them what they should be doing? Are other children seeing me and then thinking it's okay when they do the same? Will some sick person see me and then have the idea to do that to another girl? These thoughts make me so sad and fill me with fear.

I feel guilty about what happened. I know that I was so young, but why didn't I know better? Why didn't I stop my uncle? If I had stopped him, maybe there wouldn't be all those photos out there that I can never take back or erase. I feel like I have to live with it forever and that it's my fault. I don't feel worthy of anything and like a failure. What have I been good for up to this point except to be used by others over and over again? That's one of the reasons I'm unable to get a job or go back to school. I'm tired of disappointing myself. I've already had enough disappointment for the rest of my life and just don't want to fail anymore. It brings all the horrible feelings of shame and the abuse and the exploitation back. Sometimes I try to deal with my feelings and forget everything by drinking too much. I know that it's not good, but my humiliation and my anger are always with me, and sometimes I just need a way to be rid of them for a while.

I feel like I've always had to lead a double life. First I had to lie about what my uncle was doing to me. Then I had to act like it never happened because it was so unpleasant, and now I know that there's a second "little me" out there on the Internet that abusers can see. I don't want to be there, but I'm there. I wish I could turn back time and stop my uncle from taking those photos, but I can't. I'm writing this letter as a victim, even though I'm still afraid of being abused or hurt again. I want the court and the judge to know about me, what I've suffered, and how my life is. What happened to me hasn't gone away. It will never go away. I'm a real victim of child pornography, and it weighs on me every day, wherever I go.

Fig. 20 (continued)

Fig. 21 Letter to my victim(s)

Write a letter to a child who has been a victim of sexual abuse. Think of a child with whom you actually had sexual contact. If you have never had sexual contact with a child, think of a child who you have had sexual contact with in your imagination, or a child you have seen in sexualized images.

Do not send the letter. The letter should be written to help the victim(s). What would you like to say to the victim that could help them? You will discuss this letter later on with the group.

Fig. 22 Letter from my victim to me

Write a letter to yourself. The letter is from a child with whom you have had sexual contact in reality, or from a child you have seen in sexualized images. Let the child report. Describe what they say to you.

Fig. 23 Sexual development

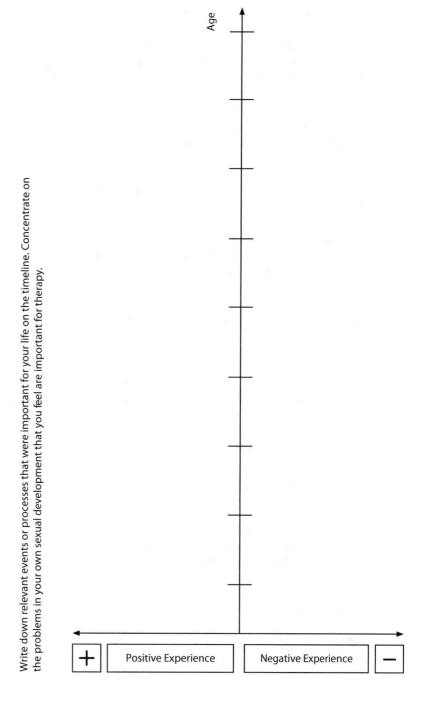

Write down relevant events or processes that were important for your life on the timeline. Concentrate on the problems in your own sexual development that you feel are important for therapy.

Age

+ Positive Experience

Negative Experience —

One can fundamentally differentiate between three types coping strategies:

1. Task-Oriented or Problem-Oriented Coping:
This category includes behavior strategies that approach or solve a problem, and cognitive strategies that either lead to a new point of view or reduce the negative consequences of a problem.

Example: You want to make amends with someone you have not spoken to for more than three months after a fight. You call the person and ask to meet with them.

2. Emotion-Oriented Coping:
Emotion-oriented coping entails an emotional response to the problem: pondering, reflecting on, and brooding over the problem, getting angry, or seeking to place blame on someone else.

Example: You want to make up with someone you have not spoken to for more than three months after a fight. But you are hurt and want the other person to get in touch first. You think about the reasons for the fight and cannot find an answer.

3. Avoidance-Oriented Coping:
Avoidance-oriented coping describes the avoidance of problems through other activities (distraction) or the search for new people (seeking out social alternatives).

Example: You want to make up with someone you have not spoken to for more than three months after a fight. You miss the person and try to block out all your thoughts about them. You have already deleted their phone number. Depressed by your sorrows, you drink a bottle of wine every night.

The first coping strategy is functional. The other two are generally dysfunctional, and increase the likelihood of becoming depressive or anxious. The latter two have the effect of making a person feel better for a short time, but in the long term they do not provide a solution to the problem.

Exercise in the group or as homework:
1.   Name three or four problems in your family, at work, or at home.
2.   How did you deal with the problem? What were the advantages and disadvantages of your strategies?
3.   What could you change by acquiring new coping strategies? What are the advantages and disadvantages of these strategies?

Reflect on and discuss the assignment as it relates to the above-mentioned coping strategies with the group.

Fig. 24 Types of coping strategies

	+	−
Short-term		
Long-term		

Fig. 25 Evaluation of consequences

Step 1. Determine the Problem and the Goal

Determine the problem or part of the problem you want to work on. Pay attention to factors in your environment that contribute to the problem. Write down the goals you would like to achieve.

....

....

....

Step 2. Gather Solutions

Write down any strategies that come to you as a solution to the problem you determined above. Do not dismiss any strategy, even if it seems awkward or absurd. Try to find at least three different approaches. Do not assess the strategies yet.

....

....

....

....

Step 3. Assess the Solution Strategies

Now assess each of the strategies you listed above. Work out the positive and negative aspects of the long-term and short-term consequences.

	+	−
Short-term		
Long-term		

	+	−
Short-term		
Long-term		

Fig. 26 Developing a solution to a problem

Step 4. Identify One or More Appropriate Strategies

Pick out the strategy that seems to promise the best results. It can also be a combination of strategies.

....

....

....

....

Step 5. Planning the Implementation

Divide up the chosen strategy/strategies into smaller steps. Each step should lead to the next. The steps should be as specific as possible, clearly demarcated, and directly attainable. It should be within your control to reach the stated goal. Try to identify and preempt possible obstacles

....

....

....

....

Step 6. Evaluating the Process

Take a look back. Did you carry out each step as planned? Did the steps work like you wanted them to? Consider every attempt you made, even if they were unsuccessful. If there were difficulties, analyze these in order to see which steps in the process should be reassessed and changed.

....

....

....

....

....

Fig. 26 (continued)

In this exercise you will draw a diagram of your whole social network. It should include all people who are in your opinion part of your social world. This might include family members (i.e. important people to whom you are related through blood, marriage, partnership, or adoption), friends, colleagues, neighbors, experts you regularly see, and every other person who is important to you. The diagram can also include people who are no longer living.

To draw the diagram, start with yourself in the middle and work your way outwards. Draw the connections between you and these other people. You can use symbols to show if you are close or distant, if you have a lot of contact or less contact with them, and how you feel about the relationship.

– Use circles to represent women and squares to represent men.

– Use a cross to represent people who are no longer living.

– In the circle or the square, write the person's age, name, and their relationship to you.

– Using a number, note next to each circle or square how much contact you have with this person: no contact (0); little contact (1); somewhat frequent contact (2); regular contact (3).

– Next to each circle/square, note your personal grade for the quality of the relationship: very comfortable (A); comfortable (B); neutral (C); problematic (D); very problematic (E).

Fig. 27 My social network

Fig. 28 My future self

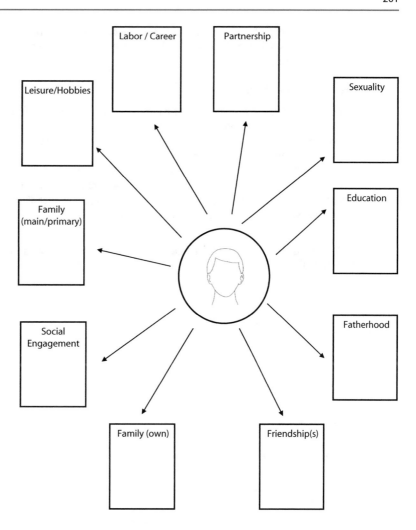

Labor / Career

Partnership

Leisure/Hobbies

Sexuality

Family
(main/primary)

Education

Social
Engagement

Fatherhood

Family (own)

Friendship(s)

Fig. 29 Evaluating the
costs and benefits of
goals

Goal (avoidance-oriented or approach-oriented?)	**Short-term Costs**	**Long-term Costs**
	Short-term Benefits	**Long-term Benefits**
Goal (avoidance-oriented or approach-oriented?)	**Short-term Costs**	**Long-term Costs**
	Short-term Benefits	**Long-term Benefits**

Risk factors are conditions that increase the likelihood of sexual contact with a child or the use of abuse images. Risk factors can be situations, feelings, thoughts, or modes of behavior.

Examples of Risk Factors:

– Situations: A visit to a playground, a visit to a swimming pool, walking past a school, financial problems, the end of a relationship, etc.
– Thoughts: "It doesn't matter to me, I've got nothing to lose," I'm not worthy of love, so I have to get love somewhere," etc.
– Feelings: Anger, sadness, emptiness, loneliness, boredom, etc.
– Behavior: Reduction of self-control through increased consumption of alcohol or other drugs, retreat from other people, not answering the telephone, spending hours on the Internetin search of sexually-arousing images, etc.

Individual Risk Factors (should there not be enough room below, please use the other side of the page)

....

....

....

....

....

....

....

....

....

....

Fig. 30 Risk factors

Warning Signs are certain conditions that have led in the past to sexual abuse or high-risk situations.

– **External Warning Signs:** Signs that are visible to others, e.g. regular alcohol abuse, unkempt appearance, provocation of arguments, retreat from others, frequent visits to playgrounds, swimming pools, or other locations where unsupervised contact with children is made easier.

– **Internal Warning Signs:** Signs that are not visible to others, e.g. thoughts, feelings, fantasies.

If you are familiar with your personal warning signs you can take timely measures. Warning signs may have different levels of danger. The more energy you put into bringing about sexual contact, the more energy necessary to stop your behavior. In the same way, it takes more energy and is more dangerous to descend a high mountain than it is to walk down a hill in the park: the air is thinner at the high elevation, it is cold, and there is no one to help. Your possibilities to act dwindle.

The closer you have come to a real abuse situation, e.g. when the child is already sitting nude on your bed, the harder it will be to halt the progress of events and stop yourself from

committing abuse. Compare that to the mountain climber: Who would stop climbing three meters below the peak, even when you can see the storm is coming?

Examples:

	External	Internal
High-risk	Retreat from others	Depression
Medium-risk	Use of images of children during masturbation	Affected by invasive sexual fantasies about children
Low-risk	Spending time with potential victims	Planning your actions

Define your own personal warning signs, and then complete the list at home. Try to assign each warning sign a number from 1-10. The larger the number, the nearer it is to sexual contact with a child.

....

....

Fig. 31 Warning signs

▮ Risk Factor   ▮ Warning Sign

....

....

What preventative measures can I take?

....

....

....

....

....

What thoughts are helpful in this situation?

....

....

....

....

What actions are helpful in this situation?

....

....

....

....

....

Fig. 32 Strategies for dealing with risk factors and warning signs

Worksheets BEDIT-A

Working Group of the Prevention Project for Juveniles

Fig. 1 WS (Worksheet) Therapy contract: patient

I agree to the following points:

1. I will take part regularly in therapy sessions.
2. I will get in touch to excuse my absence at least 24 hours before the session.
3. I will arrive to the therapy session on time.
4. I will be reliable about doing my therapy homework.
5. I will always make an effort to actively participate.
6. I will try to be honest.
7. I will take complete responsibility for my behavior.
8. I will not display any aggressive verbal or physical behavior.
9. I have been informed that I may share my sexual fantasies, previous sexual contact with children, previous offenses, as well as all private information openly, as my therapist is legally obligated to maintain therapist-patient confidentiality.
10. I am also committed to maintaining confidentiality and will not share any therapy content with a third party without permission.
11. I have been informed that the exchange of some content information with caregivers involved in the therapy process, e.g. my parents, may be necessary for the success of the therapy. My therapist will carefully assess, together with me, which information needs to be passed on, will discuss this with me in advance, and will obtain my explicit consent.
12. I have been informed that, if intent to commit an offense, particularly intent to make direct or indirect sexual contact with children, or suicidal intent is disclosed, my therapist is obligated to act in the interest of my protection and the protection of others. Any action will be discussed with me first, although in the case of acute immediate danger, decisions may be made against my will.
13. I am in agreement that my therapist will discuss any action on his/her part with me beforehand.

If I go against the agreements listed above, I am putting the success of my therapy at risk. I have been informed that this kind of therapy-jeopardizing behavior may lead to a termination of my treatment.

I consent to the above-mentioned stipulations:

______________________	______________________
Place, Date	Signature

Working Group of the Prevention Project for Juveniles
Charité – Universitätsmedizin Berlin, Corporate Member of Freie Universität Berlin, Humboldt-Universität zu Berlin, and Berlin Institute of Health, Center for Human and Health Sciences, Institute of Sexology and Sexual Medicine, Berlin, Germany
e-mail: klaus.beier@charite.de

K. M. Beier (ed.), *Pedophilia, Hebephilia and Sexual Offending against Children*,
https://doi.org/10.1007/978-3-030-61262-7_10

Fig. 2 WS Therapy
contract: therapist

I agree to the following points:

1. I will treat my patient with respect and earnestness.
2. I will not pass judgment on my patient.
3. I will make an effort to structure the work environment (collaboratively) so that my patient will be able to pursue his therapy goals in a safe context.
4. I will be available to my patient for regular therapy sessions.
5. If I am unable to make it to the session, I will cancel with at least 24 hours notice.
6. I will arrive at our agreed-upon appointments on time, focused, and prepared.
7. I will uphold the rights of my patient and will handle his written work respectfully and responsibly.
8. I will uphold therapist-patient confidentiality and will not give any information about or from my patient to any third party who is not involved in the therapy process.
9. I have informed my patient that the exchange of content information with people involved in the therapy process may be necessary for the success of the therapy. I will carefully assess, together with my patient, what information this may apply to in advance, and will obtain his explicit consent.
10. I have informed my patient that, if intent to commit an offense, particularly intent to make direct or indirect sexual contact with children, or suicidal intent is disclosed, I am obligated to act in the interests of his protection and that of others. I will discuss my actions with the patient in advance. I have informed him, however, that in the case of acute, immediate danger, decisions may or must be made against his will.
11. I will abide by ethical and professional guidelines.

With my signature, I consent to the above-mentioned stipulations:

_____   _____

Place, Date   Signature

Fig. 3 WS Therapy
goals and problem areas

Overarching goals for this therapy are…

1. learning to accept my own sexual preference and how to deal with it.
2. not to commit any acts of sexual abuse on children.
3. not to use child sexual abuse images of children.

In addition, my individual problem areas are:

1. ....
   ....
2. ....
   ....
3. ....
   ....

In therapy, I would like to learn the following:

1. ....
   ....
2. ....
   ....
3. ....
   ....

This is how I will know that I have reached my therapy goals:

1. ....
   ....
2. ....
   ....
3. ....
   ....

Fig. 4 IS (Information sheet)
Sexuality

Sexual acts are all acts that are sexually motivated. Acts are considered sexually motivated if they are in the direct service of sexual arousal or an arousing pastime and/or directly prepare the way for sexual activities.

Sexual acts can take place with or without physical contact. One can also have sex with oneself.

Sexuality has three functions that find their expression in each person to differing degrees.

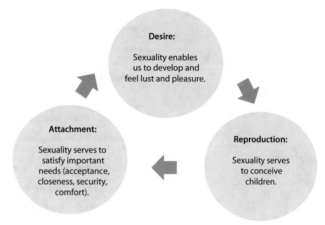

Take note: Just because someone desires closeness or wants to be loved does not mean that sex is the appropriate way to achieve this. It is important to know the difference between friendship, sex, and love, as well as not to misinterpret the desire for friendship as sexual attraction or to take advantage of it for sex.

Fig. 5 IS Dissexuality

Dissexuality or **sexual assault** or **sexual acts without mutual consent** means that one does not abide by social norms in respect to sexuality. This means that you are doing something sexual that you are NOT allowed to do!

According to § 177 of the German Penal Code (example for Germany, to be adapted to the law of each country) a **sexual assault** has occurred when **no mutual consent** has taken place.

This is the case when the person:

a) has not agreed to the situation and someone is nevertheless attempting to carry out sexual acts with him or her using force, threats, blackmail, or some other kind of manipulation. In other words, someone is trying to force someone to do something that he or she does not want to do!

b) cannot say that they are okay with it, since they do not know about the content, execution, or consequences of the sexual act or do not know how to deal with the situation. This is the case when, for example:

a. the person is too young,

b. the person is drunk or on drugs,

c. the person is intellectually disabled.

c) is in a supervisory relationship or an unequal power dynamic with the other person. A therapist may not, for example, take advantage of the position of his or her patient, and a guardian may not take advantage of the position of the person in his or her care.

Caution: Even an attempt is subject to prosecution!

Every sexual act with physical contact and without mutual consent is a **"hands-on offense."**

Every sexual act without physical contact and without mutual consent is a **"hands-off offense."** This also includes, for example, the depiction of such sexual acts.

Fig. 6 IS Child sexual
abuse

Child sexual abuse acts according to § 176 of the German Penal Code—punishable by law are:

1. sexually-motivated comments regarding a child (under 14 years), displaying pornographic images or representations, playing sound media with pornographic content in order to sexually arouse oneself, the child, or a third party;

2. sexually-motivated observations in intimate situations;

3. sexually-motivated pursuit;

4. sexually-motivated touching, caressing outside of the genital area;

5. sexually-motivated touching, caressing within the genital area (penis, vagina, breast, bottom);

6. exposing one's own genitals, with or without masturbation;

7. prompting a child to masturbate oneself;

8. prompting a child to masturbate him-or herself;

9. prompting a child to perform sexual acts on a third person or to allow a third person to perform them upon him or herself;

10. inserting one's penis, tongue, finger, or object in the vagina, rectum, or mouth;

11. offering a child for sexual acts or planning such an offense with another person.

Caution: Even an attempt is subject to prosecution!

A sexual assault is not:

Masturbating to one's own sexual fantasies about children

Looking at legal visual material

Fig. 7 IS Strategies for
dealing with risk factors.
(Note: For technical
printing reasons, the
illustration has been kept
in black-and-white. The
color gradient from
green to yellow to red is
to be taken from the
corresponding .pdf.)

IS *Sex–When and with Whom?*

AGE	< 14	14-15	16-17	18-21	> 21
< 14	☹	☹	☹	☹	☹
14-15	☹	☺	☺	😐	😐
16-17	☹	☺	☺	☺	☺
18-21	☹	😐	☺	☺	☺
> 21	☹	😐	☺	☺	☺

After: Zollorsch 2012; https://krony.de/alters-tabelle-wer-gesetzlich-mit-wem-sex-haben-darf.html

 Sex is permitted.

 Sex is punishable by law if the older person pays money or exploits the predicament the other person is in, or is a caregiver/educator.

 Sex is punishable by law if the older person pays money or exploits the predicament the other person is in, or is a caregiver/educator, or if he or she takes advantage of the sexual immaturity of the younger person.

 Sex is forbidden. The older person is committing child sexual abuse and is liable to prosecution.

Fig. 8 IS Illegal visual material

According to § 184b of the German Penal Code, a case of indirect child sexual abuse has occurred when someone acquires, possesses, distributes, shows, offers, or creates one of the representations from § 176 in the form of images, videos, sound recordings, or written materials.

In addition, the depiction of children (< **14 years of age**) in certain poses is punishable by law (according to § 184b, starting at Stage 4 or higher).

Stage	Category	Description
1	Indicative	Non-erotic or –sexualized images of children in e.g. underwear/swimsuits engaged in normal activities or in normal situations (e.g. from ads, catalogs, photo albums)
2	Nudity	Images of scantily-clad (e.g. in underwear) or naked children in normal situations (e.g. swimming pool, beach)
3	Posing	Depiction of (partially) clothed or naked children that are consciously posing or assuming an unnatural body position
4	Erotic posing	Sexualized or erotic images of (partially) clothed or naked children in provocative or unnatural poses
5	Explicit erotic posing	Sexualized depiction of (partially) clothed or naked children with an emphasis on the genital area
6	Sexual activities between children	Depiction of sexual activities between children without adults (e.g. touching, self or mutual masturbation, oral sex, sexual intercourse)
7	(Severe) child sexual abuse	Images of sexual acts by one or more children with the participation of one or more adults (e.g. touching, self or mutual masturbation, oral sex, sexual intercourse)
8	Sadism and brutality	Depiction of violent acts on children (e.g. bondage, immobilization, beating, whipping, etc.—causing pain), rape, killing, or sexual acts between children and animals.

Fig. 9 IS Sexual responsiveness to the child developmental body age

A person's sexual preference (**that is, what they are interested in sexually**) is formed along three axes, three levels, and in three forms.

Axes:

1. Gender (*male, female, any gender*)
2. Developmental body age (*child, adolescent, adult*)
3. Practice (*e.g. from in front, from behind, on top, inclusion of socks, feet etc.*)

Levels:

1. Behavior (*the things one does in regards to sex*)
2. Fantasy (*the things one imagines in regards to sex*)
3. Self-image (*how one sees oneself in regards to sex*)

Forms:

1. Genital interaction (*vaginal intercourse, anal intercourse, oral intercourse etc.*)
2. Non-genital interaction (*kissing, cuddling etc.*)
3. Masturbation (*I prefer to touch myself in this particular way/this or that often/in this or that situation in order to get myself sexually aroused*)

A sexual responsiveness to the child developmental body scheme...

- means that you feel sexually attracted to children.
- refers to children who have not yet reached puberty, that is, whose bodies still look like those of children (no pubic hair, no breast development in girls, childlike penis and testicles in boys).
- means that sexual acts with people who display a child body scheme are desired, fantasized about, and/or are carried out over a longer period of time.
- can mean that those affected are attracted not only to girls, not only to boys, but to both boys and girls.
- can be exclusive (one can only become sexually aroused by a childlike body scheme), or non-exclusive (one is not only aroused by a childlike body scheme, but can also become aroused by an adolescent and/or adult body scheme).
- can be seen in one's behavior, but doesn't have to be. Many people who feel a sexual attraction to children never commit a sexual assault.

Fig. 10 WS My sexual preference structure

Please make sure you take enough time and think again about your own sexuality. Then answer the following questions:

The Axes:

1. Which gender(s) are you interested in (*male, female, other genders*)?
   ....

2. Which developmental body age(s) are you interested in (*child, adolescent, adult*)?
   ....

3. Which sexual practices are you interested in (*Examples: from in-front, from behind, on top, feet, socks etc.*)?
   ....
   ....
   ....

The Levels:

1. My sexual behavior (*This is what I have already done or experienced sexually*):
   ....
   ....
   ....

2. My sexual fantasies (*This is what I imagine during my sexual fantasies*):
   ....
   ....
   ....

3. My sexual self-image (*This is how I see myself sexually*):
   ....
   ....
   ....

The Forms:

1. These are the genital interactions that I like (*e.g. "I like to put my penis in other people's vaginas or buttholes."*):
   ....
   ....
   ....

2. These are the non-genital interactions that I like (*e.g. "I like kissing another person."*):
   ....
   ....
   ....

3. This is the type of masturbation that I like (*e.g. "I like to rub my penis on objects in order to get myself sexually aroused."*):
   ....
   ....
   ....

A conclusive theory on the origins of sexual preferences (that is, of what someone is interested in sexually) still does not yet exist. This means that we don't yet know why some people feel sexually attracted to children.

When it comes to adult men who feel a sexual attraction to children, we know that they were often already aware of this when they were teenagers, and then afterwards nothing changed. So it may be that it always stays that way. BUT we still don't know about that in your particular case.

That is why it is important to first accept how things are NOW, and to see how your sexual preference for children might develop in the future.

Acceptance is the only way to get out of a seemingly hopeless situation. Acceptance is a decision to take this moment as it is and to get through it, and it doesn't mean that you think that it is a good thing.

In therapy, you can learn how to deal with your preference in such a way that you do not commit any hands-on or hands-off child abuse.

Sexual preference is fate, not choice!
This means that no one chooses what he or she is interested in sexually!

Acceptance is a conscious decision!

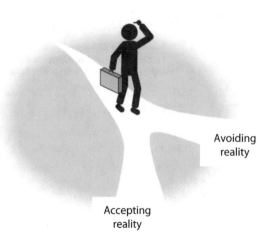

Avoiding
reality

Accepting
reality

Fig. 11 IS Can a sexual preference for children change?

Fig. 12 IS Radical
Acceptance

Acceptance means…

— not to fight against reality
— to face the facts
— to take the situation for what it is
— to not attempt to force changes where they are not possible.

Three Types of Problems:

1) solvable problems that provoke uncomfortable emotions,
2) unsolvable problems that provoke uncomfortable emotions that can be modulated,
3) unsolvable problems that provoke uncomfortable emotions that cannot be modulated.

Examine:

Can I change the situation or solve the problem? ⇨ Yes ⇨ Solve the Problem!
      (e.g. sexual preference)

⇩

No

⇩

Can I change or control the feeling?   ⇨ Yes ⇨ Control the feeling!

⇩

No

⇩

Radical acceptance is necessary!
(It is how it is. I don't think it's good but will accept it.)

Radical acceptance is necessary.
I accept that there are things I cannot change.
I accept my unpleasant feelings in response to them.

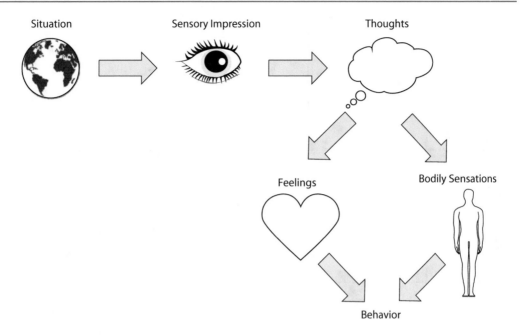

A **sensory impression** results from the reception and processing of information and environmental stimuli through the sensory organs. The human being is capable of the following kinds of perception among others:

— visual perception (seeing),

— auditory perception (hearing),

— gustatory perception (tasting),

— olfactory perception (smelling),

— vestibular perception (balancing),

— sensibility (feeling).

A **thought** is something which has been thought about or the act of thinking about something: an opinion, a perspective, a notion, or an idea.

Bodily sensations refer to all the involuntary responses of the body to feelings, such as quickened heartbeat, sweating, tingling in the hands.

Feelings refer to pleasant or unpleasant sensations that are only partially experienced consciously. Fear, joy, and surprise, for example, can be considered feelings

Behavior refers to all action that can be immediately observed by others, thus to everything that other people can see.

Fig. 13 IS Behavioral model

Situation (Where am I? What kinds of sensory impressions am I having?)	Thought (What is going through my mind?)	Feeling (How am I feeling?)	Physical sensation (What is going on in my body?)	Behavior (What am I doing? What would I maybe like to do?)

Fig. 14 WS Self-observation log for the behavioral model

Perception is a complex process of gaining information through processing environmental stimuli according to subjective criteria. Our perception of objects, people, or situations determines just a small part of their "objective" nature.

Attributes of the person doing the perceiving (e.g. your own attributes) automatically interfere in the process, such as:

■ current state of health,
■ current mood,
■ personality traits,
■ one's own attitude,
■ experiences one has already had, and many other things.

This all depends on how we evaluate something we have perceived. How we evaluate the things that we perceive has a strong influence on what we want to do in response.

We can imagine the experiences we have that form our personality, our habits, emotions, and needs as a kind of filter or glasses through which we perceive our environment.

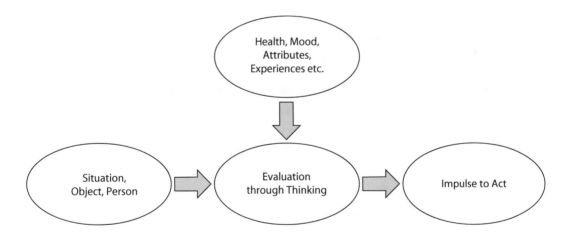

This is also the case when what we perceive is not an object but other people or situations.

Our perception usually takes place **automatically**. This means that we often do not even notice exactly what it is that we perceive.

Fig. 15 IS Perception

We humans can perceive things in two different ways:

1. **Undirected**
   - No focal point of attention
   - Attentive, but open: nothing is ignored, nothing is concentrated on
   - Perceiving without allowing oneself to be drawn in
   - General readiness to react

2. **Directed**
   - Particular focal point of attention
   - Only certain stimuli are perceived
   - Irrelevant stimuli are blurred out

The result of a perception (e.g. *"I see an apple"*) is often an action (e.g. *"I take the apple and bite into it."*).

We humans can often decide
- what we perceive,
- the perspective from which we perceive,
- when we perceive,
- what we do the perceiving with,
- how many evaluations we undertake, and
- which of the many impulses to act we subsequently follow.

The things that we are interested in sexually have an influence on the way we perceive social interactions. We are wearing rose-colored glasses.

People who are sexually oriented towards children sometimes wrongly interpret the behavior of children as a sign of sexual interest. Normal situations are sometimes perceived as sexualized.

Children never have a conscious desire for sexual contact, sexual stimulation, sexual desire etc. from/to a much older person!

Using the method of self-observation, we can make ourselves aware of what it is we perceive and learn how to direct our attention completely consciously, and thereby decide for ourselves exactly what we perceive.

What will you achieve with these perception exercises in the long term?
- You can observe yourself and others more precisely.
- You can influence how you experience things.
- You can change inappropriate behavior.

Fig. 15 (continued)

Situation (Where am I? What kinds of sensory impressions am I having?)	Thought (What is going through my mind?)	Feeling (How am I feeling?)	Physical sensation (What is going on in my body?)	Behavior (What am I doing? What would I maybe like to do?)

Fig. 16 WS Self-observation log for perception

A mistaken thought is a distorted thought or belief that has little to do with fact or reality. It is a mistake, a wrong conclusion, or a misjudgment. Errors in thinking often lead one to do things that only give pleasure, are irresponsible, and may possibly hurt oneself and others. Mistaken thoughts assist one in avoiding responsibility, persuading oneself to do something, or justifying selfish actions.

Mistaken thoughts that often accompany sexual abuse are:
1. sexual myths in connection with dissexual behavior
2. trivializations or minimizations
3. denial
4. justifications/excuses
5. shifting blame onto the victim

It is important for you to recognize your own mistaken thoughts and to replace them with functional thoughts. For this, you can use the following examination schema:

Discovering the Mistaken Thought
— Which concrete thoughts did you have in the situation? What was going through your mind?
— What did you say to yourself in the moment?

Questioning the Mistaken Thought
— Was the thought helpful? What did it do for you to think this way?
— Which advantages/disadvantages did it have for you to think exactly this way in the situation?
— Is the thought based on facts?
— Is there proof of the correctness of the thought?
— What speaks in favor of, what speaks against this thought? Is the thought logical?

Developing Appropriate, Functional Thoughts
— What could you say instead to yourself when you're once again in a similar situation?
— What do you think now, after the fact, could have been different thought in this situation?
—What do you think your mother/your friend, etc. would have thought in the same situation?
— Which interpretation of the situation now, after the fact, seems to be more realistic?

Training of Functional Thoughts
— Recite the functional thought in your mind over and over again.
— Imagine how you say the functional thought to yourself in future risk situations.
— Write down your functional thought on an index card.
— Imagine the advantages of the functional thought.

Fig. 17 IS Mistaken Thoughts

Activating Event/Situation: (What happened?)	Beliefs/Thought: (What did I think?)	Consequence/Feeling: (How do I feel?)
	Alternative Thought: (What should I think about the situation in order to experience the new feeling?)	New Feeling: (How do I want to feel in this situation?)
Activating Event/Situation: (What happened?)	Evaluative Thought: (What did I think?)	Feeling: (How do I feel?)
	Alternative Thought: (What should I think about the situation in order to experience the new feeling?)	New Feeling: (How do I want to feel in this situation?)`

Fig. 18 WS The ABC-Scheme

Please   read through the following example. First, imagine that you are wearing "rose-colored glasses." Then, consider what your perspective on the situation could be if you were instead to put on "clear glasses." Then, please write down your ideas.

1. Sexual Myths in Connection with Dissexual Behavior

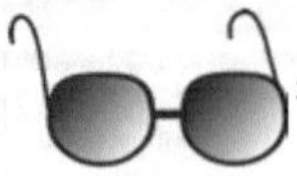

:   By having sex with adults, children can learn a lot.   .

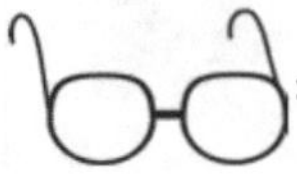

:   ....

2. Trivialization/Minimization

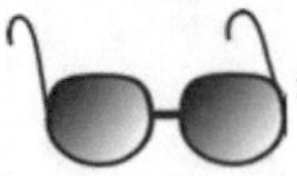

:   I didn't abuse the child; I just watched the video.

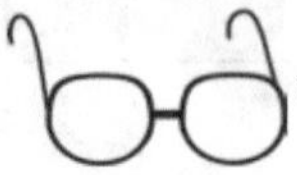

:   ....

3. Denial

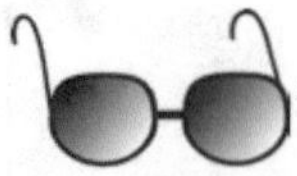

:   If that was the case, she would have said something about it by now. Nothing happened. We were only playing.

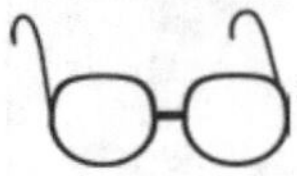

:   ....

4. Justifications/Excuses

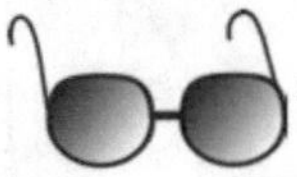

:   The girl/boy did not resist, so she/he must have wanted it.

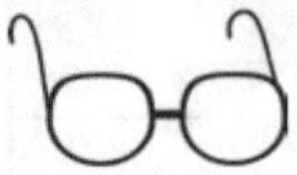

:   ....

5. Shifting Blame onto the Victim

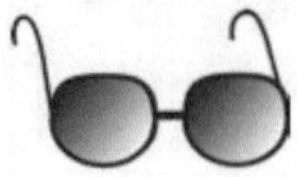

:   If she/he stands naked in front of me, then it's her/his own fault if I then sexually abuse her/him.

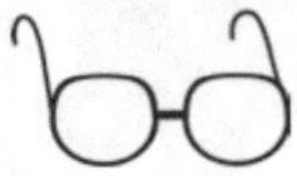

:   ....

Fig. 19 WS Mistaken thoughts in child sexual abuse

aggressive	tense	anxious
annoying	awful	frustrated
threatened	weighed down	punished
validated	thankful	lonely
determined	relieved	excited
glad	patient	heartless
bored	happy	helpless
hopeless	empty	weary
inferior	tired	nervous
depressed	powerless	provoked
in great shape	distraught	angry
impatient	sad	guilty
hostile	worried	gloomy
aloof	inhibited	disappointed
exhausted	irritated	thoughtful
miserable	confused	insecure
unstable	desperate	melancholic
unwell	content	dissatisfied

Fig. 20 IS List of feelings

Humans are born with the ability to feel. However, many people find it difficult to sense, name, and express their feelings, as well to recognize them in others.

Many people can only distinguish their feelings in terms of "good" and "bad."

Good emotional competency has a positive effect on our ability to have relationships.

It is however also important to be able regulate or control unpleasant, dangerous, or strong feelings on one's own.

It is possible to perceive feelings in oneself and others on several different levels. Among these belong:

Physical Sensations	relaxation, ease, tingling, blushing, paleness, nausea breaking out in sweat, tension
Posture	facing outward, upright, open, cowering, clenched fists, hunched over, turned away
Voice	quiet, whispering, loud, shrill, high, deep
Statements	cursing, apologizing
Thoughts	That's…great, excellent, good, awful, horrible, boring
Behavior or Behavioral Impulses	running away, fighting, hugging, crying

It is important to recognize that feelings influence one's own behavior.

Feelings are important because
— they motivate us to act,
— they activate (for example, courage) or inhibit (for example, fear) our behavior,
— they provide us with warnings and help us to orient ourselves,
— through them, we communicate and interact with others.

Fig. 21 IS The meaning of feelings

Feeling:

1. ....

2. ....

Physical Sensations:

1. ....

2. ....

Posture:

1. ....

2. ....

Voice:

1. ....

2. ....

Verbal Statements:

1. ....

2. ....

Behavior:

1. ....

2. ....

Thoughts:

1. ....

2. ....

Fig. 22 WS Perception of feelings

Below you will find several statements including a hidden feeling. Please write down the feeling that the underlined person is most likely experiencing within the space provided.

Statement	Feeling
A <u>man</u> says to a woman: "You forgot our date again!"	
A <u>mother</u> says to her son after he finishes his homework quickly and correctly: "You did this really well."	
A <u>girl</u> says to her friend: "You haven't come by to see me at all lately!"	
A student says to his <u>classmate</u>: "With so many difficulties, one could really just give up and quit!"	
A <u>woman</u> says to her husband after he comes home very late at night without telling her in advance: "Where have you been all this time?"	
A friend of yours insults you, <u>you</u> say: "We need to talk."	
A friend of yours insults you, <u>you</u> say: "I never want to see you again!"	
A father scolds his son. The <u>mother</u> says: "Don't you think he needs to be treated with bit more understanding?"	

Fig. 23 WS Identifying feelings

Fig. 24 WS Attitudes toward dealing with feelings

1. Showing feelings to others means showing weakness.

2. Feelings come and go for no reason.

3. Some feelings are false.

4. Only I can judge how I feel.

5. Others know better how I'm feeling than I do.

6. People who show their feelings lose restraint and self-control.

7. After a positivefeeling, things can only get worse.

8. Showing feelings makes oneself vulnerable to attack.

9. It is better to ignore unpleasant feelings.

10. Only women talk about feelings, not men.

11. Feelings are addictive.

12. Before taking a feeling seriously, one should first sleep on it.

13. ....

14. ....

15. ....

16. ....

17. ....

Please attempt to answer the questions accurately:

1. What kind of feelings does contact with children trigger in you?
Did you clearly identify that feeling? Try to identify one of the seven primary feelings
(fear, shame, anger, disgust, joy, love, sadness)!

....

....

....

2. What role does your relationship to the child play for your feeling?

....

....

....

3. Which thoughts about and assessments of the contact contribute to your feeling?
Typical thoughts are…/Typical feelings that will follow are…

....

....

....

4. What difference do you notice between the behavior you would like to show and the behavior that you actually show?
How would you explain the difference?

....

....

....

5. Try formulate a "motto" for every contact with a child that sums up the connection between the kind of encounter and your experience?
(e.g. "Close your eyes and get through it, when a child talks to me," "I try to help every child," etc.)

....

....

....

Fig. 25 WS Feelings in conflict situations with children

Fig. 26 IS Safety-Vault
Exercise

Now I will ask you to please seat yourself comfortably. First, feel that your body has contact with the ground. The point is only to become aware that your body is contact with its surroundings and where this contact is happening. This is not about right or wrong, but about consciously registering what is happening. Next, I would like to you to please perceive that your body is breathing and that this causes it to move. Feel these movements. Feel how your chest softly rises and falls and that your abdomen rises and falls along with it. And when you pay very close attention, you will also sense that your nostrils are making very slight movements. And remain aware of these movements that the body makes while breathing for a few moments.

The Safety-Vault Exercise makes it possible to lock away thoughts or images that are very burdensome. These images will not be pushed away with force and violence, which would only lead them to force themselves upon us again with force and violence, but instead they will be suspended for a period of time.

Imagine a safe. Imagine exactly how your own personal safe would look like…what material it's made of…pay attention to the door…the size of the safe…What does the locking mechanism look like? Is it a built-in lock or padlock? Inside this safe, you can place everything that is burdensome and that you cannot handle at the moment.

Lock the door, check the lock, and look for a place you would like to deposit the key.

Return your attention to this room.

Sometimes, one safe is not enough, so you need to use several of them. Or you can imagine safe-deposit boxes like at a bank or lockers at a train station. Banks, for example, have a lot of safe-deposit boxes.

Sometimes, it doesn't work immediately, and of course not permanently, to pack things away in the safe. Then, you must repeat the exercise again. It can initially be a huge relief to be able to lock away one's burdens for a while. It's worth it to try out this exercise often. The possibility of freeing ourselves for some time from our burdens gives us the feeling that we can do something about them. This puts control back into our own hands.

Progressive muscle relaxation (PMR) is a method that helps you to independently regulate tension that is also triggered by strong unpleasant feelings.

Preparation
I sit or lie myself down in a relaxed position—loosening everything that is restricting me—close my eyes, and loosen my shoulders as much as possible. Then I take a deep breath—hold the air tight and let it flow out again. In the process, I imagine everything unpleasant from the day streaming out of me. Every time I exhale, a bit of internal tension may be released.

Hands and Arms
I clench my dominant hand into a fist, hold it tightly, and observe the tension. Then, I release my grip again, focusing on the feeling during this transition and on the relaxation of the hand. I appreciate all the tiny sensations such as tingling, warmth and the like.

And then, I clench the other hand into a fist, hold it tightly—and release it again. How do I experience this hand today? Can I recognize any difference?

Now I turn to both hands simultaneously and clench both fists tighter and tighter. I study the sensations and then relax again.

Now, I move further to the upper-arms. I bend my elbows and push my forearms against my upper-arms. During this, I allow my hands to remain completely loose and concentrate on the tension in my bicep muscles. Then I let my arms sink down again loosely onto the floor and relax again. Then, I turn around both hands so that my palms are facing upwards. I push my arms firmly into the elbows and sense the tension from my fingertips up into my shoulders. Then I let go again and bring my arms back into a comfortable initial position. I enjoy the release. Both arms are now completely relaxed—I allow myself time to feel this.

Face
I stay calm and relaxed and now turn to my face.

First, I wrinkle my forehead so that my eyebrows are pushed up against my hairline. I feel the tension in my forehead and then release again. I flatten my forehead completely and observe the change. I feel the calm that moves outward from my forehead.

Then, I move to the region arounds my eyes: I close my eyelids tightly—observe the tension—and let go. I experience how my eyes and the area around them begin to relax, smoothing out all the wrinkles. The eyes, eyelids, and cheeks can all now relax.

Now, I move the region around my mouth. I clench my teeth tightly together—sensing the pressure and tension within my jaw muscles—and release! I open my mouth slightly and allow my lower jaw to sink downward—and feel the relief!

Fig. 27 IS Progressive muscle relaxation

I push my tongue behind my upper teeth against my gums! I observe the pressure and counter-pressure, as well as all sensations from my tongue going down to my throat. Now I let go and allow my tongue to return to a comfortable position. I allow the calmness to take effect. I observe the relaxation in the oral interior and the flow of saliva.

And now on to the lips: I press the lips tightly together! I hold the tension firmly and then release again. I pay attention to the unpleasant feeling of resolution and the warmth in the lips.

The entire face is now relaxed and calm. I allow myself to let go even more and allow the calmness to spread everywhere.

Neck, Shoulders, Upper Back
I remain calm and relaxed and focus my attention on my neck, shoulders, and upper back.

I push my head backwards so that I clearly sense my neck muscles. Then, I tense my head in a roll to the right—and then to the left, observing the shifting of the tension in the process—and then let it dangle freely. I perceive the relaxation and warmth in my neck. I let go entirely in my neck and feel a pleasant warmth streaming into the back of my head as well.

Now I pull my shoulders upwards in the direction of my ears, paying attention to the feeling of tension in the shoulder muscles—and then let my shoulders gently fall down again. I observe the relief, as my neck and shoulders ease back again. The relaxation can develop further and deepen into the shoulder belt and the throat.

If I am sitting, I let my head sink forward and push with chin gently in direction of my chest. I feel the tension in my neck and pressure in my throat and straighten my head so that it rests well at the spine. I sense closely how it feels.

If I am lying down instead, then I lift up my head, also push it downwards quickly toward the chest, perceive the sensation, and enjoy the relief.

Neck, shoulders, and upper back are now completely relaxed. I indulge myself with some time for the relaxation to take effect and spread throughout the entire body.

Chest, Stomach, Lower Back
Now I focus on my chest, my stomach, and my lower back.

I breathe freely and easily in and out and feel how, with every exhale, I relax more and more. Now I breathe in forcefully and fill my lungs as much I can—hold tension firmly—and let the air flow out. I feel how the tension subsides and breathe freely again. I allow my chest muscles to loosen completely. I enjoy how I can now continue to breathe again in my own breathing rhythm without pressure and tension.

Fig. 27 (continued)

Now I move to my stomach and pull it tightly inward. I get aware of the feeling and release. After a few deep breaths into my belly, I make my stomach muscles tight and hard, push my stomach outward, feel the sensation, and then let go. After breathing freely again for a few breaths, I pull my stomach, without breathing in the meantime, inwards—push it out again—pull it inwards again, and then release entirely. Now I enjoy my breathing in my personal rhythm and allow my entire body to rock back and forth along with it.

Now I concentrate on my lower back. I bend the small of the back into a hollow area and observe the tension in the spine, in the hips, and in the back. Then, I relax the small of the back again and focus precisely on all changes.

My body is now very relaxed and warmed-up. I allow the relaxation that I feel to spread itself all over in healing manner to all the areas where I particularly need it.

Legs
Lastly, I move to the legs, from my hips to the tips of my toes.

I tense up the gluteal and thigh muscles simultaneously, hold the tension firmly—and release it again. I pay attention to all change that happens during the process of tension and release.

And now on to the lower legs and feet: I tense up the backs of my feet, pushing my toes downward away from my face and observe any area where I can feel tension. Then I let go and sense the feeling: I put my feet back on the ground and feel the relaxation.

Now I push my toes upwards in the direction of my face until I feel tension in my shinbone—hold it firmly—and relax again. I feel the changes in my lower legs and allow my feet to relax.

Conclusion
The entire body is now relaxed. The relaxation spreads itself out and flows everywhere. Now I breathe in and out ten times while counting. With each number, I will feel myself letting go more and more until I feel at 10 completely, pleasantly relaxed: 1, 2, 3, 4, 5, 6, 7, 8, 9, 10.

Now I transform the feeling of relaxation into a freshness and rejuvenation like after a short afternoon nap, during which I count backwards from 5 to 1.
5 – I'm moving slowly towards waking up,
4 – I move my fingers and my toes slightly,
3 – I make a fist with both hands and flex my arms forcefully three times, I exhale,
2 – I open my eyes, and
1 – I am wide awake again.

Fig. 27 (continued)

I am not my feeling!
I am having a feeling.

I can always act in different way.

The following questions will help you reduce strong feelings:

1. Is my feeling justified? Check the facts!

2. Does my impulse to act in the current situation also makes sense in the long term?

3. Is my feeling in regard to the triggering experience actually appropriate and reasonable?

4. Is my impulse to act appropriate? Would most people react this way?

Avoid assumptions!
Through the gathering and evaluation of facts, it is possible to react more appropriately.

Action: If the feeling is appropriate, then act accordingly! Pay attention to how you can carry out the impulse to act a reasonable manner.

Reducing: If the feeling is not appropriate or too intense, try to reduce the feeling (for example, by creating positive experiences).

Check:

1. What is different at the moment?

2. Describe the environment in which you now find yourself.

3. Which people are involved?

4. What statements, exactly, have people made?

5. What actions, exactly, have people carried out?

6. What possibilities do you have to react today?

Fig. 28 Checking strong emotions

You can "**sense**" sexual desire within the body. This can take form of internal **sensations** (e.g. the heart beats faster, the shoulders are tensed) or external sensations (e.g. that the palms sweat or that you develop an erection). Circle the different areas, where you "**sense**" your sexual desire and write them down next to the circles.

Where do you feel sexual desire?

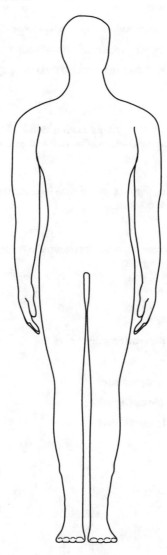

Fig. 29 WS Bodily experience with sexual desire

It is important that you know your sexual fantasies very well because…

1. Becoming an "expert"on your own sexual fantasies protects you from surprises. This reduces fear.

2. Knowledge means gaining competence, which entails a growth in self-confidence.

3. Then you can observe if fantasies change or stay the same.

4. The better you know your sexual desires and needs, the betteryou will realize when the desire arises for you to become reality. Because when fantasies just remain fantasies, no one gets hurt. But you're the only one who can make sure of this.

5. With masturbation to the most sexually arousing fantasy, you have the greatest gain in lust.

Triggers are catalysts that can increase the urge to act on fantasies about sexual contact with a child.

Internal triggers are catalysts within you that no one else can perceive (for example, unpleasant feelings such as anger, fear, hopelessness, or loneliness).

External triggers are catalysts outside of you that other people can also perceive (for example, you talking to a child).

It is very important that you know which internal and external triggers can lead to fantasies about sexual contact with a child that threaten to manifest at the behavioral level.

Fig. 30 IS Sexual fantasies

Fig. 31 WS My triggers

Please consider which of your internal triggers (inner catalysts) and external triggers (outer catalysts) amplify the urge to act on your fantasies involving sexual contact with a child and write them down in the corresponding column in the table.

Then, please estimate how likely you think it is that these triggers can also actually lead you to carry out sexual acts with a child or to use abuse images. Write down the corresponding number after each trigger.

The scale is as follows:

1	2	3	4	5
not very likely	somewhat likely	moderately likely	fairly likely	very likely

My internal triggers	My external triggers

Fig. 32 WS My sexual
fantasies with children

Please describe a sexual fantasy with a child that corresponds **exactly** to how your
imagination was and that you find especially stimulating during masturbation. Try to describe
with as much detail as possible what would happen in your ideal sexual fantasy. Describe it as
you would in a short story or a short film.

Try to formulate it using complete sentences, and avoid using just key words in order to make
your portrayal more comprehensible. Spelling and grammar mistakes are not important; only
the content of your report is relevant.

Pay attention to the following points:

1. Gender and age of the child
2. Do you know the child personally (e.g. from your circle of acquaintances, from the
neighborhood), or do you imagine a child that you don't know but have possibly seen in
pictures (magazines, television, internet)?
3. Please describe the child precisely. How does he/she look? How does he/she behave? Is
he/she quiet or lively, trusting or suspicious?
4. Where do you find yourself with the child in the fantasy? In your room, in the open, or
somewhere else?
5. Who do you say and/or what does the child say in the fantasy?
6. What do you do with the child in the fantasy? Where do you touch, caress, or hold him/her?
Do you put your finger or your penis in his/her mouth, anus, or vagina in the fantasy?
7. How does the child react? Does the child accept your contact or refuse it?
8. Where and how does the child touch or caress you?
9. Which situation or view is for you especially sexual arousing?
10. Which fantasy do you have right before you have an orgasm?
11. What are you thinking about and how do you feel before, during, and after the sexual
contact that you fantasized about?

Also make sure to answer the following 5 W-Questions:

— **Who**   (describe all individuals as precisely as possible) *is/are doing*
— **What**   (describe all sexual acts)
— **Where**   (the location)
— **When**   (the time of day), *and*
— **How**   (Who is active, who is passive? Who makes contact? Is there talking involved?
               Does eye-contact predominate? Etc.)

Also make sure to include the 5 levels within the fantasy:

1. Perception: What do you see, hear, smell, taste, feel in the fantasy?
2. Thoughts: Is anything going through your mind within the fantasy?
3. Feelings: How are you feeling during this time in the fantasy?
4: Physical sensations: What do feel inside your body within the fantasy?
5: Behavior: What exactly are you doing in the fantasy?

A consequence is a **result or an effect** of something. Every decision and every behavior have consequences that follow. These could be the reactions of other people or other kinds of results. Example: "I studied a lot (*behavior*), which is why I got an "A" on the math test (*consequence*)."

Decisions can always have positive and/or negative consequences. The short-term consequences can often be clearly distinguished from the long-term consequences.

I am doing something specific.		
	Short-Term Consequences (immediately noticeable)	**Long-Term Consequences** (only noticeable later)
Positive		
Negative		

I am *not* doing something specific.		
	Short-Term Consequences (immediately noticeable)	**Long-Term Consequences** (only noticeable later)
Positive		
Negative		

Humans often notice positive consequences directly as a result from their behavior. This is the reason why we humans frequently do things repeatedly. However, over the long-term the disadvantages begin to predominate. This is especially the case for types of behavior that can be considered problematic.

For example, after stealing something, one might quickly receive a lot of money. But later, one has to endure a prison sentence.

Thus, it is important that before acting, you always try to ask what kind of short- **AND** long-term results or consequences there could be for yourself and for others.

Fig. 33 WS Consequences of behavior

Please deal again with the possible consequences (short-and long-term) of sexual contact with children or the use of abuse images. If you already had real sexual contact with a child or used abuse images, think about what consequences this had. Write down your ideas in the corresponding column of the table.

	I have sexual contact with a child.		I use child sexual abuse images.	
	Short-term Consequences (immediately noticeable)	Long-term Consequences (only noticeable later)	Short-term Consequences (immediately noticeable)	Long-term Consequences (only noticeable later)
Positive				
Negative				

	I have *not* have sexual contact with a child.		I do *not* use child sexual abuse images.	
	Short-term Consequences (immediately noticeable)	Long-term Consequences (only noticeable later)	Short-term Consequences (immediately noticeable)	Long-term Consequences (only noticeable later)
Positive				
Negative				

Fig. 34 WS Consequences following sexual contact with children

With the journal, you can document your experiences and learn how they affect you. Every event, whether big or small, can trigger thoughts and feelings. By keeping a journal, you will discover that your thoughts and feelings and your behavior repeat themselves and form a recurring pattern. This way you will learn to anticipate unfavorable behavior und you will be able to intervene at an early stage. After a few weeks, you will get used to writing entries in your journal.

Through self-observation, you will learn…

— to pay attention to the connections between feelings, thoughts, and behavior.

— to know yourself better.

— to recognize problems in their early stages.

— to better control your actions.

— to recognize the difference between behavior and subsequent consequences to it.

— to find good solutions.

— to be aware of when the urge to act on sexual fantasies is increasing.

All of this forms the foundation for your future prevention plan!

Take notes

As soon as things happen that have to do with children, make a note of it to remind yourself of it later. Also make notes about events that preoccupy you for longer, as well as those that only slightly preoccupy you. Each note can be short (e.g. the names of the people involved, time of day, a few words describing the situation). You will then be able to utilize these notes later to write more complete entries in the pages of your journal.

Set aside time every day to work on your journal

Without a regular timeslot each day where you can sit down and fill in your journal, you will quickly lose sight of the task. If you don't make time for it every day, you will likely overlook the more subtle situations that occur repeatedly while you wait for the "big" event. You can sometimes learn the most from "smaller" events.

Structure of the journal

During each session, you will receive enough journal pages to take home with you.

Note: Keeping the journal is required for you. Your notes about the last week will from now on be discussed in every therapy session.

Fig. 35 IS The therapy journal

Fig. 36 WS My therapy journal

Please document everyday situations that are associated with your sexual interest in children. These could be real contact situations with children. But they could also be situations in which you have (sexual) fantasies about children without the children actually being there in that moment.

Date:

Situation: *(What? Who? When? Where? Describe the course of events from the beginning to the end!)*

....

....

Thoughts: *(What was going through my mind?)*

....

....

Feelings: *(What exactly was I feeling?)*

....

....

Bodily Sensations: *(What changes in my body did I perceive?)*

....

....

Reactions: *(What did I say or do? What did the others do?)*

....

....

Urge to act: *(How strong was my impulse in this situation to have actual sexual contact with a child or to use abuse images? Scale from "not at all": 0% until "very strong": 100%)*

10	20	30	40	50	60	70	80	90	100

Alternative thoughts, assessments: *(Is it possible for me to think differently about this situation afterwards?)*

....

....

Short-term consequences: *(What were the short-term effects of my behavior?)*
Positive   **negative**

....

....

Long-term consequences: *(What were the long-term effects of my behavior?)*
Positive   **negative**

....

....

Definition: Empathy is the ability to be aware of the feelings of others, to understand these feelings, to imagine how they feel, to experience these feelings, and finally to show care and concern towards these individuals. Empathy can be impaired as a result of mistaken thoughts, negative emotions, and sexual arousal.

Empathy involves:

— being able to view things from another perspective,

— being able to put yourself in someone else's place,

— being capable of understanding how someone else thinks and feels,

— being capable of understanding how one's own actions can have effects on other people.

Empathy is an important precondition for...

— being able to have relationships with others,

— being able to comprehend how a child feels and thinks. Then I can take better care not to cause any harm to a child.

Fig. 37 IS Empathy

Fig. 38 IS Letters from Victims

Letter From a Victim of Child Sexual Abuse

I am now feeling his presence in the room. Exactly at this moment, he is sitting behind me and is whispering in my ear: "I love you, Karin, I love you…" I can feel him touching me. My whole body is violated. I open my mouth, but he covers it with his hand. My scream will never be heard.

Since that first day, 12 years have gone by. He sexually molested me repeatedly for many months. Today he is still in the room, sitting behind me. He is still touching me, and I can still smell him. It still hurts, and I still cry. He is there in my waking hours and at night in my dreams. He is in my thoughts, feelings, and moods. He is still inside my body. I try to escape the memories, but there is no escape.

Are you listening to what I'm saying? This is how someone feels who has been sexually abused. I have felt this way year after year, and it will never be over.

Every day I hear of children who have been molested. I turn on the television and see them. I turn on the radio and hear about them. I open the newspaper and read about them. I hear about them from my friends, my colleagues, and my family. But who is doing anything about it? No one!

Parents, teachers, relatives, and all other adult individuals in this world should inform each other of the warning signs of sexual abuse. Children need to be informed about sexual abuse. They should know how to avoid it and what to do if they become victims. This problem should not be pushed to the side or ignored. It should be addressed and hopefully solved.

I believe that sexual abuse is worst kind of abuse that can be done to a child. Even if a child is only molested once, it can still destroy his or her life forever. The child will replay the abuse in his or her thoughts over and over again. Feelings of worthlessness, rage, fear, and filth are deeply rooted. It reaches deep into the soul of the child, and requires many years of therapy for the child to rebuild his self-esteem and feeling of self-worth.

Now I would like to speak to someone who has at some point abused a child. Some of you have been punished for it, while some have not. I don't believe that a harsh enough punishment exists for destroying a child. I want you to know that you took a small life in your hands and destroyed it forever. Always remember that they are helpless. You are too strong for them. You are not only playing with their head, but also with their soul, which makes them vulnerable to your sickening behavior.

Fig. 39 WS Report on
Letters from Victims

1. After reading this letter, what kind of thoughts did you have?

....
....
....
....
....

2. After reading this letter, what kind of feelings did you have?

....
....
....
....
....

3. How does the victim feel right after the abuse? What are the short-term consequences for the victim?

....
....
....
....
....

4. How does the victim feel after a longer period of time (weeks, months, years) after the abuse? What are the long-term consequences?

....
....
....
....
....

5. Are there differences between the short-and long-term consequences?

....
....
....
....
....

Fig. 40 Letter to my
victim(s)

Write a letter to a child that you had sexual contact with.

If you haven't ever had sexual contact with a child, write a letter to a child that you've had, or repeatedly have, sexual contact with in your fantasies.

What would you like to say to your victim? The letter should be written in such a way that it is intended to help your victim.

You will discuss this letter in the therapy session. **Do not send the letter.**

Fig. 41 IS Characteristics of a letter
from a victim

The victim could…

— express anger,
— use a hateful tone,
— describe having a good life before the abuse,
— share feelings from during the abuse
— describe the short-term and long-term consequences of the abuse
— specify the details that were felt to be the worst

Fig. 42 Letter to me
from a victim

Compose a **letter that is addressed to yourself.**The letter is from a child that you had sexual contact with in reality or in fantasy. Now let the child convey what he or she wants to say to you.

Fig. 43 Problem
Solving – New Behavior

<u>Describe a problem that you had with another person:</u>

Problem: *(What was it about? What was the triggering event? Who was affected by it? When/where did it happen?)*

....

....

Thoughts: *(What was going through your mind?)*

....

....

Reactions: *(What did you say or do? What did the others do?)*

....

....

Short-term Consequences: *(What were the short-term effects of the behavior you exhibited?)*
Positive   **negative**

....

....

Long-term Consequences: *(What were the long-term effects of the behavior you exhibited?)*
Positive   **negative**

....

....

Fig. 43 (continued)   <u>**Now think about how you could redesign the same situation:**</u>

Alternative Thoughts: *(What other kinds of thoughts could have also gone through your mind in this situation?)*

....

....

have done?)
Alternative Reactions: *(What could you have said or done instead? What could the others*

....

....

Short-term Consequences: *(What short-term effects could the newly-exhibited behavior have had?)*
Positive   **negative**

....

....

Long-term Consequences: *(What long-term effects could the newly-exhibited behavior have had?)*
Positive   **negative**

....

....

Coping strategies are thoughts and types of behavior that can be used to handle unpleasant, stressful, or overwhelming stressors. The stressors can be internal (within you and thus not visible to others) or external (outside of you and thus visible to others).

Internal Stressors   **External Stressors**

Negative feelings   Heavy workload
Deviant sexual fantasies   Argument with friends or family
Strong sexual impulses   Stress from school

There are three kinds of coping strategies:

1. **Problem-Oriented Coping:** These are strategies for really approaching the problem or solving it:
— solving the problem concretely
— seeking out support
— planning intermediate steps
— standing up for oneself
— accepting things that one cannot change
— taking on a new way ofseeing things
— **Example**: You want to make up with a good friend that you haven't spoken to for three months after you two had an argument. You call him and arrange a meeting in a café.

2. **Emotion-Oriented Coping:** These strategies involve an emotional response to the problem:
— being absorbed in oneself
— brooding
— fantasizing or imagining different scenarios
— becoming angry
— accusing other people
— expressing concern about the situation
— **Example**: You want to make up with a good friend that you haven't spoken to for three months after you two had an argument. However, you still feel offended and want him to be the first one to get in contact. You ponder a lot about what started the argument, but you still can't find a satisfying answer.

3. **Avoidance:** These strategies involve avoiding the problem:
— pursuing other activities (distraction)
— seeking out other people (social alternatives)
— **Example**: You haven't spoken with your best friend since you had an argument three months ago. You miss him and now try to strike him from memory. You already erased his number on your phone. In order to numb your sorrows a bit, you drink a bottle of red wine every night.

The first-mentioned coping mechanism is positive and effective, while the other two coping mechanisms tend not to be successful. Avoidance and emotion-oriented coping strategies usually immediately result in one feeling better. However, they do not lead to a solution and thus can even amplify the problem.

Fig. 44 IS Coping strategies

Fig. 45 WS *My coping strategies*

Name a problem you are having with your family, school, or circle of friends.

....

....

....

....

....

How have you dealt with this particular problem so far? What were the advantages and disadvantages of using that strategy?

....

....

....

....

....

....

....

....

....

Now that you have learned a bit about positive coping strategies, what could you do differently? What are the advantages and disadvantages of these new strategies?

....

....

....

....

....

....

....

....

....

Fig. 46 WS *My offense cycle*

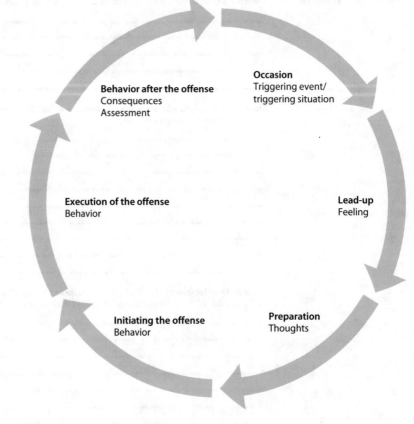

Behavior after the offense
Consequences
Assessment

Occasion
Triggering event/
triggering situation

Execution of the offense
Behavior

Lead-up
Feeling

Initiating the offense
Behavior

Preparation
Thoughts

Fig. 47 WS My offense staircase

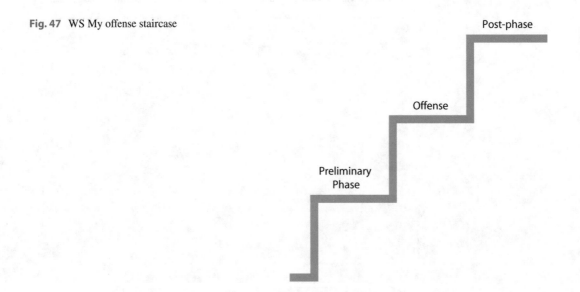

Post-phase

Offense

Preliminary
Phase

Below you will find a list of abilities that humans more or less have at their command. Assess the degree of command you believe you have for each of the abilities. Use the following scale:

0	1	2	3	4
not at all	somewhat	adequate	considerable	very good

	not at all	somewhat	adequate	considerable	very good
Confidence					
Giving compliments					
Teamwork					
Expressing needs					
Withstanding conflict					
Being responsible					
Saying no					
Expressing a different opinion					
Being ready to help					
Showing empathy					
Being tolerant					
Dealing with criticism					
Asserting yourself					
Making compromises					
Giving criticism					
Resisting temptation					
Resisting demands					

Fig. 48 WS My social competencies

	not at all	somewhat	adequate	considerable	very good
Making excuses for yourself					
Accepting compliments					
Showing feelings openly					
Admitting weaknesses					
Starting, holding, and ending conversations					
Asking for a favor					

Fig. 48 (continued)

Please fill out the following concerning your current social relationships. Mark down one of the following numbers next to each name to indicate how regularly you have contact with that person.

(0) No contact at all
(1) Infrequent contact
(2) Regular contact
(3) Very frequent contact

1. What family members do you have?

....
....
....
....
....

2. What are your male friends' names?

....
....
....
....
....

3. What are your female friends' names?

....
....
....
....
....

4. What are the names of the children with whom you are in contact?

....
....
....
....
....

Fig. 49 WS My social relationships

In the spaces below, write in the names of persons from your social environment (friends, acquaintances, family members, partners, etc.). Choose the appropriate field for each, based on how comfortable or difficult you experience your relationship to each of these people.

very enjoyable
enjoyable
neutral
difficult
very difficult

Fig. 50 WS The quality of my relationships

Fig. 51 IS Rules for
Feedback

Feedback makes sense…
when the person you are talking to
– can understand and process.
– wants feedback.
– can process the amount of information you're communicating.

when you
– refer to concrete, specific behavior.
– do not analyze.

when the feedback
– immediately follows a behavior.
– serves the purpose of communicating something.
– also encompasses positive feelings and observations.

Feedback in conflict situations requires…
– saying what bothers you in a non-accusatory way.
– paying attention to the needs and interests of the person you are talking to.
– formulating your own wishes.
– the cooperative search for solutions.

Communicate
your perceptions as your perceptions
your assumptions as your assumptions
your feelings as your feelings
when you give feedback.
Formulate I-sentences!

Before you give feedback, consider the following points:

Before the feedback:

– Be conscious of what you're feeling (happiness, admiration, pride, affection, etc.).

– Think about what concrete behavior of the other person's triggered this feeling.

– Check if the other person is ready to receive your feedback.

In the situation:

– Stick to just your feelings, such as "Right now I'm…" or "I feel…".

– Your feelings belong to you and cannot be contested by anyone else.

– Explain to the other person what brought you to say this.

– Describe the concrete instance, keeping in mind that you can only describe your own point of view.

After the situation:

– Encourage yourself for every single expression of a feeling that you achieved. The success does not consist in another person thanking you or rewarding you, but rather that you have communicated what you were feeling.

– Keep in mind that others often have very different feelings. The goal of a conversation cannot be to unite over one feeling. But you can make it understood that you want to engage with different feelings.

My positive feedback:

– Who received positive feedback from me?

....

....

– In what situation have I given positive feedback?

....

....

– What reaction have I received for my positive feedback?

....

....

– How did I feel after giving positive feedback?

....

....

Fig. 52 WS Positive feedback in relationships

Intimacy is a state of deep familiarity with another person. The concept "intimacy" is very often equated with sexual relationships, which is, however, not true.

This misunderstanding of the concept of intimacy contributes to the idea that every other kind of relationship must be **non-intimate.**

Intimacy entails…
– a feeling of security, familiarity, and emotional closeness,
– shared experiences (e.g. common free-time activities),
– caring for the other person
– to receive confirmation/acknowledgment of one's own person from the other person,
– mutual support in crisis situations,
– a feeling of a familial bond,
– functional verbal and nonverbal communication,
– opening oneself,
– the ability to solve conflicts,
– **sometimes:** shared sexuality

Depending upon whether a sexual responsiveness to the child body schema is exclusive or nonexclusive, intimacy can also be experienced in sexual relationships with age-appropriate partners.

Exclusive sexual interest in child bodies	Sexual interest in child and adult bodies
– No possibility of acting out sexual fantasies and intimate wishes (directly or indirectly) without committing child sexual abuse	– Possibility of leading intimate and sexually-fulfilling relationships with age-appropriate partners, where a part of one's sexual desires remain unfulfilled
– Factual sexual interest only in child bodies. The desire to be interested in adults "proves" a lack of sexual interest in adults	Real sexual interest in both child and adult bodies
– Fantasies during masturbation are exclusively about sexual acts with children	– Fantasies during masturbation are about sexual acts with both children and adults
– Orgasm can be reached during sexual intercourse with an age-appropriate partner mental fantasies of children are used to achieve the necessary sexual arousal and orgasm	– During sexual intercourse with an age-appropriate partner, that person or certain characteristics of theirs (e.g. breast or genital area, smell, body structure) are experienced as strongly sexually arousing

A relationship between a child and a juvenile/adult is always asymmetrical. That means it is never equal/on the same level.

Children do not yet comprehend the world of juveniles/adults.
Children live in another world.

It is not possible to be intimate with a children through sexuality, because it necessarily means committing sexual assault.
An intimate relationship with a child is impossible, even when it is strongly desired!

Fig. 53 IS Intimacy

Fig. 54 WS Intimacy in my relationships

What does your personal **ranking** of intimate relationships look like? Organize your relationships on a scale to"**very intimate**" to "**very distant.**"
very intimate
intimate
neutral
distant
very distant

Fig. 55 IS Sexual attraction to the child body age and partnership

Sexuality with a partner takes place in **three dimensions**, which are of different importance to every person:

1. **Dimension of Attachment:** Fulfillment of the basic needs of acceptance, closeness, safety, and security. Creation and expression of togetherness through physical contact, which can range from embrace to coitus. Sexuality in a partnership as communication through physical language.
2. **Dimension of Desire:** Experiencing sexual arousal, lust, sensuality, ecstasy, desiring, being desired.
3. **Dimension of Reproduction:** corresponding or differing desires to have children, disproportionate desire to have children, importance of the ability to reproduce.

Sexual Reaction Cycle:

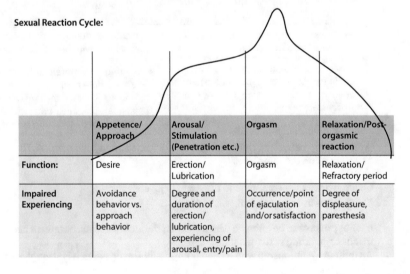

	Appetence/ Approach	Arousal/ Stimulation (Penetration etc.)	Orgasm	Relaxation/Post-orgasmic reaction
Function:	Desire	Erection/ Lubrication	Orgasm	Relaxation/ Refractory period
Impaired Experiencing	Avoidance behavior vs. approach behavior	Degree and duration of erection/ lubrication, experiencing of arousal, entry/pain	Occurrence/point of ejaculation and/or satisfaction	Degree of displeasure, paresthesia

Fig. 55 (continued)

Disruptions of the reaction cycle during sexuality with one's partner or masturbation can occur for the following reasons:
– fear of failure,
– a lack of acceptance of one's own sexuality or sexual fantasies,
– conflict with one's partner
– a lack of or insufficient communication about one's own wishes, needs, and feelings,
– insufficient physical sexual attractiveness of the partner,
– a lack of commonalities in the relationship,
– physical ailments,
– substance abuse ,
– dysfunctional beliefs,
     - simultaneous orgasm is better than staggered orgasms,
     - orgasm is the primary source of satisfaction,
     - regular sex is a duty in the relationship,
     - good sex must be varied,
     - if I regularly fantasize about children when I masturbate, I'll get used to it.

Sexual attraction to children can have different effects on the quality of a partnership:
– One has a "secret" that cannot be shared with their partner.
– One can develop feelings of guilt around their partner because, for instance, they look at child sexual abuse images on the internet, are sexually interested in children in their surroundings, or have (sexual) contact with children.
– It could become necessary to use sexual fantasies about children during sexual contact with one's partner in order to achieve sufficient sexual arousal.
– Sexual dysfunctions (e.g. erectile or orgasm dysfunctions) may develop. One may then retreat from their partner as a result.

An act of sexual abuse or the use of child sexual abuse material does not take place on impulse or in an uncontrolled way, but rather is the result of several individual steps — each of which depends on your decision.

You can picture the path to direct or indirect sexual abuse as the individual rungs of a ladder. In the case of direct or indirect sexual abuse, you have made the decision to climb up these steps. Once you reach the top, the act of sexual abuse takes place.

Your own "risk ladder" however starts off right at the bottom rung with a minimal degree of sexual arousal. The more rungs up the ladder you climb, the stronger your sexual arousal is going to be. This makes it increasingly difficult to stop the risk from developing further.

It makes a difference whether you have to take "just" one step down the ladder, (interrupting the risk development process at an early stage), or whether you have to "jump down" multiple rungs at once (interrupting the risk development process at a late stage).

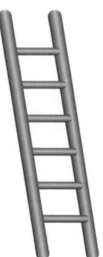

Fig. 56 IS The risk ladder – steps on the way to sexual abuse

Fig. 57 WS My risk ladder

Sexual Abuse

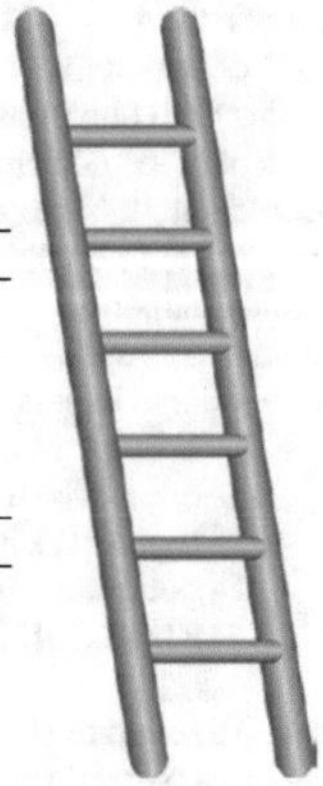

Step 6:_____
_____

Step 5:_____
_____

Step 4:_____
_____

Step 3:_____
_____

Step 2:_____
_____

Step 1:_____
_____

Fig. 58 IS Risk factors

Risk factors are conditions that increase the probability that you will initiate sexual contact with a child and commit an act of sexual abuse and/or use child abuse images.

Risk factors can be **internal** (cannot be observed by others) or **external** (can be observed by others).

Examples of risk factors are:

- **External:** End of a relationship, a fight, visiting a playground, visiting a public pool, passing by a school, surfing the Web for hours looking for sexually arousing visual material etc.
- **Internal:** Thoughts and feelings such as loneliness, boredom, rage, worthlessness; thoughts that justify child sexual abuse, such as "I don't care. It's not like I have anything to lose, anyway," "I'm not someone who gets love from people, so I guess I'll have to go out and get it myself."

When you know your own risk factors, you can steer yourself away from them in time.

Some risk factors **can be more dangerous than others.** The closer you get to coming into sexual contact with a child, the more energy you have to invest to break off from the path you've started to go down. It takes more energy and is more dangerous to climb down a 6000 m-high mountain, for example, than a hill in a city park. As the risk increases, i.e. the closer you've gotten yourself to an actual abuse situation (e.g. the child is already sitting naked on your bed), the more your will to hold yourself back from an offense (or repeat offense) will decrease.

Please write down your personal risk factors! In addition, give each of your risk factors a number, depending on how dangerous it is – i.e. how likely it is that it will result in you sexually abusing a child/using child abuse images if this risk factor is active.

The scale is as follows:

1	2	3	4	5
minimally dangerous	slightly dangerous	moderately dangerous	quite dangerous	very dangerous

Risk factor	Dangerousness
1.	
2.	
3.	
4.	
5.	
6.	
7.	
8.	
9.	
10.	

Fig. 59 WS My risk factors

Example 1:

Direct Sexual Abuse of a Child

Risk factor:

Being alone with the little boy from next-door, Matthias.

What can I do to prevent it?

Not invite Matthias over to my house.

Which thought(s) is/are helpful in this situation?

"If I go over there right now and am alone with him, I might have again the desire to touch him, then I'll be committing child sexual abuse, which I don't want. In the end, I definitely won't be doing well, since I'll have a bad conscience and will be afraid that everything will come out."

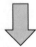

How can I behave in this situation?

When I notice that Matthias is home alone and I start to have sexual fantasies about him, I'll call a person I trust and tell them about it or I'll try to distract myself by playing sports or watching TV. I can also write my thoughts and feelings in my therapy journal. I can also masturbate.

Fig. 60 IS Examples for dealing with risk factors

Example 2:

Using child sexual abuse images

Risk factor:

Surfing online for hours, looking for child sexual abuse images of children.

What can I do to prevent it?

Cancel my internet connection.
Only surf in public internet cafes.
Ask my parents or caregiver to cut off my internet connection in the evenings.

Which thought(s) is/are helpful in this situation?

"When I spend hours surfing in the Internet, I'm just wasting my time. I could get caught consuming child pornographic material. Surfing doesn't make me happier; afterwards, I'm exhausted, annoyed, and feel unsatisfied."

How can I behave in this situation?

Call up a trusted person and tell them about it. Do sports, go jogging, or go for a walk. Write down my thoughts and feelings in my journal. Masturbate and then turn the computer off, etc.

Fig. 60 (continued)

In order to cope with risk situations, not only are problem-solving skills necessary, but also the support of confidants. This can help you in especially difficult times. Confidants can be people within your circle, such as acquaintances, friends, and family members. Confidants can also be lay support people, or even professional counselors and therapists.

These people must be informed about your sexual interest in children and about your goal of not having any sexual contact with children.

The most effective kind of support comes about when your confidants are as informed about you and your living conditions as possible.

Person's name	Phone number
1.	
2.	
3.	
4.	
5.	
6.	
7.	

Fig. 61 WS My confidants

Fig. 62 IS Coming up with a personal prevention plan

When risk situations arise, your prevention plan shows you how you can act effectively in such situations.

For each risk factor in your plan, you must consider the following:

1. How will you organize your life so that this risk factor no longer arises? What can you do as a prevention measure against this risk factor?

2. What will you say to yourself and how will you act in order to deal with this risk situation in a meaningful way (i.e. in a way that is not harmful to others)?

Formulate your strategies as detailed and concretely as possible!

Keep in mind:

- Even the best plan is useless if you don't put it into practice.

- Therapy continues at home. You must continue to practice the skills you learn in therapy in everyday life, e.g. making connections with people of your own age, dealing with your own feelings in a positive way, etc.

The following example can help you while putting together your prevention plan:

If "loneliness" represents a risk factor for you, you can combat it by widening your circle of friends and acquaintances. It is not enough to just write, "find more friends," however. You must describe exactly how you will do this, in detail (e.g. which activities you will take up, or what clubs you will join). Write down the thoughts that will help you put your plans into practice, as well. Incorporate additional strategies that can help you in moments when your motivation is low, e.g. "Call Friend X to tell him to come pick me up, so that I don't have any excuse not to go to this activity."

Fig. 63 WS Strategies for dealing with risk factors. (Note: For technical printing reasons, the illustration has been kept in black-and-white. The color gradient from green to yellow to red is to be taken from the corresponding pdf.)

My risk factor:

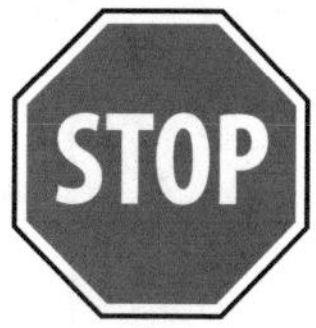

....

....

....

What can I do?

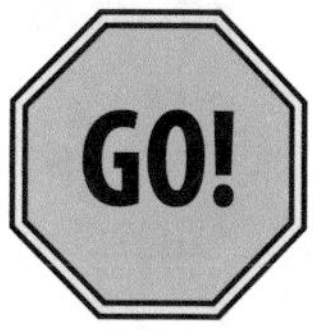

....

....

....

....

....

....

....

I know my risk situations!

I have the chance of controlling myself.

To keep control, I need support.

I will stick to my prevention plan.

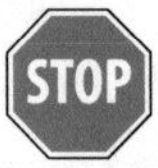

STOP	Risk factor	Coping Strategies	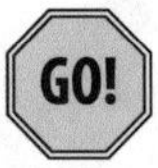 GO!

Fig. 64 WS My prevention plan

Every person has a set of strengths, attributes, skills, and resources that help him or her to reach his or her goals and to make it through tough times.

Please write down everything you can think of that could be a strength or a resource of yours on the branches of the tree.

A resource is a protective and supportive skill that a person can apply to manage adverse circumstances.

This could be things that you're good at, attributes that you like about yourself or that other people like about you, interests, successes, or the like. If you can't think of anything, ask your parents or your friends what they think.

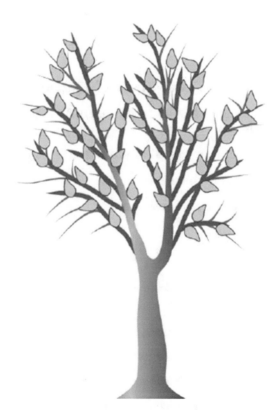

Fig. 65 WS My resources

Goals can be divided into two categories:

1. **Approach goals** help us to plan our own actions so that the desired condition is reached as directly as possible. Approach goals therefore describe what one would like to achieve (example: "I would like to eat more fruit, so that I can loseweight").

2. **Avoidance goals**, on the other hand, refer to the things that one does not want. That is, certain situations are avoided in order to contribute to the success of the actual goal (example: "I would like to snack less, so that I can lose weight").

Approach goals are often easier to achieve than avoidance goals.

It is easier to do something than to attempt to stop doing something.

As such, the goal of not committing any more acts of sexual abuse is more difficult to achieve than goals that lead to a happier and more fulfilling life and, in this way, help reduce the urge to have sexual contact with children.

When you are setting your goals, therefore, keep the following points in mind:

1. Is the goal I'm aiming for realistic? How likely is it that I will achieve my goal? When will I be able to achieve it?

2. Will this goal make me happy? How do I feel while setting this goal for myself?

3. Is this an approach or an avoidance goal?

4. Can this goal reduce the risk of child sexual abuse taking place, or could it even increase it?

Fig. 66 IS Approach and avoidance goals

Fig. 67 WS My plan   **For the next session, do a drawing on a piece of paper with your goals for the future.**
for the future

Keep in mind the following points:

1. What will I do in future (behavior, lifestyle)?

2. Where will I go in future (places, situations)?

3. How will I feel (mood, emotions)?

4. How and what will I think?

5. What is important to me in future?

In many families, there are often problems where none of the family members really knows what the best way is for them to go about solving them together. There is a simple and very effective strategy for this that you can use as a way to orient yourself. The goal is to solve problems that have caused conflicts within the family in the past *together*.

1. Defining the Problem

The current problem must be described as precisely as possible.

The following rules for conversation should be kept in mind:

- Everyone who is taking part must have the opportunity to express what is bothering or upsetting him or her.
- Only "I -messages" shall be used.
- Nobody will be insulted or blamed.
- The other members will each report back on whether they understood.

2. Developing Ideas for Solutions

Each family member says all the ideas that he or she has come up with as a solution to the problem; all suggestions will be compiled transparently for everyone.

There are three rules:

- Everything gets written down.
- Ideas do not get evaluated yet.
- Everything is allowed.

3. Evaluating approaches and Deciding on a Solution

Every idea is now examined according to the following rules:

- Each family member says what would happen if the family goes along with this approach.
- Each family member evaluates the approach with plus or minus.

At the end, all of the approaches are picked out that have been evaluated positively from each of the family members. Then the best approach is decided upon together, or different positive solutions are combined.

If there is no consensus or positive solution, a compromise must be worked out together.

4. Planning the Approach and Putting it into Action

At the end, everybody decides together who needs to do what, how, and when. You should also decide who should supervise the implementation of the solution and how you will be able to recognize if it is successful as a family. Set firm consequences together in advance that will be put into effect if the solution is implemented, as well as if it is not implemented.

Fig. 68 IS Shared problem solving

Supporting your child in his or her goal of dealing with his or her sexual particularities responsibly and not committing any acts of child sexual abuse is hugely important. This can be achieved, for example, by means of the following measures:

1. Be available to talk with your child at all times!

2. Create an atmosphere of trust for your child so that he or she feels comfortable confiding in you.

3. Set firm rules that your child must follow. Make sure that you only put rules in place that you are capable of enforcing yourself. Together with your child, decide on consequences in advance that will be put into effect if your child does not follow the rules.

4. Together with your child, consider which situations you think are associated with an increased risk for sexual abuse. Enter into a clear agreement with your child not to seek out these kinds of situations.

5. Should situations that you recognize to be risky be unavoidable, make sure that your child has sufficient adult supervision.

6. If you are having an uneasy feeling, talk to your child about it directly! Do not avoid the confrontation, but rather listen to your gut!

7. Support your child in establishing connections with people his own age, like by joining a club for youth in his age bracket, for example.

Fig. 69 IS Relapse prevention tips for parents

The following measures can be put into effect by us—as parents/as a family—in order to support our child in the goal of not sexually abusing children:

1. ....

....

2. ....

....

3. ....

....

4. ....

....

5. ....

....

Fig. 70 IS Our prevention measures

Selective Serotonin Reuptake Inhibitors (SSRIs)

Mechanism: Medication developed for the treatment of depression and anxiety, which increases the concentration of the messenger serotonin in the brain. This results in a slower "flood" of emotional states.

Effects: Reduction of sexual desire, erectile, and orgasmic function. This does not occur in every case, however, and the effect is considerably less marked than with antiandrogens (see below).

Side Effects: Gastrointestinal problems such as nausea, dry mouth, loss of appetite, diarrhea, constipation, headaches, insomnia, disturbances in thinking.

Preliminary and Follow-up Examinations: Regular blood tests

Dosage: Best-researched: Fluotexine. Median dosage 40-60 mg/day, onset of effects after 2 to 4 weeks, maximal efficacy after 2 to 3 months.

Alternatives: Fluvoxamine (Fevarin® 200-300 mg/day) and Paroxetine (Seroxat®, Tagonis® 20-40 mg/day).

Advantages: Improvement of mood in the case of depression.

Disadvantages: Only slight reduction of sexual desire; see side effects.

Antiandrogen Medications I: Cyproterone Acetate (Brand Name: Androcur®)

Mechanism: Testosterone loses its effect in the brain (hence the reduction of sexual desire and sexual fantasies) and at other parts in the body (e.g. reduction of beard and chest hair, though not scalp hair) because the receptor sites are occupied by the medication.

Effects:

Almost always: Reduction of sexual desire and sexual fantasies, impaired erectile and orgasmic function.

Often: Greater perception of the needs for affection and attention.

Very rarely (less than 0.1%): Sexual desire and sexual fantasies remain unaffected.

Side Effects: Increased liver values, fatigue, concentration problems, depressive moods, breast growth, weight gain, disturbance of the fat metabolism, disturbance of blood sugar levels, thromboses, disturbance of semen production.

Preliminary and Follow-up Examinations: Regular blood tests.

Dosage: 300-600 mg by injection every 2 weeks or 50-100 mg daily as a tablet; The injection is always recommended because of lower strain on the liver.

Advantages: Reliable reduction of sexual desire and sexual fantasies, tried and tested medication, generally good tolerability.

Disadvantages: See side effects.

Fig. 71 IS Pharmacological treatment options

Antiandrogen Medications II: GnRH-Analogues (Brand Names: Salvacy®, Decapeptyl®, Enantone®, Trenantone®)

Mechanism: The testicles are normally instructed by the brain via a messenger (hormone) to produce testosterone. The medication works through decreasing or stopping the production of this messenger. The testicles thus cease to receive signals to produce more testosterone.

Effects:

Almost always: Reduction of sexual desire and sexual fantasies, impaired erectile and orgasmic function.

Often: Greater perception of the needs for affection and attention.

Very infrequently (less than 0.1%): Sexual desire and sexual fantasies remain unaffected.

Side Effects: Increased perspiration, hot flashes, bone pain, weight gain, increased mammary tissue, disturbance of fat metabolism, disturbance of blood sugar levels, fatigue, joint or back pain, muscle weakness, disturbance of sperm production.

Distinctive Feature: At the beginning of treatment too much testosterone is produced. Cyproterone acetate (see above) must thus be taken supplementarily for 6 weeks.

Preliminary and Follow-up Examinations: Bone density tests at the beginning of therapy, regular blood tests.

Dosage: Ca. 3-10 mg via injection every 3 months.

Advantages: Reliable reduction of sexual desire and sexual fantasies, generally stronger than with cyproterone acetate. Generally good tolerability.

Disadvantages: See side effects.

Opioid Antagonists (Brand Names: Adepend®, Nemexin®)

Mechanism: Medication developed for the treatment of alcohol addiction. The body's own reward compounds (opioids) lost their effect in the brain (via a lower sensation of reward after sexual behavior, e.g. masturbation) because receptor sites are occupied by the medication. Also displays effects in the case of "sex addiction" (hypersexuality).

Effects: Reduction of sexual desire and sexual fantasies, impaired erectile and orgasmic function, delayed seminal discharge.

Side effects: Headache, insomnia, listlessness, nausea, irritability, loss of appetite, sensation of thirst, change in blood pressure, joint and muscle pain, fatigue.

Preliminary and Follow-up Examinations: Exclusion of opioid addiction or use (e.g. heroin), regular blood tests.

Dosage: 100-200 mg daily as a tablet; the injection is always recommended because of lower strain on the liver.

Advantages: Reduction of sexual desire and sexual fantasies.

Disadvantages: See side effects.

Fig. 71 (continued)

Bibliography

Abel G, Becker J, Cunningham-Rathner J. Complications, consent, and cognitions in sex between children and adults. Int J Law Psychiatry. 1984;7:89–103.

Abel GG, Becker JV, Mittelman M, Cunningham-Rathner J, Rouleau JL, Murphy WD. Self-reported sex crimes of nonincarceratedparaphiliacs. J Interpers Violence. 1987;2(1):3–25.

Abel GG, Osborn CA, Twigg DA. Sexual assault throughout the life span: adult offenders with juvenile histories. In: Barbaree H, Marshall W, Hudson S, editors. The juvenile sex offender. New York: Guilford Press; 1993. p. 104–17.

Ahlers CJ, Schaefer GA, Beier KM. Das Spektrum der Sexualstörungen und ihre Klassifizierbarkeit in DSM-IV und ICD-10. Sexuologie. 2006;12(3/4):120–52.

Ahlers CJ, Schaefer GA, Mundt IA, Roll S, Englert H, Willich S, Beier KM. How unusual are the contents of paraphilias – prevalence of Paraphilia-Associated Sexual Arousal Patterns (PASAPs) in a community-based sample of men. J Sex Med. 2011;8(5):1362–70. https://doi.org/10.1111/j.17436109.2009.01597.x.

Alanko K, Salo B, Mokros A, Santtila P. Evidence for heritability of adult men's sexual interest in youth under age 16 from a population-based extended twin design. J Sex Med. 2013;10(4):1090–9. https://doi.org/10.1111/jsm.12067.

Alby B, Schmidt-Bucher KJ. Modelllernen. In: Borg-Laufs M, editor. Lehrbuch der Verhaltenstherapie mit Kindern und Jugendlichen. Band II: Diagnostik und Intervention. 2nd ed. Tübingen: dgvt; 2007. p. 453–86.

Allam J, Middleton D, Browne K. Different clients, different needs? The practice issues in community-based treatment for sex offender. Crim Behav Ment Health. 1997;7(1):69–84.

Amelung T, Kuhle LF, Konrad A, Pauls A, Beier KM. Androgen deprivation therapy of self-identifying, help-seeking pedophiles in the Dunkelfeld. Int J Law Psychiatry. 2012;35(3):176–84.

American Psychiatric Association. Diagnostic and statistical manual of mental disorders, 5th edition: DSM-5. Washington, DC: American Psychiatric Association; 2013.

Andrews DA, Bonta J. The psychology of criminal conduct. 4th ed. Cincinnati: Anderson; 2006.

Anna Konrad, Till Amelung & Klaus M. Beier. Misuse of Child SexualAbuse Images: Treatment Course of a Self-Identified Pedophilic Pastor, J Sex Marital Ther. 2018;44:3:281–294, https://doi.org/10.1080/00926 23X.2017.1366958.

Archer R, Forbes Y, Metcalfe C, Winter D. An investigation of the effectiveness of a voluntary sector psychodynamic counselling service. Br J Med Psychol. 2000;73(3):401–12. https://doi.org/10.1348/000711200160499.

Arkowitz S, Vess J. An evaluation of the Bumby RAPE and MOLEST scales as measures of cognitive distortions with civilly committed sexual of-fenders. Sex Abuse J Res Treat. 2003;15:237–49.

Armbrust M, Ehrig C. Skillstraining für Patienten mit Borderline-Störung. PPmP – Psychotherapie·Psychosomatik·Medizinische Psychologie. 2016;66(07):283–98.

Awad GA, Saunders EB. Adolescent child molesters: clinical observations. Child Psychiatry Hum Dev. 1989;19(3):195–206.

Babchishin KM, Hanson RK, Hermann CA. The characteristics of online sex offenders: A meta-analysis. Sex Abuse J Res Treat. 2011;23:92–123.

Baekeland F, Lundwall L. Dropping ou of treatment: a critical review. Psychol Bull. 1975;82:738–83. https://doi.org/10.1037/h0077132.

Banse R. Untersuchung zu Ursachen pädophilen sexuellen Interesses. Zwischenbericht Januar 2012. 2012.

Banse R, Schmidt AF, Clarbour J. Indirect measures of sexual interest in child sex offenders: A multi-method approach. Crim Justice Behav. 2010;37(3):319–35.

Banse R. Sexueller Missbrauch von Kindern. Was sind die Ursachen? Vortrag im Symposium: 5. Internationales Symposium für Forensische; 2013.

Bartling G, Echelmeyer L, Engberding M. Problemanalyse im psychotherapeutischen Prozess: Leitfaden für die Praxis. Stuttgart: Kohlhammer; 2008.

Basson R, Althof S, Davis S, Fugl-Meyer K, Goldstein I, Leiblum S, et al. Summary of the recommenda-

© The Author(s), under exclusive license to Springer Nature Switzerland AG 2021
K. M. Beier (ed.), *Pedophilia, Hebephilia and Sexual Offending against Children*,
https://doi.org/10.1007/978-3-030-61262-7

tions on sexual dysfunctions in women. J Sex Med. 2004;1(1):24–34.

Baumrind D. The influence of parenting style on adolescent competence and substance use. J Early Adolesc. 1991;11(1):56–95.

Beck JS. Cognitive therapy: basics and beyond. New York: Guilford; 1995.

Becker JV. Treating adolescent sexual offenders. Prof Psychol Res Pract. 1990;21(5):362.

Beckstead AL. Can we change sexual orientation? Arch Sex Behav. 2012;41:121–34. https://doi.org/10.1007/s10508-012-9922-x.

Beech A, Fordham AS. Therapeutic climate of sexual offender treatment programs. Sex Abuse. 1997;9(3):219–37.

Beier KM. Dissexualität im Lebenslängsschnitt. Theoretische und empirische Untersuchungen zu Phänomenologie und Prognose begutachteter Sexualstraftäter. Heidelberg: Springer; 1995.

Beier KM. Differential typology and prognosis for dissexual behavior – a follow-up study of previously expert-appraised child molesters. Int J Leg Med. 1998;111(3):133–41.

Beier KM. Sexuelle Präferenzstörungen und Bindungsprobleme. Sexuologie. 2010;17(1):24.

Beier KM, Amelung T, Kuhle L, Grundmann D, Scherner G, Neutze J. Hebephilie als sexuelle Störung. Fortschritte der Neurologie Psychiatrie. 2013;81(03):128–37.

Beier KM, Amelung T, Grundmann D, Kuhle LF. Pädophilie und Hebephilie im Kontext sexuellen Kindesmissbrauchs. Sexuologie. 2015a;22(3-4): 127–36.

Beier KM, Amelung T, Kuhle LF, Grundmann D, Scherner G, Neutze J. Hebephilia as a sexual disorder. Fortschritte der Neurologie. 2015b;83(2): e1–9.

Beier KM, Amelung T, Pauls A. Antiandrogene Therapie als Teil der Prävention von sexuellem Kindesmissbrauch im Dunkelfeld. Forensische Psychiatrie, Psychologie, Kriminologie. 2010;1:49–57.

Beier KM, Bosinski HAG, Loewit K. Sexualmedizin: Grundlagen und Praxis. 2th ed. München: Elsevier, Urban und Fischer; 2005.

Beier KM, Grundmann D, Kuhle LF, Scherner G, Konrad A, Amelung T. The German Dunkelfeld project: a pilot study to prevent child sexual abuse and the use of child abusive images. J Sex Med. 2015;12(2):529–42.

Beier KM, Loewit K. Syndyastic sexual therapy – concept and foundations. Sexuologie. 2011;18(1-2): 85–94.

Beier KM, Loewit K. Sexual medicine in clinical practice. New York: Springer; 2013.

Beier KM, Neutze J, Mundt IA, Ahlers CJ, Goecker D, Konrad A, Schaefer GA. Encouraging self-identified pedophiles and hebephiles to seek professional help: First results of the Berlin Prevention Project Dunkelfeld (PPD). Child Abuse Negl. 2009;33:545–9.

Beier KM, Oezdemir UC, Hellenschmidt T. Pharmakotherapie bei sexu-ellen Präferenz- und Verhaltensstörungen. In: Bilke-Hentsch O, Sevecke K, editors. Aggressivität – Impulsivität – Delinquenz. Von gesunden Aggressionen bis zur forensischen Psychiatrie bei Kindern und Jugendlichen. Stuttgart: Georg Thieme Verlag; 2016a.

Beier KM, Oezdemir UC, Schlinzig E, Groll A, Hupp E, Hellenschmidt T. "Du träumst von ihnen" – Das Projekt Primäre Prävention von sexuellem Kindesmissbrauch durch Jugendliche (PPJ). Sexuologie. 2015c;22: 2–18.

Beier KM, Oezdemir UC, Schlinzig E, Groll A, Hupp E, Hellenschmidt T. "Just dreaming of them": The Berlin Project for Primary Prevention of Child Sexual Abuse by Juveniles (PPJ). Child Abuse Negl. 2016b; 52:1–10.

Beier KM, Schaefer GA, Goecker D, Neutze J, Ahlers ChJ. Prevention Project Dunkelfeld – Treating pedophiles in the community to improve child protection in Germany; Presentation at the IASR-Meeting 2007, Vancouver, Canada, abstracts on http://www.iasr.org. 2007.

Beier KM, Scherner G, Gieseler H, Siegel S, Wagner J, Kossow S, Amelung T, Grundmann D, Kuhle LF. Primärpräventive Therapieangebote bei Pädophilie und Hebephilie – Teil der Prävention sexuellen Kindesmissbrauchs im Dunkelfeld. Interdisziplinäre Fachzeitschrift. 2015d;18(2):140–59.

Beier KM. Sexualität und Geschlechtsidentität – Entwicklung und Störungen. In: Fegert JM, Eggers JM, Resch F, editors. Psychiatrie und Psychotherapie des Kindes- und Jugendalters. Heidelberg: Springer; 2012. p. 735–85.

Bem B, Daryl J. Exotic becomes erotic: a developmental theory of sexual orientation. Psychol Rev. 1996;103(2):320–35.

Bennett R, Marshall E. Group work with parents of adolescent sex offenders: intervention guidelines. Adv Soc Work. 2005;6(2):276–89.

Bensley LS, Van Eenwyk J, Simmons KW. Self-reported childhood sexual and physical abuse and adult HIV-risk behaviors and heavy drinking. Am J Prev Med. 2000;18(2):151–8.

Berner W, Briken P, Hill A, editors. Sexualstraftäter behandeln mit Psychotherapie und Medikamenten. Köln: Deutscher Ärzte-Verlag; 2007.

Berliner Institut für Sexualwissenschaft und Sexualmedizin. BEDIT – The Berlin Dissexuality Therapy Program. Weimar: Gutenberg. 2013.

Berthelot N, Godbout N, Hébert M, Goulet M, Bergeron S. Prevalence and correlates of childhood sexual abuse in adults consulting for sexual problems. J Sex Marital Ther. 2014;40(5):434–43. https://doi.org/10.1080/0092623X.2013.772548.

Bessler C. Jugendliche SexualstraftÄter – Persönlichkeitsmerkmale, Beurteilungsverfahren und Behand- lungsansÄtze. In: Steinhausen H-C, Bessler C, editors. Jugenddelinquenz. Stuttgart: Kohlhammer; 2008. p. 176–99.

Bieneck S, Stadler L, Pfeiffer C, Niedersachsen KF. Erster Forschungsbericht zur Repräsentativerhebung Sexueller Missbrauch 2011. Hannover: Kriminologisches Forschungsinstitut Niedersachsen (KFN); 2011.

Blake E, Gannon T. Social perception deficits, cognitive distortions, and empathy deficits in sex offenders. Trauma Violence Abuse. 2008;9(1):34–55. https://doi.org/10.1177/1524838007311104.

Blanchard R, Klassen P, Dickey R, Kuban ME, Blak T. Sensitivity and specificity of the phallometric test for pedophilia in nonadmitting sex offenders. Psychol Assess. 2001;13(1):118–26. https://doi.org/10.1037//1040-3590.13.1.118.

Blanchard R, Kuban ME, Blak T, Cantor JM, Klassen P, Dickey R. Phallometric comparison of pedophilic interest in nonadmitting sexual offenders against stepdaughters, biological daughters, other biologically related girls, and unrelated girls. Sex Abuse J Res Treat. 2006;18:1–14.

Blanchard R, Cantor JM, Robichaud LK. Biological factors in the development of sexual deviance and aggression in males. In: Barbaree HE, Marshall WL, editors. The juvenile sex offender. 2nd ed. New York: Guilford Press; 2008. p. 77–105.

Blanchard R, Lykins AD, Wherett D, Kuban ME, Cantor JM, Blak T, Klassen PE. Pedophilia, hebephilia, and the DSM-V. Arch Sex Behav. 2009;38(3):335–50. https://doi.org/10.1007/s10508-008-9399-9.

Blasingame GD. Practical strategies for working with youth with intellectual disabilities who have sexual behavior problems. In: Bromberg DS, O'Donohue WT, editors. Toolkit for working with juvenile sex offenders (practical resources for the mental health professional). Waltham: Academic Press; 2014. p. 479–506.

Bode H, Heßling A. Jugendsexualität 2015. Die Perspektive der 14- bis 25-Jährigen. Ergebnisse einer aktuellen Repräsentativen Wiederholungsbefragung. Köln: Bundeszentrale für gesundheitliche Aufklärung; 2015.

Boonmann C, van Vugt ES, Jansen LM, Colins OF, Doreleijers TA, Stams GJJ, Vermeiren RR. Mental disorders in juveniles who sexuallyoffended: a meta-analysis. Aggress Violent Behav. 2015;24:241–9.

Bordin ES. The generalizability of the psychoanalytic concept of the working alliance. Psychother Theory Res Pract. 1979;16(3):252–60.

Borduin CM, Schaeffer CM. Multisystemic treatment of juvenile sexual offenders: a progress report. J Psychol Hum Sex. 2002;13(3–4):25–42.

Borg-Laufs M, Hungerige H. Selbstmanagementtherapie mit Kindern. Ein Praxishandbuch. In: Stuttgart: Klett-Cota; 2005.

Borg-Laufs M. Erstkontakt und Beziehungsgestaltung mit Kindern und Jugendlichen. In: Schneider S, Margraf J, editors. Lehrbuch der Verhaltenstherapie, Band 3: Störungen im Kindes- und Jugendalter. Heidelberg: Springer; 2009. p. 183–92.

Bosley JT, Hiscox S. Documenting treatment for sexually abusive youth. In: Bromberg DS, O'Donohue WT, editors. Toolkit for working with juvenile sex offenders (practical resources for the mental Health professional). Waltham: Academic Press; 2014. p. 449–78.

Bradford JMW, Pawlak A. Double-blind placebo crossover study of cyproterone acetate in the treatment of the paraphilias. Arch Sex Behav. 1993;22:383–402.

Bradford JMW, Greenberg DM. Pharmacological treatment of deviant sexual behavior. Annu Rev Sex Res. 1996;7:283–306.

BRAVO. Dr. Sommer-Studie 2016: Die erste Diät mit Elf. Die ersten Selfies im Netz mit Zwölf. Der erste Sex mit 17. 2016. http://www.bauermedia.com/presse/archiv/artikel/dr-sommer-studie-2016-die-erste-diaet-mit-elf-die-ersten-selfies-im-netz-mit-zwoelf-der-erste-sex-mit-17-bravoveroeffentlicht-studie-zu-aufklaerung-liebe-koerper-und-sexualitaet/controller/2016/1/25/.

Brezo J, Paris J, Vitaro F, Hébert M, Tremblay R, Turecki G. Predicting suicide attempts in young adults with histories of childhood abuse. Br J Psychiatry J Ment Sci. 2008;193(2):134–9.

Briken P, von Franqué F, Berner W. Paraphilie und hypersexuelle Störungen. In: Briken P, Berner W, editors. Praxisbuch sexuelle Störungen. Stuttgart: Thieme; 2013. p. 239–48.

Bundeskriminalamt. Polizeiliche Kriminalstatistik Bundesrepublik Deutschland. Berichtsjahr 2016. Wiesbaden. 2017. https://www.bka.de/DE/AktuelleInformationen/StatistikenLagebilder/PolizeilicheKriminalstatistik/PKS2016/pks2016_node.html.

Bumby KM. Assessing the cognitive distortions of child molesters and rapists: development and validation of the MOLEST and RAPE scales. Sex Abuse J Res Treat. 1996;8:37–54.

Bumby KM, Hansen DJ. Intimacy deficits, fear of intimacy, and loneliness among sexual offenders. Crim Justice Behav. 1997;24:315–31.

Bundeskinderschutzgesetz. In der Fassung der Bekanntmachung vom 22. Dezember 2011 (BGBl. 2011 I, S. 2975-2982). 2011. Online unter: http://www.bag-kjs.de/media/raw/BGBl_BKischG_28_12_2011.pdf.

Bundeskriminalamt. Polizeiliche Kriminalstatistik. Bundesrepublik Deutschland, Jahrbuch 2014. 2015. Online unter: https://www.bka.de/SharedDocs/Downloads/DE/Publikationen/PolizeilicheKriminalstatistik/2014/pks2014Jahrbuch.pdf?__blob=publicationFile&v=1.

Bundesministerium der Justiz und für Verbraucherschutz. Strafgesetzbuch. Dreizehnter Abschnitt. Straftaten gegen die sexuelle Selbstbestimmung. 2016. Online unter: https://www.gesetze-im-internet.de/stgb/BJNR001270871.html#BJNR001270871BJNG005002307.

Bundeskriminalamt. Polizeiliche Kriminalstatistik Bundesrepublik Deutschland. Berichtsjahr 2016. Wiesbaden. 2017. https://www.bka.de/DE/AktuelleInformationen/StatistikenLagebilder/PolizeilicheKriminalstatistik/PKS2016/pks2016_node.html.

Bundschuh C. Pädosexualität: Entstehungsbedingungen Und Erscheinungsformen. 1st ed. Opladen: Leske + Budrich Verlag; 2001.

Carson DK, Foster MJ, Tripathi N. Child sexual abuse in India: current issues and research. Psychol Stud. 2013;58(3):318–25. https://doi.org/10.1007/s12646-013-0198-6.

Cantor JM, Kabani N, Christensen BK, Zipursky RB, Barbaree HE, Dickey R, et al. Cerebral white matter deficiencies in pedophilic men. J Psychiatr Res. 2008;42(3):167–83. https://doi.org/10.1016/j.jpsychires.2007.10.013.

Cantor JM, Lafaille S, Soh DW, Moayedi M, Mikulis DJ, Girard TA. Diffusion tensor imaging of pedophilia. Arch Sex Behav. 2015;44(8):2161–72. https://doi.org/10.1007/s10508-015-0629-7.

Chen LP, Murad MH, Paras ML, Colbenson KM, Sattler AL, Goranson EN, Elamin MB, Seime RJ, Shinozaki G, Prokop LJ, Zirakzadeh A. Sexual abuse and lifetime diagnosis of psychiatric disorders: systematic review and meta-analysis. Mayo Clin Proc. 2010;85(7):618–29.

Cohen LJ, Galynker I. Clinical features of pedophilia and implications for treatment. J Psychiatr Pract. 2002;8(5):276–89.

Cortoni F, Marshall WL. Sex as a coping strategy and its relationship to ju-venile sexual history and intimacy in sexual offenders. Sex Abuse J Res Treat. 2001;13:27–43.

Cougle JR, Timpano KR, Sachs-Ericsson N, Keogh ME, Riccardi CJ. Examining the unique relationships between anxiety disorders and childhood physical and sexual abuse in the national comorbidity survey-replication. Psychiatry Res. 2010;177(1–2):150–5.

Davis RA. A cognitive-behavioral model of pathological Internet use. Comput Hum Behav. 2001;17:187–95.

Dember WN. William James on sensation and perception. Psychol Sci. 1990;1(3):163–6.

Dennison SM, Stough C, Birgden A. The Big 5 dimension personality approach to understanding sex offenders. Psychol Crime Law. 2001;7:243–61.

Dolan RJ. Emotion, cognition, and behavior. Science. 2002;298(5596):1191–4.

Dombert B, Schmidt AF, Banse R, Briken P, Hoyer J, Neutze J, Osterheider M. How common is men's self-reported sexual interest in prepubescent children? J Sex Res. 2015;53:214–23. https://doi.org/10.1080/00224499.2015.1020108.

Duff S, Willis A. At the precipice: Assessing a non-offending client's potential to sexually offend. J Sex Aggress. 2006;12(1):45–51.

Dunsieth NW, Nelson EB, Brusman-Lovins LA, Holcomb JL, Beckman D, Welge JA, et al. Psychiatric and legal features of 113 men convicted of sexual offenses. J Clin Psychiatry. 2004;65(3):293–300.

Dyshniku F, Murray ME, Fazio RL, Lykins AD, Cantor JM, editors. Minor physical anomalies as a window into the prenatal origins of Pedophilia. Arch Sex Behav. 2015;44(8):2151–9. https://doi.org/10.1007/s10508-015-0564-7.

Egle UT, Hoffmann SO, Steffens M. Psychosoziale risiko-und schutzfaktoren in kindheit und jugend als prädisposition für psychische störungen im erwachsenenalter gegenwärtiger stand der forschung. Nervenarzt. 1997;68(9):683–95.

Eke AW, Seto MC, Williams J. Examining the criminal history and future offending of child pornography offenders: An extended prospective follow-up study. Law Hum Behav. 2011;35(6):466–78. https://doi.org/10.1007/s10979-010-9252-2.

Ekman P. Emotion in the human face. Cambridge, UK: Cambridge University Press; 1982.

Elliott IA, Beech AR, Mandeville-Norden R, Hayes E. Psychological pro-files of Internet sexual offenders: comparisons with contact sexual offenders. Sex Abuse J Res Treat. 2009;21:76–92.

Elliott M, Browne K, Kilcoyne J. Child sexual abuse prevention: What offenders tell us. Child Abuse Negl. 1995;19(5):579–94.

Ellis A. Die rational-emotive Therapie. Das innere Selbstgespräch bei seelischen Problemen und seine Veränderung. München: Pfeiffer; 1977.

Ellis A, Hoellen B. Die Rational-Emotive Verhaltenstherapie – Reflexionen und Neubestimmungen. München: Pfeiffer; 1997.

Engelhardt L, Willers B, Pelz L. Sexual maturation in East German girls. Acta Paediatr. 1995;84:1362–5.

Fagan EJ, Wise TN, Schmidt CW, Ponticas Y, Marshall RD, Costa PT Jr. A comparison of five-factor personality dimensions in males with sexual dys-functions and males with paraphilia. J Pers Assess. 1991;5:434–48.

Faistbauer S. Dissexualitätsbehandlung im einzeltherapeutischen Setting zur Prävention sexueller Übergriffe auf Kinder. (Dissertationsschrift). 2011. Online unter: http://www.diss.fu-berlin.de/diss/receive/FUDISS_thesis_000000020741.

Feelgood S, Cortoni F, Thompson A. Sexual coping, general coping and cog-nitive distortions in incarcerated rapists and child molesters. J Sex Aggress. 2005;11:157–70.

Feelgood S, Hoyer J. Child molester or pedophile? sociolegal versus psychopathological classification of sexual offenders against children. J Sex Aggress. 2008;14(1):33–43. https://doi.org/10.1080/13552600802133860.

Fernandez YM, Marshall WL, Lightbody S, O'Sulli-van C. The child molester empathy measure: description and examination of its reliability and validity. Sex Abuse. 1999;11(1):17–31.

Fernandez Y, Harris AJ, Hanson RK, Sparks J. Stable-2007 coding manual revised 2012. Unpublished manuscript. Public Safety Canada; 2012.

Fiedler P. Verhaltenstherapie in und mit Gruppen. Psychologische Psychotherapie in der Praxis. Weinheim: Beltz; 1996.

Finkelhor D, Lewis IA. An epidemiologic approach to the study of child molestation. Ann N Y Acad Sci. 1988;528(1):64–78.

Finkelhor D, Kendall-Tackett K. A developmental perspective on the childhood impact of crime, abuse, and violent victimization. In: Cicchetti D, Toth SL, editors. Developmental perspectives on trauma: theory, research, and intervention. Rochester symposium on developmental psychology, vol. 8. Rochester: University of Rochester Press; 1997. p. 1–32.

Finkelhor D. What's wrong with sex between adults and children: ethics and the problem of sexual abuse. Am J Orthopsychiatry. 1979;49:692–7.

Finkelhor D. Child sexual abuse: new theory and research. New York: Free Press; 1984.

Finkelhor D. Current information on the scope and nature of child sexual abuse. Future Child. 1994;4(2): 31–53.

Finkelhor D. The prevention of childhood sexual abuse. Future Child. 2009;19(2):169–94.

Fliegel S. Rollenspiele. In: Margraf J, editor. Lehrbuch der Verhaltenstherapie, vol. Bd. 1. Berlin, Heidelberg, New York: Springer; 1996. p. 353–9.

Franke GH. BSI: Brief symptom inventory von LR Derogati; (Kurzform der SCL-90-R). Göttingen: Beltz Test; 2000.

Freud S. Über Psychoanalyse. In: Fünf Vorlesungen gehalten zur 20-jährigen Gründungsfeier der Clark University in Worcester, Massachusetts, September 1909. Leipzig und Wien: Franz Deuticke; 1910.

Freund K, McKnight CK, Langevin R, Cibiri S. The female child as a surrogate object. Arch Sex Behav. 1972;2(2):119–33.

Fuhrer U. Jugendalter: Entwicklungsrisiken und Entwicklungsabweichungen. In: Petermann F, editor. Lehrbuch der klinischen Kinderpsychologie. Göttingen: Hogrefe; 2013. p. 119–36.

Gaffney G, Berlin F. Is there hypothalamic-pituitarygonadal dysfunction in paedophilia? A pilot study. Br J Psychiatry. 1984;45:657–60.

Gerwinn H, Pohl A, Granert O, van Eimeren T, Wolff S, Jansen O, et al. The (in)consistency of changes in brain macrostructure in male paedophiles: A combined T1-weighted and diffusion tensor imaging study. J Psychiatr Res. 2015;68:246–53. https://doi.org/10.1016/j.jpsychires.2015.07.002.

Görgen T, Rauchert K, Fisch S. Langfristige Folgen sexuellen Missbrauchs Minderjähriger. Forensische Psychiatrie, Psychologie, Kriminologie. 2012;6(1):3–16.

Görlitz G. Psychotherapie für Kinder und Familien. Übungen und Materialien für die Arbeit mit Eltern und Bezugspersonen. 3th ed. Stuttgart: Klett –Cotta; 2010a.

Görlitz G. Psychotherapie für Kinder und Familien. Übungen und Materialien für die Arbeit mit Eltern und Bezugspersonen. 3th ed. Stuttgart: Klett –Cotta; 2010b.

Grawe K. Verhaltenstherapie in Gruppen. München: Urban & Schwarzberg; 1980.

Grawe K. Psychologische Therapie. 2nd ed. Goettingen: Hogrefe; 2000.

Gray AS, Pithers WD. Relapse prevention with sexually aggressive adolescents and children: expanding treatment and supervision. In: Barbaree HE, Marshall WL, Hudson SM, editors. The juvenile sex offender. New York: Guilford Press; 1993. p. 289–319.

Greenberg DM, Bradford JM. Treatment of the paraphilic disorders: a review of the role of the selective serotonin reuptake inhibitors. Sex Abuse. 1997;9(4): 349–60.

Grubin D. Medical models and interventions in sexual deviance. In: Laws DR, O'Donohue WT, editors. Sexual deviancy: theory, assessment and treatment. New York: The Guildford Press; 2008. p. 595–610.

Grundmann D, Krupp J, Scherner G, Amelung T, Beier KM. Stability of self-reported arousal to sexual fantasies involving children in a clinical sample of pedophiles and hebephiles. Arch Sex Behav. 2016;45(5):1153–62. https://doi.org/10.1007/s10508-016-0729-z.

Guay DR. Drug treatment of paraphilic and nonparaphilic sexual disorders. Clin Ther. 2009;31(1):1–31.

Habetha S, Bleich S, Sievers C, Marschall U, Weidenhammer J, Fegert JM. Deutsche Traumafolgekostenstudie. Kiel: Schmidt & Klaunig; 2012.

Hartmann K. Theoretische und empirische Beiträge zur Verwahrlosungsforschung. Berlin: Springer; 1970.

't Hart-Kerkhoffs LA, Boonmann C, Doreleijers TA, Jansen LM, van Wijk AP, Vermeiren RR. Mental disorders and criminal re-referrals in juveniles who sexually offended. Child Adolesc Psychiatry Ment Health. 2015;9(1):4.

Häuser W, Schmutzer G, Brähler E, Glaesmer H. Maltreament in childhood and adolescence – results from a survey of a representative sample of the German population. Dtsch Arztebl Int. 2011;108(17):287–94. https://doi.org/10.3238/arztebl.2011.0287.

Hall GCN, Hirschmann R. Sexual aggression against children: a conceptual perspective of etiology. Crim Justice Behav. 1992;19:8–23.

Hames R, Blanchard R. Anthropological data regarding the adaptiveness of hebephilia. Arch Sex Behav. 2012;41:745–7. https://doi.org/10.1007/s10508-012-9972-0.

Halse A, Grant J, Thornton J, Indermaur D, Stevens G, Chamarette C. Intrafamilial adolescent sex offenders' response to psychological treatment. Psychiatr Psychol Law. 2012;19(2):221–35.

Hanson RK, Bussiere MT. Predicting relapse: a meta-analysis of sexual offender recidivism studies. J Consult Clin Psychol. 1998;66(2):348–62.

Hanson RK, Harris AJR. Where should we intervene? dynamic predictors of sexual assault recidivism. Crim Justice Behav. 2000;27:6–35.

Hanson RK, Gordon A, Harris A, Marques J, Murphy W, Quinsey V, Seto M. First report of the collaborative outcome data project on the effectiveness of psychological treatment for sex offenders. Sex Abuse J Res Treat. 2002;14:169–94.

Hanson RK, Harris AJR, Scott T-L, Helmus L. Assessing the risk of sexual offenders on community supervision: the dynamic supervision project (User Report 2007-05). Ottawa: Public Safety Canada; 2007.

Hanson RK, Morton-Bourgon KE. Predictors of sexual recidivism: An updated meta-analysis (Research Report No. 2004-02). Ottawa: Public Safety and Emergency Preparedness Canada; 2004.

Hanson RK, Morton-Bourgon EM. The characteristics of persistent sexual offenders: a meta-analysis of recidivism studies. J Consult Clin Psychol. 2005;73:1154–63.

Harris A, Phenix A, Hanson RK, Thornton D. Static 99: coding rules revised 2003. Ottawa, Ontario: Solicitor General Canada; 2003.

Haselton MG, Nettle D, Andrews PW. The evolution of cognitive bias. In: Buss DM, Murray DR, editors. The handbook of evolutionary psychology. Hoboken: John Wiley & Sons Inc.; 2005. p. 724–46.

Hautzinger M, editor. Kognitive Verhaltenstherapie bei psychischen Störungen. 3rd ed. Weinheim: Psychologie Verlags Union; 2000.

Hautzinger M, Eimecke S, Mattejat F. Lern- und ognitionspsychologische Grundlagen. In: Mattejat F, editor. Das große Lehrbuch der Psychotherapie, vol. 4: Verhaltenstherapie mit Kindern, Jugendlichen und ihren Familien. München: CIP-Medien; 2006. p. 35–52.

Hayashino DS, Wurtele SK, Klebe KJ. Child molesters: an examination of cognitive factors. J Interpers Violence. 1995;10:106–16.

Hayes SC, Luoma JB, Bond FW, Masuda A, Lillis J. Acceptance and commitment therapy: model, processes and outcomes. Behav Res Ther. 2006; 44:1–25.

Hayes SC, Strosahl K, Wilson KG. Acceptance and commitment therapy: understanding and treating human suffering. New York: Guilford Press; 1999.

Heim C, Mayberg HS, Mletzko T, Nemeroff CB, Pruessner JC. Decreased cortical representation of genital somatosensory field after childhood sexual abuse. Am J Psychiatry. 2013;170:616–23.

Heiman M. Helping parents address their child's sexual behavior problems. J Child Sex Abus. 2002a;10(3):35–57.

Heiman M. Helping parents address their child's sexual behavior problems. J Child Sex Abus. 2002b;10(3):35–57.

Herdt G. Rituals of manhood: male initiation in Papua New Guinea. Berkeley: University of California Press; 1982.

Henry F, McMahon P. What survivors of child sexual abuse told us about the people who abused them. Paper presented at the National Sexual Violence Prevention Conference. Texas: Dallas; 2000.

Hill A, Briken P, Kraus C, Strohm K, Berner W. Differential pharmacological treatment of paraphilias and sex offenders. Int J Offender Ther Comp Criminol. 2003;47(4):407–21.

Hofmann SG. An introduction to modern CBT: psychological solutions to mental health problems. West Sussex: Wiley-Blackwell; 2012.

Holmes M. Damit aus Fantasien keine Taten werden! PiD-Psychotherapie im Dialog. 2006;7(03):338–9.

Holt-Lunstad J, Smith TB, Layton JB. Social relationships and mortality risk: a meta-analytic review. PLoS Med. 2010;7(7):e1000316.

Hunter JA, Figueredo AJ, Malamuth NM, Becker JV. Juvenile sex offenders: toward the development of a typology. Sex Abuse. 2003;15(1):27–48.

Iffland JA, Berner W, Dekker A, Briken P. What keeps them together? Insights into sex offender couples using qualitative content analyses. J Sex Marital Ther. 2016;42(6):534–51.

Institute for Sexology and Sexual Medicine. BEDIT – The Berlin dissexuality therapy program. Weimar: Gutenberg; 2013.

Internet Watch Foundation (IWF) Annual Report 2018. https://www.iwf.org.uk/report/2018-annual-report.

Irish L, Kobayashi I, Delahanty DL. Long-term physical health consequences of childhood sexual abuse: a meta-analytic review. J Pediatr Psychol. 2010;35:450–61.

Jahnke S, Philipp K, Hoyer J. Stigmatizing attitudes towards people with pedophilia and their malleability among psychotherapists in training. Child Abuse Negl. 2015;40:93–102. https://doi.org/10.1016/j.chiabu.2014.07.008.

Jespersen AF, Lalumière ML, Seto MC. Sexual abuse history among adult sex offenders and non-sex offenders: a meta-analysis. Child Abuse Negl. 2009;33(3):179–92. https://doi.org/10.1016/j.chiabu.2008.07.004.

Jones S. Parents of adolescents who have sexually offended: providing support and coping with the experience. J Interpers Violence. 2015;30(8):1299–321.

Joyal CC, Cossette A, Lapierre V. What exactly is an unusual sexual fantasy? J Sex Med. 2015;12:328–40. https://doi.org/10.1111/jsm.12734.

Kafka MP, Hennen J. A DSM-IV Axis I comorbidity study of males (n = 120) with paraphilias and paraphiliarelated disorders. Sex Abuse. 2002;14(4):349–66.

Kahl H, Schaffrath Rosario A. Pubertät im Wandel – wohin geht der Trend? Sexuelle Reifeentwicklung von Kindern und Jugendlichen in Deutschland. BZgA Forum. 2007;3:19–25.

Kahn TJ, Chambers HJ. Assessing reoffense risk with juvenile sexual offenders. Child Welf J Policy Pract Program. 1991;70(3):333–45.

Kanfer FH, Phillips JS. Lerntheoretische Grundlagen der Verhaltenstherapie. München: Kindler; 1975.

Kanfer FH, Reinecker H, Schmelzer D. Selbstmanagement-Therapie: Ein Lehrbuch für die klinische Praxis. Berlin: Springer; 2000.

Kast V. Trauern. Phasen und Chancen des psychischen Prozesses. Stuttgart: Kreuz; 1982.

Kear-Colwell J, Pollock P. Motivation or confrontation: which approach to the child sex offender? Crim Justice Behav. 1997;24(1):20–33.

Kelly G. The psychology of personal constructs. New York: Norton; 1955.

Kramer R. The DSM and the stigmatization of people who are attracted to minors. In Pedophilia, minor-attracted persons, and the DSM: issues and controversies. Symposium conducted at the meeting of the

B4U-ACT, Inc., Westminster, MD. 2011. http://www. b4uact.org/science/symp/2011/Proceedings.pdf.

Klüver H, Bucy P. Preliminary analysis of functions of the temporal lobes in monkeys. Arch Neurol Psychiatry. 1939;42(6):979–1000. https://doi.org/10.1001/archneurpsyc.1939.02270240017001.

Konrad A, Amelung T, Beier KM. Misuse of child sexual abuse images: treatment course of a self-identified pedophilic pastor. J Sex Marital Ther. 2018;44(3):281–94. https://doi.org/10.1080/0092623X.2017.1366958.

Konrad A, Haag S, Scherner G, Amelung T, Beier KM. Previous judicial detection and paedophilic sexual interest partially predict psychological distress in a non-forensic sample of help-seeking men feeling inclined to sexually offend against children. J Sex Aggress. 2017b;23(3):266–77.

Konrad A, Kuhle LF, Amelung T, Beier KM. Is emotional congruence with children associated with sexual offending in pedophiles and hebephiles from the community?. Sexual Abuse. 2015. 1079063215620397.

Konrad A, Kuhle LF, Amelung T, Beier KM. Is emotional congruence with children associated with sexual offending in pedophiles and hebephiles from the community? Sex Abuse. 2018;30(1):3–22.

Kreutzmann AC. Psychische Gesundheit von Jugendlichen mit einer sexuellen Präferenz für das kindliche Körperschema – Ergebnisse aus dem Dunkelfeld. Unveröffentlichte Masterarbeit. Universität Osnabrück, Deutschland; 2017.

Krohne HW, Pulsack A. Das Erziehungsstil-Inventar (ESI). Beltz test; 1995.

Kuhle L, Grundmann D, Beier KM. Missbrauchstäter und -täterinnen. Sexueller Missbrauch von Kindern: Ursachen und Verursacher. In: Fegert JM, Hoffmann U, König E, Niehues J, Liebhardt H, editors. Sexueller Missbrauch von Kindern und Jugendlichen. Berlin, Heidelberg: Springer; 2015. p. 109–29.

Kuhle LF, Konrad A, Beier KM. Variability in sexual preference and use of sexually explicit and non-explicit images of children. Toronto: Paper presented at the 30th Annual Conference of the Association for the Treatment of Sexual Abusers; 2011.

Kuhle LF, Kossow SB, Beier KM. Das Präventionsprojekt Dunkelfeld. Informationsveranstaltung zum Präventionsprojekt Dunkelfeld. Berlin; 2015.

Kuhle LF, Schlinzig E, Beier KM. Prävention der Nutzung von Missbrauchsabbildungen. Sexuologie. 2015;22(3–4):185–90.

Kuhle LF, Schlinzig E, Kaiser G, Amelung T, Konrad A, Röhle R, Beier KM. The association of sexual preference and dynamic risk factors with undetected child pornography offending. J Sex Aggress. 2017;23(1):3–18.

Kuhle LF, Schmidt RC, Beier KM. Static risk factors for child sexual offending in undetected pedohebephiles. Paper presented at the 35th Annual Conference of the Association for the Treatment of Sexual Abusers, Orlando, Florida, USA; 2016.

Kuhle LF, Neutze J, Amelung T, Grundmann D, Scherner G, Konrad A, Beier KM. Treatment change in child pornography offending in pedophiles and hebephiles in the Prevention Project Dunkelfeld. In: Paper presented at the 12th meeting of the International Association for the Treatment of Sexual Offenders. Germany: Berlin; 2012.

Kuhle LF, Kossow SB, Beier KM. Das Präventionsprojekt Dunkelfeld. Berlin: Informati-onsveranstaltung zum Präventionsprojekt Dunkelfeld; 2015a.

Kuhle LF, Schlinzig E, Beier KM. Prävention der Nutzung von Missbrauchsabbildungen. Sexuologie. 2015b;22(3-4):185–90.

Lanning KV. Child molesters: A behavioral analysis. Arlington: National Center for Missing and Exploited Children; 2001.

Laulik S, Allam J, Sheridan L. An investigation into maladaptive personality functioning in Internet sex offenders. Psychology, Crime & Law. 2007;13:523–35.

Lauth GW, Mackowiak K. Kognitive Verfahren. In: Schneider S, Markgraf J, editors. Lehrbuch der Verhaltenstherapie, Band 3 Störungen im Kindes- und Jugendalter. Heidelberg: Springer; 2009. p. 221–32.

Laws DR, Marshall WL. A conditioning theory of the etiology and maintenance of deviant sexual preference and behavior. In: Marshall WL, Laws DR, Barbaree HE, editors. Handbook of sexual assault. New York: Plenum Press; 1990. p. 209–30.

Lazarus RS, Folkman S, editors. Stress, appraisal, and coping. New York: Springer Publishing Company; 1984.

Lazarus R. Psychological stress and the coping process. New York: McGraw-Hill; 1966.

Leeb RT, Lewis T, Zolotor AJ. A review of physical and mental health consequences of child abuse and neglect and implications for practice. Am J Lifestyle Med. 2011;5:454–68. https://doi.org/10.1177/1559827611410266.

Letourneau EJ, Schoenwald SK, Sheidow AJ. Children and adolescents with sexual behavior prob-lems. Child Maltreat. 2004a;9(1):49–61.

Letourneau EJ, Schoenwald SK, Sheidow AJ. Children and adolescents with sexual behavior problems. Child Maltreat. 2004b;9(1):49–61.

Linehan MM. Trainingsmanual zur Dialektisch-Behavioralen Therapie der Borderline-Persönlichkeitsstörung. CIP-Medien. 1996.

Liu H, Umberson DJ. The times they are a changin': marital status and health differentials from 1972 to 2003. J Health Soc Behav. 2008;49(3):239–53.

Lösel F, Schmucker M. The effectiveness of treatment for sexual offenders: a comprehensive meta-analysis. J Exp Criminol. 2005;1(1):117–46.

Longo RE, Groth AN. Juvenile sexual offenses in the histories of adult rapists and child molesters. Int J Offender Ther Comp Criminol. 1983;27(2):150–5.

Maccoby E, Martin JA. Socialization in the context of the family: parent-child interaction. In: Mavis Hetherington E, editor. Handbook of child psychology: socialization, personality, and social development. 4th ed. New York: John Wiley & Sons; 1983. p. 1–102.

Machlitt K. Perspektiven der Behandlung sexuell grenzverletzender Jugendlicher – Überlegungen zu einem integrativen Behandlungskonzept. In Deutsches Jugendinstitut e. V. IKK-Nachrichten 1–2: Sexualisierte Gewalt durch Minderjährige; 2004. p. 11–16.

Mann RE, Hanson RK, Thornton D. Assessing risk for sexual recidivism: Some proposals on the nature of psychologically meaningful risk factors. Sex Abuse J Res Treat. 2010;22:191–217. https://doi.org/10.1177/1079063210366039.

Margraf J, Schneider S, editors. Lehrbuch der Verhaltenstherapie. Band 1: Grundlagen, Diagnostik, Verfahren, Rahmenbedingungen. Heidelberg: Springer; 2008.

Marlatt GA, Gordon JR. Relapse prevention. New York: Guilford; 1985.

Marsa F, O'Reilly G, Carr A. Attachment styles and psychological profiles of child sex offenders in Ireland. J Interpers Violence. 2004;19:228–51.

Marshall WA, Tanner JM. Variations in pattern of pubertal changes in girls. Arch Dis Child. 1969;44(235):291–303.

Marshall WA, Tanner JM. The variations in the pattern of pubertal changes in boys. Arch Dis Child. 1970;45(239):13–23.

Marshall WL. The relationship between self-esteem and deviant sexual arousal in nonfamilial child molesters. Behav Modif. 1997;21(1):86–96. https://doi.org/10.1177/01454455970211005.

Marshall WL, Champagne F, Brown C, Miller S. Empathy, intimacy, loneliness, and self-esteem in non-familial child molesters: a brief report. J Child Sex Abus. 1998a;6(3):87–98.

Marshall WL, Champagne F, Brown C, Miller S. Empathy, intimacy, loneliness, and self-esteem in nonfamilial child molesters: a brief report. J Child Sex Abus. 1998b;6(3):87–98.

Marshall WL, Cripps E, Anderson D, Cortoni F. Self-esteem and coping strategies in child molesters. J Interpers Violence. 1999;14(9):955–62.

Marshall WL. Are pedophiles treatable? evidence from North American studies. Seksuologia Polska (Polish Sexology). 2008;6(1):39–43.

Marshall WL, Barbaree HE. An integrated theory of the etiology of sexual offending. In: Marshall WL, Laws DR, Barbaree HE, editors. Handbook of sexual assault: Issues, theories, and treatment of the offender. New York: Plenum Press; 1990. p. 257–75.

Marshall WL, Barbaree HE, Eccles A. Early onset and deviant sexuality in child molesters. J Interpers Violence. 1991;6(3):323–35.

Marshall WL, Hamilton K, Fernandez Y. Empathy deficits and cognitive dis-tortions in child molesters. Sex Abuse J Res Treat. 2001;13:123–30.

Marshall WL, Hudson SM, Hodkinson S. The importance of attachment bonds in the development of juvenile sex offending. In: Barbaree HE, Marshall WL, Hudson SM, editors. The Juvenile Sex Offender. New York: Guilford Press; 1993. p. 164–81.

Marshall LE, Marshall WL, Moulden HM, Serran GA. The prevalence of sexual addiction in incarcerated sexual offenders and matched community nonoffend-ers. Sex Addict Compuls. 2008;15:271–83.

Marshall WL, Marshall LE, Serran GA. Strategies in the treatment of paraphilias: a critical review. Annu Rev Sex Res. 2006;17:162–82.

Marshall WL, Serran GA, Cortoni FA. Childhood attachments, sexual abuse, and their relationship to adult coping in child molesters. Sex Abuse J Res Treat. 2000;12:17–26.

Marshall WL, Serran GA, Moulden H, Mulloy R, Fernandez YM, Mann R, Thornton D. Therapist features in sexual offender treatment: their reliable identification and influence on behaviour change. Clin Psychol Psychother. 2002;9(6):395–405.

Marshall WL, Serran GA, Fernandez YM, Mulloy R, Mann RE, Thornton D. Therapist characteristics in the treatment of sexual offenders: tentative data on their relationship with indices of behaviour change. J Sex Aggress. 2003;9(1):25–30.

Marques JK, Day DM, Nelson C, Miner MH. The sex offender treatment and evaluation project. California's relapse prevention program. In: Laws DR, editor. Relapse prevention with sex offenders. New York: Guilford Press; 1989.

Maruna S, Mann RE. A fundamental attribution error? rethinking cognitive distortions. Legal Criminol Psychol. 2006;11(2):155–77.

McElvaney R. Disclosure of child sexual abuse: delays, non-disclosure and partial disclosure. What the research tells us and implications for practice.Child. Abuse Rev. 2013;24(3):159–69.

McGrath R, Cumming G, Burchard B, Zeoli S, Ellerby L. Current practices and emerging trends in sexual abuser management: The Safer Society 2009 North American Survey. Brandon: Safer Society Press; 2010.

McGuire RJ, Carlisle JM, Young BG. Sexual deviations as conditioned behaviour: a hypothesis. Behav Res Ther. 1964;2(2–4):185–90. https://doi.org/10.1016/0005-7967(64)90014-2.

Metzke CW, Steinhausen HC. BewÄltigungsstrategien im Jugendalter. Zeitschrift für Entwicklungspsychologie und pÄdagogische Psychologie. 2002;34(4):216–26.

Middleton D, Mandeville-Norden R, Hayes E. Does treatment work with internet sex offenders? emerging findings from the internet sex offender treatment programme (i-SOTP). J Sex Aggress. 2009;15(1):5–19. https://doi.org/10.1080/13552600802673444.

Miller WR, Rollnick S. Motivational interviewing: helping people change. New York: Guilford Press; 2013.

Mohnke S, Müller S, Amelung T, Krüger THC, Ponseti J, Schiffer B, et al. Brain alterations in paedophilia: a critical review. Prog Neurobiol. 2014;122:1–23. https://doi.org/10.1016/j.pneurobio.2014.07.005.

Moreno JL. The concept of sociodrama. Sociometry. 1943;4:434–49.

Müller K, Curry S, Ranger R, Briken P, Bradford J, Fedoroff JP. Changes in sexual arousal as measured by penile plethysmography in men with pedophilic sexual interest. J Sex Med. 2014;11:1221–9.

Neutze J, Goecker D, Ahlers CJ, Schaefer GA, Beier KM. Berliner Gruppentherapie zur Prävention sexueller Übergriffe auf Kinder. Berlin: Unveröffentlichtes Manuskript. Institut für Sexualwissenschaft und Sexualmedizin; 2005.

Neutze J, Goecker D, Ahlers CJ, Schaefer GA, Beier KM. Berliner Gruppentherapie zur Prävention sexueller Übergriffe auf Kinder – revidierte Fassung. Berlin: Unveröffentlichtes Manuskript. Institut für Sexualwissenschaft und Sexualmedizin; 2008.

Neutze J, Grundmann D, Scherner G, Beier KM. Undetected and detected child sexual abuse and child pornography offenders. Int J Law Psychiatry. 2012;35(3):168–75. https://doi.org/10.1016/j.ijlp.2012.02.004.

Neutze J, Seto MC, Schaefer GA, Mundt IA, Beier KM. Predictors of child pornography offenses and child sexual abuse in a community sample of pedophiles and hebephiles. Sex Abuse J Res Treat. 2011;23(2):212–42. https://doi.org/10.1177/1079063210382043.

Noll JG, Trickett PK, Susman EJ, Putnam FW. Sleep disturbances and childhood sexual abuse. J Pediatr Psychol. 2006;31(5):469–80.

O'Donohue W, Plaud JJ. The conditioning of human sexual arousal. Arch Sex Behav. 1994;23(3):321–44. https://doi.org/10.1007/BF01541567.

O'Donohue WT. Assessing and modifying denial in juvenile sexual offenders. In: Bromberg DS, O'Donohue WT, editors. Toolkit for working with juvenile sex offenders (practical resources for the mental health pro-fessional). Waltham: Academic Press; 2014. p. 187–200.

Olver ME, Stockdale KC, Wormith JS. A meta-analyis of predictors of offender treatment attrition and ist relationship to recidivism. J Consult Clin Psychol. 2011;79:6–21. https://doi.org/10.1037/a0022200.

O'Reilly G. Assessment and intervention with young people who sexually offend. In: Bromberg DS, O'Donohue WT, editors. Toolkit for working with juvenile sex offenders (practical resources for the mental health professional). Waltham: Academic Press; 2014. p. 313–38.

Otto H. Grundkurs Strafrecht: Die einzelnen Delikte(7.Aufl.) § 66. Delikte gegen die sexuelle Selbstbestimmung. Berlin: De Gruyter Lehrbuch; 2005. p. 369–84.

Paolucci EO, Genuis ML, Violato C. A meta-analysis of the published research on the effects of child sexual abuse. J Psychol. 2001;135(1):17–36.

Pagé CA, Tourigny M, Renaud P. A comparative analysis of youth sex offenders and non-offender peers: is there a difference in their coping strategies? Sexologies. 2010;19(2):78–86.

Paras ML, Murad MH, Chen LP, Goranson EN, Sattler AL, Colbenson KM, Elamin MB, Seime RJ, Prokop LJ, Zirakzadeh A. Sexual abuse and lifetime diagnosis of somatic disorders: a systematic review and meta-analysis. JAMA. 2009;302:550–61.

Pierce S. The lived experience of parents of adolescents who have sexually offended: I am a survivor. J Forensic Nurs. 2011;7(4):173–81.

Pfäfflin F, Ross T. Begutachtung und Behandlung von Sexualstraftätern. Bundesgesundheitsblatt – Gesundheitsforschung – Gesundheitsschutz. 2007; 50(1):44–51.

Pfaus JG, Kippin TE, Centeno S. Conditioning and sexual behavior: a review. Horm Behav. 2001;40(2):291–321. https://doi.org/10.1006/hbeh.2001.1686.

Pithers WD. Relapse prevention with sexual aggressors: A method for maintaining therapeutic gain and enhancing external supervision. In: Marshall WL, Laws DR, Barbaree HE, editors. Handbook of sexual assault: issues, theories and treatment of the offender. New York: Plenum; 1990. p. 343–61.

Polisois-Keating A, Joyal CC. Functional neuroimaging of sexual arousal: A preliminary meta-analysis comparing pedophilic to non-pedophilic men. Arch Sex Behav. 2013;42(7):1111–3. https://doi.org/10.1007/s10508-013-0198-6.

Ponseti J, Granert O, Jansen O, Wolff S, Beier KM, Neutze J, Bosinski HAG. Assessment of pedophilia using hemodynamic brain response to sexual stimuli. Arch Gen Psychiatry. 2012;69(2):187–94. https://doi.org/10.1001/archgenpsychiatry.2011.130.

Prentky RA, Knight RA. Identifying critical dimensions for discriminating among rapists. J Consult Clin Psychol. 1991;59:643–61.

Prochaska JO, DiClemente CC. The transtheoretical approach: towards a systematic eclectic framework. Homewood: Dow Jones Irwin; 1984.

Psychiatrie Z. Abgerufen Januar 2018, von. http://docplayer.org/45631469-Sexueller-missbrauch-von-kindern-was-sind-die-ursachen.html.

Pullman L, Leroux E, Motayne G, Seto M. Examining the developmental trajectories of adolescent sex offenders. Child Abuse Negl. 2014;38:1249–58.

Quayle E, Taylor M. Pedophiles, pornography and the internet: assessment issues. Br J Soc Work. 2002;32:863–75.

Quayle E, Taylor M. Model of problematic internet use in people with a sexual interest in children. Cyber Psychol Behav. 2003;6:93–106.

Rauchfleisch U. Dissozial. Entwicklung, Struktur und Psychodynamik dissozialer Persönlichkeiten. Göttingen: Vandenhoeck; 1981.

Raymond NC, Coleman E, Ohlerking F, Christenson GA, Miner M. Psychiatric comorbidity in pedophilic sex offenders. Am J Psychiatry. 1999;156: 786–8.

Raymond NC, Grant JE, Kim SW, Coleman E. Treatment of compulsive sexual behaviour with naltrexone and serotonin reuptake inhibitors: two case studies. Int Clin Psychopharmacol. 2002;17(4):201–5.

Reitzle M. D-ZKE (vormals ZKE). Zürcher Kurzfragebogen zum Erziehungsverhalten (deutsche Neunormierung). Diagnostische Verfahren für Beratung und Therapie von Paaren und Familien. Göttingen: Hogrefe; 2015.

Rice ME, Harris GT. Is androgen deprivation therapy effective in the treatment of sex offenders? Psychol Public Policy Law. 2011;17(2):315–32. https://doi.org/10.1037/a0022318.

Riegel DL. Effects on boy-attracted pedosexual males of viewing boy erotica [Letter to the Editor]. Arch Sex Behav. 2004;33:321–3. https://doi.org/10.1023/B:ASEB.0000029071.89455.53.

Righthand S, Welch C. Characteristics of youth who sexually offend. J Child Sex Abus. 2004;13(3–4):15–32.

Rinck M, Becker ES. Lernpsychologische Grundlagen. In: Wittchen H-U, Hoyer J, editors. Klinische Psychologie & Psychotherapie. Berlin Heidelberg: Springer; 2011. p. 108–26.

Rogers CR. Die klientenzentrierte Gesprächspsychotherapie. Fischer: Frankfurt am Main; 1999.

Ryback RS. Naltrexone in the treatment of adolescent sexual offenders. J Clin Psychiatry. 2004;65:982–6.

Salter D, McMillan D, Richards M, Talbot T, Hodges J, Bentovim A, et al. Development of sexually abusive behaviour in sexually victimised males: a longitudinal study. The Lancet. 2003;361(9356):471–6. https://doi.org/10.1016/S0140-6736(03)12466-X.

Santtila P, Antfolk J, Räfsä A, Hartwig M, Sariola H, Sandnabba NK, Mokros A. Men´s sexual interest in children: one-year incidence and correlates in a population-based sample of Finnish Male Twins. J Child Sex Abus. 2015;24:115–34. https://doi.org/10.1080/10538712.2015.997410.

Schaefer GA, Mundt IA, Feelgood S, Hupp E, Neutze J, Ahlers CJ, Beier KM. Potential and Dunkelfeld offenders: two neglected target groups for prevention of child sexual abuse. Int J Law Psychiatry. 2010;33(3):154–63.

Scherner G, Konrad A, Grundmann D. Therapie im Präventionsprojekt Dunkelfeld. Sexuologie. 2015;22(3-4):165–74.

Schiffer B, Amelung T, Pohl A, Kaergel C, Tenbergen G, Gerwinn H, et al. Gray matter anomalies in pedophiles with and without a history of child sexual offending. Transl Psychiatry. 2017;7(5):e1129. https://doi.org/10.1038/tp.2017.96.

Schlinzig E, Peter A, Beier KM. Primäre Prävention von sexuellem Kindesmiss-brauch durch Jugendliche (Zwischenbericht an das BMFSFJ). Berlin: Charité – Universitäts-medizin Berlin, Institut für Sexualwissenschaft und Sexualmedizin; 2017.

Schmid S. Integrating families into treatment for adolescents with illegal sexual behavior. In: Bromberg DS, O'Donohue WT, editors. Toolkit for working with juvenile sex offenders (practical resources for the mental health professional). Waltham: Academic Press; 2014. p. 507–32.

Schmidt AF, Banse R, Imhoff R. Indirect measures in forensic contexts. Behavior-based assessment in psychology: going beyond self-report in the personality, affective, motivation, and social domains. 2015. p. 173–194.

Schmucker M, Lösel F. The effects of sexual offender treatment on recidivism: an international meta-analysis of sound quality evaluations. J Exp Criminol. 2015;11(4):597–630.

Schuler M, Mohnke S, Amelung T, Dziobek I, Lemme B, Borchardt V, Gerwinn H, Kärgel C, Kneer J, Massau C, Pohl A, Tenbergen G, Weiß S, Wittfoth M, Waller L, Beier KM, Walter M, Ponseti J, Schiffer B, Walter H. Empathy in pedophilia and sexual offending against children: A multifaceted approach. Journal of Abnormal Psychology. 2019. https://doi.org/10.1037/abn0000412.

Schuler M, Gieseler H, Schweder K, von Heyden M, Beier KM. Troubled Desire - An Online Self-Management Application for Individuals with Sexual Interest in Children. JMIR Mental Health. https://doi.org/10.2196/22277 (forthcoming/in press).

Schuler M, Mohnke S, Walter H. Empathy. In: Hess U, Fischer A, editors. Facial mimicry in social context. Cambridge University Press: Cambridge; 2016. p. 192–221.

Schwarze C, Hahn G. Herausforderung Pädophilie. Beratung, Selbsthilfe, Prävention. Köln: Psychiatrie Verlag; 2016.

Seidman BT, Marshall WL, Hudson SM. An examination of intimacy and loneliness in sex offenders. J Interpers Violence. 1994;9:518–34.

Seiffge-Krenke I. Depression bei Kindern und Jugendlichen: Prävalenz, Diagnostik, Ätiologische Faktoren, Geschlechtsunterschiede, therapeutische Ansätze. Prax Kinderpsychol Kinderpsychiatr. 2007;56(3):185–205.

Seligman MEP. On the generality of the laws of learning. Psychol Rev. 1970;77:406–18.

Seto MC, Lalumière ML. What is so special about male adolescent sexual offending? A review and test of explanations through meta-analysis. Psychol Bull. 2010;136(4):526.

Seto MC. Pedophilia and sexual offending against children: theory, assessment, and intervention. 2nd ed. Washington, DC: American Psychological Association; 2008.

Seto MC. Pedophilia. Ann Rev Clin Psychol. 2009;5:391–407. https://doi.org/10.1146/annurev.clinpsy.032408.153618.

Seto MC. Is pedophilia a sexual orientation? Arch Sex Behav. 2012;41(1):231–6. https://doi.org/10.1007/s10508-011-9882-6.

Seto M, Cantor J, Blanchard R. Child pornography offenses are a valid diagnostic indicator of pedophilia. J Abnorm Psychol. 2006;115(3):610–5.

Seto MC. Internet sex offenders. Washington, DC: American Psychological Association; 2013.

Seto MC, Kingston DA, Bourget D. Assessment of the paraphilias. Psychiatr Clin North Am. 2014;37(2):149–61.

Seto MC, Lalumiere ML. What is so special about male adolescent sexual offending? a review and test of explanations through meta-analysis. Psychol Bull. 2010;136(4):526.

Siegel S, Kuhle LF, Amelung T. Medikamentöse Therapie im Präventionsprojekt Dunkelfeld. Sexuologie. 2015;22(3-4):175–80.

Smith DW, Saunders BE. Personality characteristics of father/perpetrators and nonoffending mothers in incest families: individual and dyadic analyses. Child Abuse Negl. 1995;19(5):607–17.

Steen C, Bromberg DS. Relapse prevention as a treatment modality for juvenile sex offenders. In: Bromberg DS, O'Donohue WT, editors. Toolkit for working with juvenile sex offenders (practical resources for the mental health professional). Waltham: Academic Press; 2014. p. 201–30.

Steine IM, Harvey AG, Krystal JH, Milde AM, Grønli J, Bjorvatn B, Nordhus IH, Eid J, Pallesen S. Sleep disturbances in sexual abuse victims: a systematic review. Sleep Med Rev. 2012;16(1):15–25.

Stiels-Glenn M. The availability of outpatient psychotherapy for paedophiles in Germany. Recht Psychiatr. 2010;28(2):74–80.

Stinson JD, Becker JV, Tromp S. A preliminary study on findings of psy-chopathy and affective disorders in adult sex offenders. Int J Law Psychiatry. 2005;28:637–49.

Stiglmayr CE, Lammers C-H, Bohus M. Acht-samkeit und Akzeptanz in der Dialektisch-Behavioralen Therapie der Borderline-Persönlichkeitsstörung. Psyochotherapie im Dialog. 2006;7(3):280–5.

Stoltenborgh M, IJzendoorn MH, Euser EM, Bakermans-Kranenburg MJ. A global perspective on child sexual abuse: meta-analysis of prevalence around the world. Child Maltreat. 2011;16:79–101.

Stuyvesant R, Mercier DC, Haidle A. An outpatient treatment response for youth assessed as LOW to moderate risk. In: Bromberg DS, O'Donohue WT, editors. Toolkit for working with juvenile sex offenders (practical resources for the mental health professional). Waltham: Academic Press; 2014. p. 231–62.

Swift JK, Greenberg RP. Premature discontinuation in adult psychotherapy: a meta-analysis. J Consult Clin Psychol. 2012;80(4):547–59. https://doi.org/10.1037/a0028226.

Taylor M, Holland G, Quayle E. Typology of pedophile picture collections. Police J. 2001;74:97–107.

Tenbergen G, Wittfoth M, Frieling H, Ponseti J, Walter M, Walter H, et al. The neurobiology and psychology of pedophilia: recent advances and challenges. Front Hum Neurosci. 2015;9:344. https://doi.org/10.3389/fnhum.2015.00344.

Tierney DW, McCabe MP. An evaluation of self-report measures of cognitive distortions and empathy among Australian sex offenders. Arch Sex Behav. 2001;30(5):495–519.

Thibaut F, Barra FDL, Gordon H, Cosyns P, Bradford JMW. The World Federation of Societies of Biological Psychiatry (WFSBP) guidelines for the biological treatment of paraphilias. World J Biol Psychiatry. 2010;11(4):604–55. https://doi.org/10.3109/15622971003671628.

Thibaut F, Bradford JMW, Briken P, De La Barra F, Häßler F, Cosyns P. The World Federation of Societies of Biological Psychiatry (WFSBP) guidelines for the treatment of adolescent sexual offenders with paraphilic disorders. World J Biol Psychiatry. 2016;17(1):2–38.

Thibaut G, Cordier B, Kuhn JM. Effect of a longlasting gonadotrophin hormone-releasing hormone agonist in six cases of severe male paraphilia. Acta Psychiatr Scand. 1993;87:445–50.

Thornton D, Beech AR. Integrating statistical and psychological factors through the structured risk assessment model. Poster presented at the 21st Association for the treatment of Sexual Abusers Conference, Montreal. 2002.

Thornton JA, Stevens G, Grant J, Indermaur D, Chamarette C, Halse A. Intrafamilial adolescent sex offenders: family functioning and treatment. J Fam Stud. 2008;14(2–3):362–75.

Trickett PK, Noll JG, Putnam FW. The impact of sexual abuse on female development: Lessons from a multigenerational, longitudinal research study. Dev Psychopathol. 2011;23:453–76.

Turner D, Basdekis-Jozsa R, Briken P. Prescription of testosterone-lowering medications for sex offender treatment in German forensic-psychiatric institutions. J Sex Med. 2013;10(2):570–8.

University of Rochester Press. BEDIT (2013): Berliner Institut für Sexualwissenschaft und Sexualmedizin (2013). BEDIT – The Berlin Dissexuality Therapy Program. Weimar: Gutenberg.

Urbaniok F. Der deliktorientierte Therapieansatz in der Behandlung von StraftÄtern – Konzeption, Metho- dik und strukturelle Rahmenbedingungen im Zürcher PPD-Modell. Psychotherapie-Wissenschaft. 2003;11(4):202–13.

Urbaniok F, Endrass J. Therapeutische Arbeit mit deliktrelevanten Phantasien. Schweiz Arch Neurol Psychiatr. 2006;157(1):15–22.

Walker EA, Unutzer J, Rutter C, Gelfand A, Saunders K, VonKorff M, et al. Costs of health care use by women HMO members with a history of childhood abuse and neglect. Arch Gen Psychiatry. 1999;56(7):609. https://doi.org/10.1001/archpsyc.56.7.609.

Ward T. Sexual offenders' cognitive distortions as implicit theories. Aggress Violent Behav. 2000;5:491–507.

Ward T, Beech A. An integrated theory of sexual offending. Aggress Violent Behav. 2006;11:44–63.

Ward T, Gannon AT. Rehabilitation, etiology and self-regulation: The comprehensive good lives model of treatment for sexual offenders. Aggress Violent Behav. 2006;11(1):77–94.

Ward T, Hudson SM. A self-regulation model of relapse prevention. In: Laws DR, Hudson SM, Ward T, editors. Remaking relapse prevention with sex offenders: a sourcebook. Thousand Oaks: Sage; 2000. p. 79–101.

Ward T, Hudson SM, Keenan T. A self-regulation model of the sexual offense process. Sex Abuse J Res Treat. 1998;10:141–57.

Ward T, Hudson SM, Marshall WL. Attachment style in sex offenders: a preliminary study. J Sex Res. 1996;33:17–26.

Ward T, Hudson SM, Marshall WL, Siegert R. Attachment style and inti-macy deficits in sex offenders: a theoretical framework. Sex Abuse J Res Treat. 1995;7:317–35.

Ward T, Polaschek D, Beech AR. Theories of sexual offending. Chichester: John Wiley & Sons; 2006.

Ward T, Siegert RJ. Toward a comprehensive theory of child sexual abuse: a theory knitting perspective. Psychology Crime Law. 2002;8:319–51.

Warschburger P. Gruppentherapeutische Methoden mit Kindern und Jugendlichen. In: Mattejat F, editor. Das große Lehrbuch der Psychotherapie, Band 4: Verhaltenstherapie mit Kindern, Jugendlichen und ihren Familien. Muenchen: CIP-Medien; 2006. p. 383–90.

Weber H. Ärger. Psychologie einer alltÄglichen Emotion. Juventa: Weinheim; 1994.

Wetzels P. Zur Epidemiologie physischer und sexueller Gewalterfahrungen in der Kindheit: Ergebnisse einer repräsentativen retrospektiven Prävalenzstudie für die BRD. (KFN-Forschungsberichte No. 59). Hannover: Kriminologisches Forschungsinstitut Niedersachsen e.V; 1997.

Wierzbicki M, Pekarik G. A meta-analysis of psychotherapy dropout. Prof Psychol Res Pract. 1993;24(2):190–5. https://doi.org/10.1037/0735-7028.24.2.190.

Wilken B. Methoden der kognitiven Umstrukturierung. Ein Leitfaden für die psychotherapeutische Praxis. 4th ed. Stuttgart: Kohlhammer; 2008.

Willers B, Engelhardt L, Pelz L. Sexual maturation in East German boys. Acta Paediatr. 1996;85:785–8.

Wilson GD, Cox DN. The child-lovers: a study of paedophiles in society. London: Peter Owen; 1983.

Wilson RJ. Emotional congruence in sexual offenders against children. Sex Abuse J Res Treat. 1999;11:33–47.

Wolpe J. Psychotherapy by reciprocal inhibition. Stanford: Stanford University Press; 1958.

World Health Organization. The ICD-10 classification of mental and behavioral disorders. Clinical descriptions and guidelines. Geneva: World Health Organization; 1992.

World Health Organization. ICD-10 Version: 2010. ICD-10 Version. 2010.

World Health Organization. European report on preventing child maltreatment. 2013. Online unter: http://www. euro.who.int/__data/assets/pdf_file/0019/217018/ European-Report-on-Preventing-Child-Maltreatment. pdf.

World Health Organization. International Statistical Classification of Diseases and Related Health Problems (Eleventh Revision). WHO 2018. https:// www.who.int/classifications/icd/en/.

Worling JR. Adolescent sibling-incest offenders: differences in family and individual functioning when compared to adolescent nonsibling sex offenders. Child Abuse Negl. 1995;19(5):633–43.

Worling JR, Langström N. Risk of sexual recidivism in adolescents who offend sexually. In: Barbaree HE, Marshall WL, editors. The juvenile sex offender. New York: Guilford; 2006. p. 219–47.

Worling JR, Langton CM. Assessment and treat-ment of adolescents who sexually offend: clinical issues and implications for secure settings. Crim Justice Behav. 2012;39(6):814–41.

Wortley R, Smallbone S. Child pornography on the Internet. 2006. Online unter: www.cops.usdoj.gov/ files/RIC/Publications/e04062000.pdf.

Yalom ID, Leszcz M. The theory & practice of group psychotherapy. 5th ed. New York: Basic Books; 2005.

Zarbock G. Praxisbuch Verhaltenstherapie: Grundlagen und Anwendungen biografisch-systemischer Verhaltenstherapie. 4th ed. Lengerich: Pabst Science Publishers; 2014.

Index